Handbook of
Gastrointestinal Drug Therapy

Handbook of Gastrointestinal Drug Therapy

Edited by

Michael M. Van Ness, M.D., F.A.C.P., F.A.C.G.
Associate Professor of Internal Medicine, Northeastern Ohio Universities College of Medicine, Rootstown, Ohio; Attending Physician, Canton Affiliated Hospitals, Canton, Ohio

Michael S. Gurney, M.D.
Assistant Professor of Internal Medicine, Uniformed Services University of the Health Sciences, F. Edward Hébert School of Medicine; Attending Physician, Gastroenterology Division, Naval Hospital, Bethesda, Maryland

Foreword by Stanley B. Benjamin, M.D.
Chief, Division of Gastroenterology, and Professor of Medicine, Georgetown University School of Medicine, Washington, D.C.

Little, Brown and Company
Boston/Toronto/London

Copyright © 1989 by Michael Van Ness and Michael Gurney

First Edition

SmithKline 2

All rights reserved. No part of this book may be reproduced in any form or by any electronic or mechanical means, including information storage and retrieval systems, without permission in writing from the publisher, except by a reviewer who may quote brief passages in a review.

Library of Congress Catalog Card No. 89-83787

ISBN 0-316-89724-8

Printed in the United States of America

FG

To

Hyman J. Zimmerman, M.D., Professor of Medicine, Georgetown University School of Medicine, and Distinguished Physician, Veterans Administration Medical Center, Washington, D.C.

and

Frank Ruddle, Ph.D., Professor of Biology, Yale University, New Haven, Connecticut

whose dedication to the art and science of clinical medicine and basic science research has been an inspiration to all who have been privileged to know and work with them

Contents

Foreword	xiii
Preface	xv
Contributing Authors	xvii

I. ANTI-ULCER AND ANTIGASTROESOPHAGEAL REFLUX DISEASE DRUGS — 1

1. Antacids — 7
Michael M. Van Ness

2. H2-Antagonists — 13
Margaret Andrea and Michael M. Van Ness

Cimetidine	13
Ranitidine	29
Famotidine	35
Nizatidine	38

3. Cytoprotective Agents — 59
Thomas Dorsey

Sucralfate	59
Misoprostol	63

4. Bismuth — 72
Margaret Andrea, James King, and Michael M. Van Ness

5. Metoclopramide — 77
David G. Litaker

6. Omeprazole — 83
Michael Carboni

II. INFLAMMATORY BOWEL DISEASE DRUGS — 91

7. Corticosteroids — 99
W. Zack Taylor and Michael M. Van Ness

8. Sulfasalazine — 112
Michael Canty

9. Antimetabolites — 119
Michael M. Van Ness

10. Metronidazole — 125
Thomas Dorsey

11. 5-ASA and 4-ASA 134
Edward Fox

5-ASA 134
4-ASA 137

12. Total Parenteral Nutrition 143
Joel Sabangan, Steven Swartz, and
Michael M. Van Ness

III. ACUTE INFECTIOUS GASTROINTESTINAL DISEASE DRUGS 157

13. Bacterial Infections 161
John Malone and Michael S. Gurney

Salmonella 161
Shigellosis 164
Vibrio Cholera 166
Campylobacter 169
Clostridia Difficile 171

14. Fungal Infections 178
Marsha G. Pierdinock

Nystatin and Clotrimazole 178
Ketoconazole 179
Amphotericin B 181

15. Viral Infections 184
Marsha G. Pierdinock

Acyclovir 184
Ganciclovir 185

16. Protozoal Infections 188
Marsha G. Pierdinock

Giardiasis 188
Cryptosporidiosis 190

17. Amebiasis 193
Marsha G. Pierdinock

Metronidazole (Flagyl) 193
Iodoquinol 195

18. Intestinal Nematodes 197
David G. Litaker

Ascaris lumbricoides 197
Trichuris trichiura 199
Hookworm 200
Strongyloides stercoralis 200

19.	**Chemoprophylaxis of Traveler's Diarrhea** Lee R. Mandel	**203**
	Trimethoprim-Sulfamethoxazole	203
	Doxycycline	204
	Bismuth Subsalicylate	205
	Norfloxacin	206
	Final Recommendations	207
20.	**Ciprofloxacin** John Malone	**210**
21.	**Acute Diverticulitis** Michael M. Van Ness	**215**

IV. LIVER AND PANCREATIC DISEASE DRUGS — 223

22.	**Corticosteroids** Michael M. Van Ness	**227**
23.	**Azathioprine** Michael M. Van Ness	**234**
24.	**Heavy Metal Antagonists** Michael M. Van Ness	**240**
25.	**Colchicine** Michael M. Van Ness	**246**
26.	**Vitamin K** Margaret Andrea and Michael M. Van Ness	**254**
27.	**Vaccination Agents** Ira Knepp	**257**
28.	**Disulfiram** Galen Grayson	**262**
29.	**Lactulose** Frank A. Hamilton	**266**
30.	**Gallstone Therapeutic Agents** Michael S. Gurney	**271**
	Chenodiol	271
	Ursodeoxycholic Acid (Ursodiol)	275
	Monooctanoin (Moctanin)	276
31.	**Pancrealipase** Michael S. Gurney	**282**

V. MOTILITY DISORDER DRUGS — 287

32.	**Antidiarrheal Agents** Michael S. Gurney	**291**

Kaolin and Pectin	291
Loperamide	292

33. Bile Salt Binders — 298
Michael S. Gurney

34. Anticonstipation Agents — 303
Michael Carboni and Michael S. Gurney

Bulk-Forming Agents	303
Contact Laxatives	309
Anthraquinones	309
Diphenylmethane Derivatives	311
Ricinoleic Acid	312
Docusate (Dioctyl Sulfosuccinate)	313
Lubricants	314

35. Smooth-Muscle Relaxants — 320
William F. Siebert, Jr.

Nitroglycerin	320
Calcium Channel-Blocking Agents	322
Dicyclomine Hydrochloride	324
Belladonna and Similar Antimuscarinics	325

36. Prokinetic Agents — 330
Thomas Dorsey

Domperidone	330
Cisapride	332

VI. GASTROENTEROLOGY PROCEDURE–RELATED DRUGS — 339

37. Bacteremia Prophylaxis Agents — 341
Eugene Killeavy

Bacteremia	341

38. Purgatives — 349
Thomas A. Dowgin

Polyethylene Glycol Electrolyte Lavage Solutions	349

39. Tranquilizers — 355
Michael Canty

Benzodiazepines	355
Diazepam	355
Midazolam	359

40. Sclerosing and Hemostatic Agents — 365
David A. Johnson

Sodium Tetradecyl Sulfate (STS)	**365**
Sodium Morrhuate	**366**
Absolute Alcohol	**367**
Epinephrine	**367**
Vasopressin	**369**

41. Antimotility Agents — **375**
Robert Dolan and Michael S. Gurney

Atropine	**375**
Glucagon	**376**

42. Iodinated Contrast Agents — **379**
John Mehegan

43. Naloxone Hydrochloride — **383**
Robert Dolan

VII. OTHER AGENTS — **387**

44. Somatostatin — **389**
Michael S. Gurney

45. Antiserotonin Agents — **397**
Michael S. Gurney

Cyproheptadine (Periactin)	**397**
Methysergide (Sansert)	**398**

46. Cyclosporine — **401**
Tho D. Le

Appendix: Drugs and Pregnancy — **407**
Michael M. Van Ness

Index — **413**

Foreword

The application of pharmacologic principles to gastrointestinal drug therapy is required for the safe and effective treatment of diseases of the gastrointestinal tract. Given the ubiquitous nature of disorders of the gastrointestinal tract, all physicians, from the primary-care provider to the subspecialty consultant, need a complete and thorough understanding of the drugs available. This text not only provides a solid foundation for the family practitioner, internist, or general surgeon, but it goes beyond a review of approved agents and indications and provides an up-to-date analysis of some promising experimental drugs. Lastly, the authors look at non-FDA approved uses of currently available agents and examine the potential benefit of some nonapproved drug applications.

The editors, Drs. Michael M. Van Ness and Michael S. Gurney, are uniquely qualified to provide this type of analysis. They have worked in the rich environment of Bethesda Naval Hospital, have conducted their own research, and have benefitted from a referral system that places Bethesda at the focus of a worldwide medical network as well as daily contact with colleagues at the National Institutes of Health, the National Cancer Institute, Georgetown University, and the Armed Forces Institute of Pathology.

They are to be congratulated for preparing a useful and informative text that provides physicians at all levels of practice with current and practical guidelines on gastrointestinal drug therapy.

Stanley B. Benjamin, M.D.

Preface

This book was inspired by our participation in teaching conferences in the Gastroenterology Division of the Department of Internal Medicine at Bethesda Naval Hospital, Bethesda, Maryland. The stimulus of young, aggressive, and eager Fellows in gastroenterology caused us to review and update our knowledge of medications useful in the treatment of gastrointestinal diseases.

Although many of the agents discussed are well known to students and practicing physicians, the application of these drugs in a thoughtful and consistent manner to routine and not-so-routine situations demands a conscientious approach to the mechanism of action and pharmacodynamics of each agent.

We have not steered away from newer agents with narrow applications, nor have we avoided discussion of drugs with utility outside the Food and Drug Administration guidelines. The latter situation demands a thorough understanding of the risks and benefits inherent in the use of the drug in question. To keep as current as possible in this regard, we have focused considerable attention on the most recent literature available for review as well as our own experiences.

It is a testimony to the Gastroenterology Division at Bethesda Naval Hospital as well as the Department of Internal Medicine that this work was produced by two of its members while we continued to provide outstanding care, perform quality research, and support the needs of a large and growing beneficiary population.

Our special thanks to our editors, Susan Pioli and Laurie Anello of Little, Brown and Company. Without their constant support and encouragement, this work would never have been completed in a timely manner.

Invaluable assistance and encouragement were provided by Mr. Jerry Meyers and his staff at the Stitt Library, Bethesda Naval Hospital.

The house officers and secretarial staff of the Department of Internal Medicine, Northeastern Ohio Universities College of Medicine, under the direction of Andrew Ognibene, Brigadier General, U.S. Army Medical Corps (ret.), at Aultman Hospital and Timken Mercy Medical Center, supported and advanced this effort enthusiastically.

Last, without the patience and love of our wives, Jean and Pamela, and our children, Emma, Claire, Elliott, Kaitlin, Emily, Evan, Tessa, and Travis, this book could not have been written.

M.M.V.N.
M.S.G.

Contributing Authors

Margaret Andrea, R.N., C.G.C.
Gastrointestinal Assistant and Clinical Research Coordinator, Gastroenterology Associates, Canton, Ohio

Michael Canty, M.D.
Instructor in Medicine, Uniformed Services University of the Health Sciences, F. Edward Hébert School of Medicine; Senior Fellow, Gastroenterology Division, Naval Hospital, Bethesda, Maryland

Michael Carboni
Fourth-year medical student, Northeastern Ohio Universities College of Medicine, Rootstown, Ohio

Robert P. Dolan, M.D.
Instructor in Medicine, Uniformed Services University of the Health Sciences; F. Edward Hébert School of Medicine; Chief Resident, Department of Internal Medicine, Naval Hospital, Bethesda, Maryland

Thomas Dorsey, M.D.
Assistant Professor of Medicine, Uniformed Services University of the Health Sciences, F. Edward Hébert School of Medicine; Staff Physician, Gastroenterology Division, Naval Hospital, Bethesda, Maryland

Thomas A. Dowgin, M.D.
Instructor in Medicine, Uniformed Services University of the Health Sciences, F. Edward Hébert School of Medicine, Bethesda, Maryland; Staff Internist, Naval Hospital, Yokosuka, Japan

Edward P. Fox, M.D.
Clinical Instructor, Internal Medicine, Uniformed Services University of the Health Sciences, F. Edward Hébert School of Medicine; Attending Physician, Naval Hospital, Bethesda, Maryland

Galen Grayson, M.D.
Fellow, Department of Surgical Research, The Children's Hospital and Harvard Medical School; Intern, Department of Medicine, Lemuel Shattuck Hospital, Boston

Michael S. Gurney, M.D.
Assistant Professor of Internal Medicine, Uniformed Services University of the Health Sciences, F. Edward Hébert School of Medicine; Attending Physician, Gastroenterology Division, Naval Hospital, Bethesda, Maryland

Frank A. Hamilton, M.D., M.P.H.
Director, Gastrointestinal Diseases Programs, Division of Digestive Diseases and Nutrition, National Institutes of Health; Senior Staff Physician, Gastroenterology Division, Naval Hospital, Bethesda, Maryland

David A. Johnson, M.D., F.A.C.P., F.A.C.G.
Assistant Professor of Medicine, Uniformed Services University of the Health Sciences, F. Edward Hébert School of Medicine; Staff Gastroenterologist, Department of Internal Medicine, Naval Hospital, Bethesda, Maryland

Eugene Killeavy, M.D.
Instructor of Internal Medicine, Baylor University; Post-Doctoral Fellow, Cardiology, Texas Heart Institute, Houston, Texas

James King, M.D.
Chairman, Gastroenterology Section, Northeastern Ohio Universities College of Medicine, Rootstown, Ohio; Medical Director, Gastroenterology Unit, Timken Mercy Medical Center, Canton, Ohio

Ira G. Knepp, M.D.
Fellow, Gastroenterology Division, Naval Hospital, Bethesda, Maryland

Tho D. Le, M.D.
Resident, Department of Internal Medicine, Naval Regional Medical Center, San Diego, California

David G. Litaker, M.D.
Instructor, Department of Internal Medicine, Medical University of South Carolina College of Medicine; Staff Physician, Department of Internal Medicine, Naval Regional Medical Center, Charleston, South Carolina

John Malone, M.D.
Instructor, Uniformed Services University of the Health Sciences, F. Edward Hébert School of Medicine; Fellow, Division of Infectious Diseases, Naval Hospital, Bethesda, Maryland

Lee R. Mandel, M.D., F.A.C.P.
Assistant Professor of Medicine, Uniformed Services University of the Health Sciences, F. Edward Hébert School of Medicine; Head, General Medicine Division, Department of Internal Medicine, Naval Hospital, Bethesda, Maryland

John P. Mehegan, M.D.
Assistant Professor of Medicine, Uniformed Services University of the Health Sciences, F. Edward Hébert School of Medicine; Staff, Department of Internal Medicine, Naval Hospital, Bethesda, Maryland

Contributing Authors

Marsha G. Pierdinock, M.D.
Assistant Professor of Medicine, Uniformed Services University of the Health Sciences, F. Edward Hébert School of Medicine; Staff, Department of Internal Medicine, Naval Hospital, Bethesda, Maryland

Joel Sabangan, M.D.
Resident in Internal Medicine, Canton Affiliated Hospitals, Canton, Ohio

William F. Siebert, Jr., D.O.
Teaching Fellow, Department of Medicine, Uniformed Services University of the Health Sciences, F. Edward Hébert School of Medicine; Fellow, Gastroenterology Division, Naval Hospital, Bethesda, Maryland

Steven E. Swartz, M.D.
Senior Surgical Resident, Department of Surgery, Naval Hospital, Houston, Texas; Teaching Fellow, Uniformed Services University of the Health Sciences, F. Edward Hébert School of Medicine, Bethesda, Maryland

Michael M. Van Ness, M.D., F.A.C.P., F.A.C.G.
Associate Professor of Internal Medicine, Northeastern Ohio College of Medicine, Rootstown, Ohio; Attending Physician, Canton Affiliated Hospitals, Canton, Ohio

W. Zack Taylor, M.D.
Staff Gastroenterologist, Naval Hospital, Portsmouth, Virginia

Handbook of
Gastrointestinal Drug Therapy

Notice The indications and dosages of all drugs in this handbook have been recommended in the medical literature and conform to the practices of the general medical community. The medications described do not necessarily have specific approval by the Food and Drug Administration for use in the diseases and dosages for which they are recommended. The package insert for each drug should be consulted for use and dosage as approved by the FDA. Because standards for usage change, it is advisable to keep abreast of revised recommendations, particularly those concerning new drugs.

Anti-Ulcer and Antigastroesophageal Reflux Disease Drugs

Treatment of Acid-Peptic Disease

Over the past decade, the treatment of peptic ulcer and gastroesophageal reflux disease has been revolutionized by the development of effective drugs for suppression of acid secretion, the widespread use of endoscopic instruments giving precise diagnostic information, and the acceptance of newer invasive methods like esophageal manometry and 24-hour pH probe monitoring. With these advances, new challenges arise such as how to treat early recurrence of peptic ulcer disease, how best to give prophylaxis of stress mucosal ulceration and bleeding, and what to do with the rare patient with refractory acid-peptic disease.

Historical Perspective

Until the introduction of competitive H2-receptor antagonists in 1978, medical therapy of peptic ulcer disease was limited to antacid therapy with dietary and life-style regulation. In 1915, Sippy introduced a powder consisting of calcium carbonate, sodium bicarbonate, magnesium oxide, and bismuth subcarbonate. Approximately 60 percent of ulcers healed on his "sippy diet," but serious life-style disruptions and occasional complications of the alkaline diet like the milk-alkali syndrome occurred in up to one-third of patients. Severe metabolic alkalosis, azotemia, and hypercalcemia caused death in rare (<5%) cases.

As late as 1974, Menguy stated that the ulcer patient needed to "lead a stereotyped existence" so as not to stimulate the sensitive "ulcer-prone" stomach.

The problems of recurrent and recalcitrant ulcers and complications like bleeding, perforation, and gastric outlet obstruction provided the impetus to surgeons to develop innovative procedures to deal with these problems. In

1881, Woffler performed the first gastrojejunostomy for an obstructing carcinoma of the stomach, and in the same year Billroth accomplished the first successful gastric resection by performing a gastroduodenostomy for a pyloric carcinoma.

The incidence of dumping in the two- to five-year period after surgery ranges from 27 percent for selective vagotomy and drainage, to 4 percent for parietal cell vagotomy. Diarrhea is reported in 17 percent of the total vagotomy and drainage patients, compared to only 3 percent of the parietal cell vagotomy patients. Ulcer recurrence is seen in 16 percent of the parietal cell vagotomy patients, 14.9 percent of the selective vagotomy and drainage patients, and 9.6 percent of the total vagotomy and drainage patients.

Uncontrollable bleeding, perforation, and refractory gastric outlet obstruction remain clear and compelling reasons for surgical intervention. The costs and consequences of surgical intervention remain strong incentives for use of effective medical therapy.

Currently, H2-receptor antagonists as a class are the "gold standard" by which agents effective in the treatment of acid-peptic disease are measured. To review, acid secretion results from parietal cell receptor stimulation by one or more secretagogues: histamine, acetylcholine, or gastrin. Agents that block interaction of these agonists with the H2-histamine receptor, the M1-cholinergic receptor, and the gastrin receptor decrease the acidity and volume of gastric secretions. At the present time, four H2-receptor antagonists are approved by the Food and Drug Administration for treatment of duodenal ulcer disease: cimetidine (introduced in 1977), ranitidine (introduced in 1982), famotidine (introduced in 1987), and nizatidine (introduced in 1988). The agents differ in chemical structure, potency, and dosage. All are remarkably safe and effective. The use of one or all of these agents can be justified in a number of other conditions, including gastroesophageal reflux disease, prophylaxis against and treatment of acute allergic drug reactions, stress mucosal ulceration prophylaxis, acute acetaminophen overdose, pill-induced esophagitis, and as an adjunct in the treatment of acute upper gastrointestinal hemorrhage.

The most powerful suppressor of acid secretion currently undergoing clinical trials is the substituted benzimidazole omeprazole. It inhibits the action of the hydrogen ion/potassium (H+/K+)−ATPase present on the luminal portion of the parietal cell membrane, thereby markedly decreasing basal and pentagastrin-stimulated acid secretion. Although not approved by the Food and Drug Administration for peptic ulcer disease, omeprazole heals duodenal ulcers more rapidly and with prompter pain relief than the H2-receptor antagonists cimetidine and ranitidine. In one trial omeprazole healed 100 percent of peptic ulcers refractory to treatment with H2-receptor antagonists, colloidal bismuth, or sucralfate alone and in combination. Omeprazole is known to cause enterochromaffinlike cell hyperplasia and carcinoid tumors in rats. Its use may be limited to short-duration therapy of patients with refractory peptic ulcer disease.

Agents that enhance mucosal defenses are also available. Sucralfate, a basic aluminum salt of sucrose octasulfate, becomes viscous and adhesive at a pH less than 4 and binds to ulcerated mucosa. It protects gastric mucosa by an increase in intramucosal prostaglandin E2, by inhibition of pepsin, and by absorption of bile acids. It accelerates healing of mucosal lesions compared to placebo therapy and is approved for the short-term treatment of acute duodenal ulcer. Like the H2-receptor antagonists, its use can be justified from evidence in the medical literature for a number of other conditions, such as prophylaxis against stress-induced mucosal ulceration, bile reflux gastritis, refractory peptic ulcer disease, and drug-induced gastritis (from aspirin, other nonsteroidal anti-inflammatory agents, and alcohol).

Another class of compounds that enhance mucosal defenses are the prostaglandins. These compounds, derivatives of arachidonic acid, are found in most mammalian tissues and have many biologic properties. In the gastric mucosa, the endogenous prostaglandins E2 and I2 decrease gastric acid secretion and accelerate ulcer healing. Exogenous prostaglandinlike drugs appear to act by a "cytoprotective" mechanism at low doses and an antisecretory mechanism at higher doses. Although controversy exists as to the components of cytoprotection (thickened gastric mucous, decreased epithelial cell exfoliation, maintenance of gastric blood flow, or restoration of the hydrophobic nonwetable surface of the gastric mucosa), use of these agents (misoprostol, enprostil) in doses that suppress acid secretion is effective in the treatment of peptic ulcer.

Renewed interest in an infectious component to the pathogenesis and early recurrence of peptic ulcer disease has sparked interest in the anti-ulcer effects of bismuth. The organism *Campylobacter pylori* is associated with acute and chronic gastritis and a susceptibility to antral ulceration. This organism is most effectively eradicated by a combination of bismuth and antimicrobial agents. The utility of bismuth alone or in combination with antimicrobial agents for treatment of duodenal ulcers has been shown. Eradication of the organism was associated with recurrence of ulcers in only 20 percent of cases, compared to ulcer recurrence in nearly 50 percent of cases treated with cimetidine alone. The role of bismuth remains to be clearly defined, but its potential uses are generating considerable interest and excitement.

Michael M. Van Ness

References

1. Behar, J, et al. Efficacy of sucralfate in the prevention of recurrence of duodenal ulcer. Gastroenterology 1986; 90:1343 (abstr).

    Sucralfate, 1 gram pc bid, was found to decrease the duodenal ulcer relapse rate (35%, N = 30) at 1 year compared to placebo (81%, N = 31).

2. Buchman, E, et al. Unrestricted diet in the treatment of duodenal ulcer. Gastroenterology 1969; 56:1016–1020.

    Dietary modification plays no significant role in the healing rates of patients with duodenal ulcer disease.

3. Christiansen, J, et al. Prospective controlled vagotomy trial for duodenal ulcer. Ann Surg 1981; 193:49–55.

    A prospective evaluation of the effectiveness, morbidity, mortality, and ulcer recurrence rate after parietal cell vagotomy, truncal vagotomy and drainage, and selective gastric vagotomy and drainage. Complications were least but ulcer recurrences highest in the parietal cell vagotomy group.

4. Hamilton, I, et al. Healing and recurrence of duodenal ulcer after treatmment with tripotassium dicitrato bismuthate (TDB) tablets or cimetidine. Gut 1986; 27:106–110.

The patient cohort treated with TDB had a recurrence rate of 25% at 12 months, compared to a recurrence rate of 68% in the cimetidine-treated group.
5. Hasan, M, and Sircus, V. The factors determining success or failure of cimetidine treatment of peptic ulcer. J Clin Gastro 1981; 3:225–229.

   Drinking up to five pints of beer a day did not interfere with duodenal ulcer healing in British patients.
6. Lam, S-K, et al. Prostaglandin El (misoprostol) overcomes the adverse effect of chronic cigarette smoking on duodenal ulcer healing. Dig Dis Sci 1986; 31 (Feb suppl.):68S–74S.

   Misoprostol overcame the adverse effects of cigarette smoking on duodenal ulcer healing.
7. Marshall, B J, and Warren, J R. Unidentified curved bacilli in the stomach of patients with gastritis and peptic ulceration. *Lancet* 1984; i:1311–1315.

   The authors noted curved, gram-negative rods in the stomach of gastritis patients and were motivated to fulfill Koch's postulates in a subsequent report. A new and provocative line of research was initiated based on these observations and may explain the cause of refractory ulcer disease in a subset of chronically achlorhydric patients.
8. Menguy, R B. Stomach. In Schwartz, S I (ed.), *Principles of Surgery*. New York: McGraw-Hill, 1974.

   A comprehensive review of the state-of-the-art treatment of peptic ulcer disease immediately prior to the introduction of H2-receptor antagonists into clinical practice.
9. Ostensen, H, et al. Smoking, alcohol, coffee, and familial factors: Any associations with peptic ulcer disease? Scand J Gastro 1981; 20:1227–1235.

   In a Norwegian population, neither coffee nor alcohol intake correlated with peptic ulcer incidence, while tobacco smoking and family history increased the relative risk between 25 and 100%.
10. Sontag, S, et al. Cimetidine, cigarette smoking, and recurrence of duodenal ulcer. NEJM 1984; 311:689–693.

    Continued cigarette smoking during the time of treatment to prevent recurrent ulcer negated the benefits of cimetidine therapy. Optimal prophylaxis against ulcer recurrence requires cessation of smoking.
11. Walan, A, et al. Effect of omeprazole and ranitidine on ulcer healing and relapse rates in patients with benign gastric ulcer. NEJM 1989; 320:69–75.

    In a study of 602 patients with benign gastric ulcer, healing rates at four weeks were 80% in the 40 mg omeprazole group and 59% in the ranitidine group. In a subgroup of 68 patients taking concurrent NSAIAs, the healing rates were 81% in the 40 mg omeprazole group and 32% in the ranitidine group.

Antacids

Michael M. Van Ness

Even with the widespread availability of H2-receptor antagonists, sucralfate, and other effective agents, antacids still have a place in the treatment of acid-peptic disease. Antacids work by neutralizing gastric acid. The neutralizing capacity, sodium content, monthly cost of therapy, and number of tablets containing 140 milliequivalents of acid-neutralizing capacity vary widely (Table 1–1). Unlike sodium bicarbonate (baking soda), none of the acid-neutralizing compounds listed in Table 1–1 is absorbed into the systemic circulation.

The different agents—aluminum hydroxide, magnesium hydroxide, calcium carbonate, and aluminum phosphate—have several distinguishing features. The aluminum-containing compounds (aluminum hydroxide and aluminum phosphate) tend to be constipating and hence are frequently combined with agents that tend to produce diarrhea, such as magnesium hydroxide. When taken in 4 to 8 gram/day dosages, Fordtran and Barreras have shown that calcium carbonate, a very effective acid-neutralizing drug, causes nearly a 50 percent increase in acid output (4 mEq/hr to 7 mEq/hr), with a fall in gastric pH from a baseline of 1.7 to 1.2. This acid rebound is felt to be secondary to contact of the small bowel mucosa with calcium, not antral alkalinization or elevated serum total calcium levels, despite an average rise of serum calcium levels of 0.7 milligram/deciliter.

Brody and Bachrach have advanced the idea that the rapid acid-neutralizing capacity of liquid antacids (<15 minutes) makes them superior to the slower acid-neutralizing action of tablets.

INDICATIONS

Antacids are indicated in the treatment of common heartburn (pyrosis), symptomatic hiatal hernia and peptic esophagitis (gastroesophageal reflux disease), gastritis, and peptic ulcer.

Peterson showed that 30 milliliters of a Mylanta-like antacid (capable of neutralizing 154 mEq of acid), given 7 times a day (1 and 3 hours postcibal and at bedtime), resulted in a duodenal ulcer healing rate of 78 percent after 4 weeks of therapy, compared to a 45 percent healing rate in patients treated with placebo. The daily acid-neutralizing action of the dosages used in the study was 1078 milliequivalents.

Fordtran has reinforced the notion that adequate quantities of liquid antacids must be taken to optimize duodenal ulcer healing rates and that failure to heal duodenal ulcers with antacids may result simply from inadequate dosing. Other authors disagree. In a study from Norway, Berstad found that 2 antacid tablets 7 times a day for 4 weeks resulted in a healing of peptic ulcers in 81 percent of patients

Table 1–1. Comparison of liquid and tablet antacids

	Acid-neutralizing capacity (mEq/ml)	Volume containing 140 mEq (ml)	Sodium content (mg/5 ml)	Monthly cost of therapy ($)
Antacids (liquid)				
Aluminum hydroxide, Magnesium hydroxide				
Maalox TC	4.2	33	1.2	44
Delcid	4.1	34	1.5	57
Aluminum hydroxide, Magnesium hydroxide, Simethicone				
Maalox Plus	2.3	61	2.5	68
Mylanta II	3.6	39	1.1	63
Gelusil	2.2	64	0.7	80
Gelusil II	3.0	47	1.3	74
Riopan Plus	1.8	78	0.7	78
Calcium carbonate, Glycine				
Titralac	4.2	33	11.0	35

	Acid-neutralizing capacity (mEq/tablet)	Volume containing 140 mEq (tablets)	Sodium content (mg/tablet)	Monthly cost of therapy ($)
Antacids (tablets)				
Aluminum hydroxide, Magnesium hydroxide				
Camalox	16.7	8	1.5	54
Aluminum hydroxide, Magnesium hydroxide, Simethicone				
Maalox Plus	5.7	25	1.4	106
Mylanta II	11.0	39	1.1	63
Gelusil II	8.2	17	2.1	107
Riopan Plus	10.0	14	0.3	76
Calcium carbonate				
Tums	10.5	13	2.7	56
Alka-2	10.5	13	2.0	58
Calcium carbonate, Glycine				
Titralac	9.5	15	0.3	57
Aluminum carbonate				
Rolaids	6.9	20	53.0	86
Aluminum hydroxide				
Amphogel	2.0	70	7.0	360

(N = 78) despite only 280 milliequivalents of daily acid-neutralizing capacity. Interestingly, Berstad found that the anticholinergic drug pirenzepine, a new M1-muscarinic receptor antagonist, in combination with a low dose of antacids, was equivalent to a double dose of antacid in the healing of duodenal ulcers. He believes the combination of pirenzepine and low-dose antacids may improve patient compliance compared to high-dose antacids alone.

Priebe has demonstrated the utility of an intensive antacid regimen in the prevention of stress mucosal ulceration and acute gastrointestinal bleeding. Mylanta II, at an initial dose of 30 milliliters/hour via NG tube, was compared to a cimetidine regimen, at an initial dose of 300 milligrams intravenously every 6 hours. Both regimens were titrated to a gastric pH greater than 3.5. The highest hourly quantity of antacid was 120 milliliters. The most intensive cimetidine regimen was 400 milligrams every 4 hours. Upper gastrointestinal bleeding was defined by the presence of frank blood on NG aspirate or a series of three positive guaiac tests. Of the 37 patients treated with antacids, no bleeding was noted. Of the 38 patients treated with cimetidine, seven bled. Four of the antacid patients developed diarrhea, one exhibited hypermagnesemia, and one experienced persistent metabolic alkalosis (6 of 37, or a 16% complication rate). Cost, patient comfort, and staff hours for drug administration were not commented on in the report. Although this study remains a landmark report, more recent data on continuous infusion H2-receptor antagonist therapy for prevention of stress mucosal ulceration and bleeding suggests certain advantages to this form of therapy compared to antacids.

One study, performed by Rydning, has shown a positive benefit of low-dose antacids, one tablet with 30 milliequivalents of acid-neutralizing capacity, on healing of gastric ulcers. A total of 67 percent of 42 gastric ulcers were healed at 4 weeks, compared to 25 percent of 44 gastric ulcers in patients given placebo.

Simethicone is often added to antacid formulations. It has trivial acid-neutralizing capability and is included only for its so-called antigas characteristics. Simethicone works better on Madison Avenue than in the gastrointestinal tract.

Antacids are particularly useful in treatment of patients with chronic renal failure. Blood loss as high as 6 milliliters/day can occur from the gastrointestinal tract of uremic patients. Gastritis and duodenitis are present in 60 to 80 percent of patients with chronic renal failure. Postdialysis gastric acid hypersecretion is common (15–20% of patients). Aluminum hydroxide not only neutralizes gastric acid but blocks absorption of phosphate. Hyperphosphatemia is common when serum creatinine approaches 3 milligrams/deciliter and is best prevented by the administration of aluminum-containing antacids. Once serum phosphate levels are demonstrated to be normal, calcium-containing antacids like calcium carbonate can be added to maintain serum calcium levels and to minimize osteomalacia. Constipation can occur with aluminum hydroxide.

Magnesium-containing antacids can precipitate hypermagnesemia in patients with chronic renal failure and are to be avoided in these patients.

CONTRAINDICATIONS

There are few contraindications to the use of antacids. As emphasized in the previous discussion, adequate dosing to ensure ulcer healing requires a high degree of patient compliance. Magnesium-containing antacids should be avoided in patients with chronic renal failure as central nervous system depression, skin irritation, and, rarely, muscle paralysis with respiratory failure can occur.

Concurrent use of antacids and tetracycline is contraindicated. Calcium binds and prevents absorption of tetracycline. Although one might think that aluminum- or magnesium-based antacids would be useful in this situation, these ions chelate tetracycline as efficiently as calcium. Furthermore, by raising gastric pH, these agents ionize tetracycline, thereby further impairing its absorption.

Antacids are well recognized for their ability to decrease the absorption of iron and cimetidine.

ADMINISTRATION

For treatment of acute peptic ulcer disease, it is recommended that 30 milliliters of a single-strength antacid (e.g., Maalox or Mylanta) or 15 milliliters of a double-strength antacid (e.g., Maalox Plus or Mylanta II) be administered 1 and 3 hours after meals and at bedtime for a total of 4 weeks. Despite Berstad's data from Norway, this amount of antacid is probably required to ensure optimal healing of duodenal ulcer.

For treatment of other acid-related conditions such as gastroesophageal reflux disease, symptomatic hiatal hernia, and heartburn, administration of antacid is on an as-needed basis, not to exceed four to six doses a day.

In the patient with chronic renal failure, dosages must be adjusted on an individual basis. For control of hyperphosphatemia, 30 milliliters with each meal is an appropriate starting dose.

PEARLS AND PITFALLS

1. Magnesium-containing antacids are contraindicated in patients with chronic renal failure.
2. Adequate acid-neutralizing capacity (as much as 1000 mEq) is required to ensure optimal duodenal ulcer healing.
3. Tetracycline, iron, and all H2-receptor antagonist absorption is inhibited by aluminum-, magnesium-, and calcium-containing antacids.
4. Simethicone is virtually useless in the treatment of acid-peptic disease.
5. Aluminum-containing antacids tend to be constipating. Magnesium-containing antacids tend to be laxatives.

6. In chronic renal failure patients, administration of aluminum-containing antacids for phosphate binding is best at mealtime.

References

1. Barreras RF. Acid secretion after calcium carbonate in patients with duodenal ulcer. NEJM 1970; 282:1402–1405.

   Excessive rebound of acid output is seen after calcium carbonate ingestion. In the third hour after calcium carbonate ingestion, the mean acid output in a cohort of 20 men was 11.4 mEq/hour (basal acid output 5.3 mEq/hr).

2. Berstad A, et al. Controlled clinical trial of duodenal ulcer healing with antacid tablets. Scand J Gastro 1982; 17:953–959.

   A provocative study indicating that a low-dose antacid regimen may be efficacious in the treatment of duodenal ulcer disease.

3. Berstad A, Weberg R. Antacids in the treatment of gastroduodenal ulcer. Scand J Gastro 1986; 21:385–391.

   A comprehensive review of the clinical trials involving antacids in the treatment of peptic ulcer disease.

4. Brody M, Bachrach WH. Antacids I. Comparative biochemical and economic considerations. Am J Dig Dis 1959; 4:435–458.

   These authors demonstrated the superiority of liquid antacids over tablets in terms of capacity to rapidly neutralize gastric acid.

5. Chobanian MC, Chobanian SJ. Hollow organ and liver disease in the chronic dialysis and transplant patient. In Manual of clinical problems in gastroenterology, ed. S. J. Chobanian and M. M. Van Ness. Boston: Little, Brown, 1988.

   An up-to-date review of the use of antacids in patients with chronic renal failure.

6. Fordtran JS. Acid rebound. NEJM 1968; 279:900–905.

   Calcium carbonate, both 4 and 8 g doses, induces gastric acid hypersecretion.

7. Fordtran JS, Morawski SG, Richardson CT. In vivo and in vitro evaluation of liquid antacids. NEJM 1973; 288:923–928.

   As shown in Table 1–1, different antacids vary markedly in their in vivo and in vitro acid-neutralizing capacity.

8. Peterson WL, et al. Healing of duodenal ulcer with an antacid regimen. NEJM 1977; 297:341–345.

   The first clear demonstration of efficacy of a large-dose antacid regimen in the healing of duodenal ulcer. After 4 weeks of therapy with 30 mls of antacid 7 times a day (1080 mEqs of acid-neutralizing capacity), ulcers were healed completely in 28 of the 36 antacid-treated patients, compared to 17 of the 38 placebo-treated patients. This article remains the standard against which other antacid trials must be compared.

9. Priebe HJ, et al. Antacid versus cimetidine in preventing acute gastrointestinal bleeding. NEJM 1980; 302:426–430.

   A landmark study demonstrating that an intensive antacid regimen can decrease the incidence of upper gastrointestinal bleeding in an intensive care unit. In comparison to a regimen of intermittent cimetidine therapy, less upper gastrointestinal tract bleeding was noted in the antacid group. Complications occurred in 16% of the antacid-treated cohort. No side effects from cimetidine were noted even though it was used in doses as high as 400 mgs intravenously every 4 hours.

10. Rydning A, et al. Healing of benign gastric ulcer with low-dose antacids and fiber diet. Gastroenterology 1986; 91:56–61.

A 6-week, low-dose aluminum–magnesium antacid regimen, 120 mEq/day, in combination with low- and high-fiber diets was associated with a 67% gastric ulcer healing rate (28 of 42 patients), compared to a 25% healing rate (11 of 44 patients) treated with placebo. The amount of fiber did not correlate with ulcer healing.

2

H2-Antagonists

Margaret Andrea and Michael M. Van Ness

Cimetidine

Cimetidine, the first histamine type 2-receptor antagonist, has had a marked impact on the practice of gastrointestinal medicine. Medical and surgical approaches to duodenal ulcer disease, gastric ulcer disease, gastric acid hypersecretory states, and other conditions related to the secretion of gastric acid, like gastroesophageal reflux disease and stress-related mucosal bleeding, are dramatically different since the introduction of cimetidine in 1977 as the pioneer in this new class of agents.

MECHANISM OF ACTION

Cimetidine is a structural analogue of histamine with an aliphatic side chain attached to an imidazole ring (Fig. 2–1). It binds reversibly with the H2-receptor, thereby inhibiting the accumulation of intracellular cyclic AMP. Although H2-receptors have been identified in the uterus, the cardiac atria, the cutaneous vascular bed, and on T-suppressor cells, the primary locus of cimetidine action is in the stomach, where parietal cell acid secretion is suppressed.

Cimetidine is a moderately potent inhibitor of parietal cell acid secretion. Basal acid output is decreased 90 percent for the 6 hours after a 300 milligram dose. Nocturnal acid output is reduced by 67 percent. Pepsin concentration in gastric secretions is not reduced by cimetidine. However, by decreasing the total volume of gastric secretion, total pepsin secretion is likewise reduced. Furthermore, as depicted in Table 2–1, elevations in gastric pH decrease the activity of pepsin, a useful fact in the treatment of acid-peptic diseases.

The pharmacokinetic properties of cimetidine are outlined in Table 2–2. Cimetidine is a weak imidazole base that is well absorbed from the small intestine, with peak blood levels reached 60 to 90 minutes after ingestion. The drug's half-life is about 2 hours. Because 50 to 70 percent of an oral dose is excreted unchanged by the kidneys, renal failure markedly prolongs the half-life of cimetidine to 3.5 hours and dosage reductions are appropriate.

Cimetidine absorption is modestly inhibited by concurrent antacid dosing. Antacids (Mylanta II, Maalox, Alterna Gel, or milk of magnesia) decrease peak serum concentrations and total cimetidine absorption by one-third. A more sustained rise in nocturnal intragastric pH is achieved by cimetidine administration alone at bedtime as compared to cimetidine and antacids together.

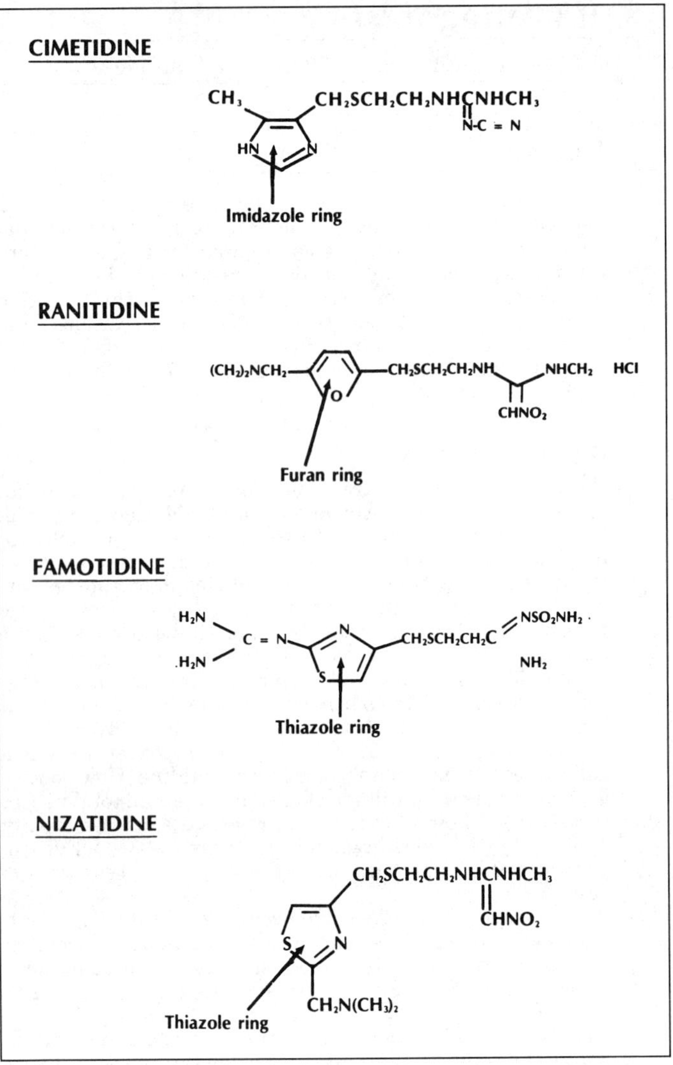

CIMETIDINE

CH₃ — [Imidazole ring] — CH₂SCH₂CH₂NHCNHCH₃
                                   ‖
                                   N-C≡N

Imidazole ring

RANITIDINE

(CH₃)₂NCH₂ — [Furan ring] — CH₂SCH₂CH₂NH   NHCH₃   · HCl
                                          \\ /
                                           C
                                           ‖
                                          CHNO₂

Furan ring

FAMOTIDINE

H₂N\
     C = N — [Thiazole ring] — CH₂SCH₂CH₂C⟨NSO₂NH₂ / NH₂⟩
H₂N/

Thiazole ring

NIZATIDINE

[Thiazole ring] — CH₂SCH₂CH₂NHCNHCH₃
                         ‖
                        CHNO₂

CH₂N(CH₃)₂

Thiazole ring

Fig. 2–1. Structure and formula of available H2-receptor antagonists.

Table 2–1. Significance of intragastric pH values

pH	Significance
>3.5	Decreased frequency of bleeding
>4.5	Pepsin inactivated
5	99.9% of acid neutralized
<5-7	Abnormalities in coagulation time, platelet aggregation, polymerization of fibrinogen
>7	Decreased frequency of rebleeding
>8	Pepsin destroyed

Source: From DA Peura, Recognizing, setting therapeutic goals, and selecting therapy for the prevention and treatment of stress-related mucosal damage. Pharm 1987; 7:95S–103S.

INDICATIONS

Cimetidine is indicated for the short-term treatment of active duodenal ulcer disease, for short-term maintenance against recurrence of duodenal ulcer disease, for the short-term treatment of active benign gastric ulcer disease, and for the treatment of pathologic hypersecretory conditions like Zollinger-Ellison syndrome, as outlined in Table 2–3.

Cimetidine is the most widely studied H2-receptor antagonist in the treatment of active duodenal ulcer disease. It is clearly superior to placebo in the treatment of duodenal ulcer disease. Cimetidine is equivalent to intensive antacid regimens in terms of duodenal ulcer healing rates. Fedeli conducted a prospective, randomized study of 51 uncomplicated duodenal ulcer patients. He demonstrated equal efficacy of cimetidine, 200 milligrams 3 times a day and 400 milligrams at bedtime, and Maalox, 30 milliliters 1 and 3 hours after meals and at bedtime. After 4 weeks of therapy, 78 percent of the cimetidine-treated patients and 75 percent of the Maalox-treated patients had healed duodenal ulcers.

In trial after trial, the duodenal ulcer healing rate by endoscopic criteria after 4 weeks of therapy with cimetidine, 300 milligrams orally 4 times a day, has been over 70 percent. Pain relief and decreased antacid consumption are clearly achieved as early as 5 to 7 days into therapy.

In an effort to increase patient compliance, simplified dosing regimens have been studied. Based on the studies of nocturnal acid output by Gledhill and Isenberg, which demonstrated a significant reduction in 24-hour acid output and nocturnal acid output by once-a-day dosing with cimetidine, Capurso and his colleagues, performing a prospective, double-blind study of 187 acute duodenal ulcer patients in seven medical centers, compared the ulcer healing rates of cimetidine, 400 milligrams twice a day and 800 milligrams at bedtime. After 4 weeks of therapy, 65 of the 96 patients (68%) receiving 400 milligrams of cimetidine twice a day and 76 of the 91 patients (84%) receiving 800 milligrams of cimetidine at bedtime were healed.

Table 2–2. Pharmacokinetic properties of intravenous H2-receptor antagonists in patients with normal renal function

	Cimetidine	Ranitidine	Famotidine	Nizatidine
Volume of distribution (l/kg)	0.8–2.1	1.2–1.9	1.1–1.4	0.8–1.5
Plasma protein binding (percent)	13–25	15	15–20	35
Elimination half-life (hr)	1.6–2.1	1.6–2.1	2.5–3.5	1.0–2.0
Renal clearance (ml/min)	293–486	489–512	304	500
Plasma clearance (ml/min)	442–702	568–709	412	666–1000

Adapted and reproduced with permission from Ostro, MJ. Pharmacodynamics and pharmacokinetics of parenteral histamine (H2)-receptor antagonists. Am J Med 1987; 83 (suppl 6A):15–20.

Table 2–3. Indications and dosage for H2-receptor antagonists

Drug	Indications	Dosage Oral	Parenteral
Cimetidine	Duodenal ulcer		
	• active	800 mg qhs, 400 mg bid, or 300 mg qid	300 mg q6-8h
	• maintenance	400 mg qhs	
	Gastric ulcer		
	• active	300 mg qid	300 mg q6-8h
	Zollinger-Ellison	300 mg qid	300 mg qid
		with dosage adjustment as necessary	
Ranitidine	Duodenal ulcer		
	• active	150 mg bid, or 300 mg qhs	50 mg q6-8h
	• maintenance	150 mg qhs	
	Gastric ulcer		
	• active	150 mg bid	50 mg q6-8h
	GERD*	150 mg bid	
	Zollinger-Ellison	150 mg bid	150 mg bid
		with dosage adjustment as necessary	
Famotidine	Duodenal ulcer		
	• active	20 mg bid, or 40 mg qhs	20 mg q12h
	• maintenance	20 mg qhs	
	Zollinger-Ellison	20 mg bid	20 mg q12h
		with dosage adjustment as necessary	
Nizatidine	Duodenal ulcer		
	• active	150 mg bid, or 300 mg qhs	
	• maintenance	150 mg qhs	

*GERD = Gastroesophageal Reflux Disease

In a similar study of nocturnal ulcer therapy, DeLattre found the healing rate for 420 patients receiving 400 milligrams of cimetidine twice a day for 8 weeks to be 94 percent, compared to the healing rate for 428 patients receiving 800 milligrams of cimetidine at bedtime of 92 percent.

Not all patients with duodenal ulcer disease heal with cimetidine. The factors determining success or failure of cimetidine were examined by Hasan and Sircus in 1981. They found that early age of onset of the disease, smoking cigarettes, continued use of nonsteroidal anti-inflammatory agents, and heavy alcohol intake (> 5 pints of beer per day) correlated independently with treatment failure. Hasan and Sircus also found that the maximum acid output of these recalcitrant ulcer patients was no different than that of control patients.

Other authors find that significant differences do exist in basal acid output between these refractory duodenal ulcer patients and normals. Collen found that approximately 5 percent of duodenal ulcer patients have basal acid outputs greater than 15 milliequivalents/hour. In a study of 43 patients with duodenal ulcer disease, 31 patients healed after 8 weeks of standard therapy had a mean basal acid output of 5.5 milliequivalents/hour. The mean basal acid output of the 12 patients with refractory duodenal ulcers on standard therapy was 19.6 milliequivalents/hour. These 12 patients required 600 to 900 milligrams of ranitidine to heal their duodenal ulcers. These results were confirmed by Yokoya, who found elevations of both basal acid output and maximal acid output in patients with refractory duodenal ulcer.

Cimetidine is effective for the prevention of recurrent duodenal ulcer disease. Sontag has shown that, whereas the recurrence rate for duodenal ulcer in patients receiving placebo is approximately 48 percent at 6 months and 50 percent at 12 months, the recurrence rate for patients receiving cimetidine, 400 milligrams at bedtime, is 17 percent at 6 months and 28 percent at 12 months.

Cimetidine also benefits those patients who have suffered a perforated duodenal ulcer. Simpson evaluated the postoperative course of 60 patients with perforated duodenal ulcer treated by simple closure with an omental patch and cimetidine. Re-operation, rebleeding, and recurrent peptic symptoms were significantly lower in the cimetidine-treated group compared to the control group.

Cigarette smoking negates the benefit of cimetidine prophylaxis against recurrent duodenal ulcer disease. Sontag showed that among nonsmokers receiving cimetidine prophylaxis, the recurrence rate of symptomatic duodenal ulcer after 1 year of observation was 4 percent. Among nonsmokers receiving placebo the recurrence rate of symptomatic duodenal ulcer was 13 percent, compared to a recurrence rate of 22 percent for smokers receiving cimetidine. The duodenal ulcer recurrence rate for smokers receiving placebo was 51 percent.

There are other possible explanations for duodenal ulcer recurrence. Hansky has shown a modest but statistically significant increase in basal and food-stimulated gastrin levels in treated duodenal ulcer patients. Before treatment with cimetidine, 400 milligrams twice a day, the mean basal gastrin level in a cohort of 16 duodenal ulcer patients was 27.5 picomoles/liter and the mean food-stimulated gastrin level was 1.67 nanomoles/liter. After 6 months of therapy, the mean basal gastrin level was 38.5 picomoles/liter and the mean food-stimulated gastrin level was 4.36 nanomoles/liter. Whether this increased gastrin stimulates excessive acid output with cessation of cimetidine therapy remains to be worked out.

Another explanation of the high duodenal ulcer recurrence rate on maintenance cimetidine therapy is Marshall's intriguing observation that *Campylobacter pylori,* a gram-negative spiral-shaped rod, can cause acute and chronic antral gastritis. It is now known that chronic gastritis is associated with duodenal ulcer disease in up to 100 percent of cases. Dooley has shown that cimetidine has little effect on *C. pylori* colonization of the gastric mucosa. In a study of 54 patients with duodenal ulcer (90% of whom had *C. pylori* on antral biopsy), half were treated with cimetidine, 400 milligrams orally twice a day, and half were treated with colloidal bismuth subcitrate, 15 milliliters orally 4 times a day. Colloidal bismuth subcitrate is known to be bactericidal to *C. pylori* in vitro. After 6 weeks of treatment, 77 percent of the cimetidine-treated patients had healed duodenal ulcers, but no reduction in *C. pylori* colonization was observed. Among the colloidal-bismuth subcitrate-treated patients, 86 percent of the ulcers were healed and nearly half were clear of histologic or microbiologic evidence of *C. pylori* infection.

Cimetidine is effective in the treatment of benign gastric ulcer. Hentschel studied the effect of cimetidine in a double-blind, multicenter trial. Of 130 patients who completed the initial 8 weeks of cimetidine therapy, 200 milligrams 3 times a day with 400 milligrams at bedtime, 112 (86%) healed. Of these 112, 84 then remained in the trial for one year. They received either cimetidine, 400 milligrams, or placebo at bedtime. On maintenance therapy, 72 of the 84 (86%) remained healed after one year, compared to only 45 percent on placebo.

Some gastric ulcer patients are resistant to therapy. Continued cigarette smoking and use of nonsteroidal anti-inflammatory agents are well recognized to inhibit healing of benign gastric ulcers. Other gastric ulcer patients are simply resistant to cimetidine therapy. In a study of 18 gastric ulcer patients who failed to heal after 12 weeks of cimetidine, 800 milligrams daily, Yokoya showed an increased ID50, the cimetidine dose required for 50 percent inhibition of pentagastrin-induced maximum acid output.

Cimetidine is effective in the treatment of Zollinger-Ellison syndrome and other hypersecretory states (short bowel syndrome, systemic mastocytosis, and endogenous hyperhistaminemia from basophilic leukemia). Cimetidine provided the first medical treatment alternative to total gastrectomy. McCarthy reported the initial series of Zollinger-Ellison syndrome patients in 1978. Of 61 patients, 40 had relief of symptoms with cimetidine, 300 milligrams 4 times a day. Daily doses were increased in the other 21 patients as necessary to control symptoms and ranged as high as 600 milligrams 4 times a day. Symptoms of pain, nausea, vomiting, and diarrhea were either completely or markedly improved in all patients. Patients in this study were on the drug as long as 18 months. No patient rejected the drug although six of them developed gynecomastia. Tumor progression was not affected by cimetidine. Saeed has demonstrated a clear correlation between the total daily oral dose of cimetidine and the continuous intravenous dose required to decrease basal acid output to less than 10 milliequivalents/hour. In 47 Zollinger-Ellison syndrome patients undergoing operation, this degree of acid suppression allowed an uncomplicated perioperative course.

A survey of cimetidine-prescribing practices was performed by Cocco in 1981. The survey found that cimetidine is used as adjunctive therapy for a number of conditions related to gastric acid secretion, including upper gastrointestinal hemorrhage, stress mucosal ulceration prophylaxis, and gastroesophageal reflux disease. Since that time, other clinical situations have emerged that may justify cimetidine use, such as acetaminophen overdose and Menetrier's disease (hypertrophic hypersecretory gastropathy).

Better control of upper gastrointestinal hemorrhage is believed to result from neutralization of gastric acid. Increasing gastric pH results in (1) inactivation of pepsin and (2) normalization of coagulation time, platelet aggregation, and polymerization of fibrinogen. Early studies like La Brooy's in 1979 showed little benefit of cimetidine and antacids over placebo and antacids in upper gastrointestinal hemorrhage. The drug regimens employed were 10 milliliters of antacids every 2 hours (273 mEq of acid-neutralizing capacity a day) with and without cimetidine, 400 milligrams every 6 hours intravenously. He found that bleeding continued or recurred in 11 of 51 (21.5%) patients on cimetidine and antacid, and in 12 of 50 (24%) patients on placebo and antacid. The inclusion of actively bleeding patients in La Brooy's study may have masked the potential benefit of cimetidine in prevention of rebleeding. Also, Collen has shown that patients with bleeding duodenal ulcers are more likely to have gastric acid hypersecretion, requiring increased dosages of H2-receptor antagonists to effectively neutralize it. The type of regimen employed by La Brooy in 1979 is not considered the type of intensive H2-receptor therapy required for patients with recent upper gastrointestinal hemorrhage from duodenal ulcer in 1988.

The benefits of continuous infusion cimetidine in the treatment of patients with upper gastrointestinal hemorrhage include less rebleeding and lower mortality. Rather than intermittent bolus injections of cimetidine, continuous infusion therapy is recommended. Ostro has shown that continuous infusion administration achieves gastric pH above 6 in 80 percent of patients, with little fluctuation in serum concentration. Siepler found that 50 milligrams of cimetidine every hour intravenously combined with 30 milliliters of antacid every two hours, compared to 300 milligrams of cimetidine intravenously every 6 hours combined with 30 milliliters of antacid every 2 hours, decreased rebleeding (3 of 15 versus 17 of 30) and mortality (6.6% versus 23.8%) in an indigent population admitted to an intensive care unit.

Because (1) stress-related mucosal damage occurs in patients with trauma, burns, and serious medical illness (Table 2–4), (2) stress reduces duodenal bicarbonate secretion

(Fig. 2–2), and (3) gastric acid is essential for the development of stress-related mucosal damage, investigations were initiated soon after cimetidine's release to study its efficacy in the prophylaxis of stress-related mucosal ulcerations. In one of the first studies, Halloran found that only two of 26 cimetidine-treated patients suffering severe head injury experienced upper gastrointestinal bleeding serious enough to require blood transfusion, whereas eight of 24 placebo-treated patients did require blood transfusion for stress-related mucosal bleeding.

Although Priebe found that a program of intensive antacids (as much as 120 mls of Mylanta II every hour) was superior to intermittent cimetidine therapy, Kingsley found the lowest frequency of stress-related mucosal bleeding in patients receiving continuous infusion therapy. In a prospective study of 249 critically ill patients randomized to receive either bolus antacids (90 mls every 3 hours), bolus cimetidine (300 mgs every 6 hours), continuous infusion antacids (60 mls every hour), or continuous infusion cimetidine (50 mgs every hour), the frequency of bright red nasogastric aspirates was 9 of 61 (15%) in the antacid bolus group, 2 of 64 (3%) in the antacid drip group, 5 of 65 (7.7%) in the cimetidine bolus group, and 1 of 59 (1.7%) in the continuous infusion cimetidine group. Continuous infusion cimetidine therapy is superior to intermittent cimetidine or antacid therapy for the prevention of stress-related mucosal injury and bleeding.

The benefit of continuous infusion cimetidine therapy as compared to intermittent therapy was confirmed by Ostro in 1985 when he showed no bleeding from the upper gastrointestinal tract in a cohort of 23 acutely ill patients, at risk for stress-related mucosal bleeding, treated with 50 milligrams of cimetidine intravenously every hour.

Table 2–4. Natural history of stress-related mucosal damage

Author(s), year	Population	Number of patients	Percent with lesions	Percent bleeding
Lucas, 1971	Trauma	42	100	21
Czaja, 1974	Burns	32	86	22
LeGall, 1976	ICU			
	sepsis	14	100	21
	no sepsis	16	48	0
Kamada, 1977	Head injury		75	17
Peura, 1985	ICU	18	83	39
Poleski, 1986	MICU		60	

Source: Adapted from DA Peura. Stress-related mucosal damage. Am J Med 1987; 83 (suppl 6A):4–11.

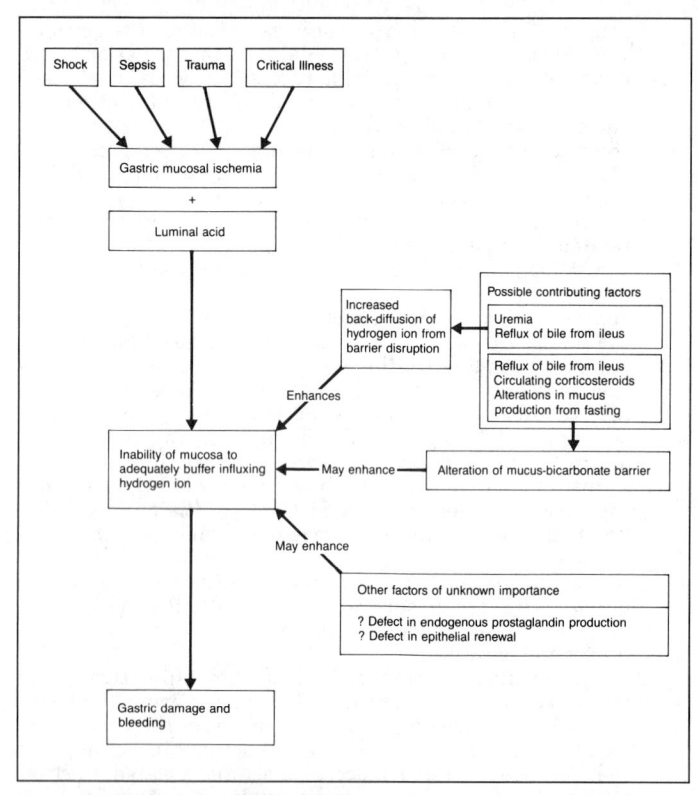

Fig. 2–2. Schematic representation of the various factors thought to be responsible for the pathogenesis of stress-related mucosal damage. (From TA Miller, Stress erosive gastritis. In: Moody FG, ed. *Surgical Treatment of Digestive Disease*. Chicago: Yearbook, 1986; 203–215.)

Cimetidine therapy is also of benefit to patients who develop stress-related mucosal bleeding. As shown by Peura, endoscopic signs of bleeding cleared or did not develop in 20 of 21 patients treated with cimetidine.

Frank has demonstrated that a bolus of 300 milligrams of cimetidine with a continuous infusion of 37.5 milligrams of cimetidine/hour (total drug, 900 mg a day after the first day of therapy) is equivalent in terms of maintenance of gastric pH above 4 to a total of 1200 milligrams/day given by intermittent bolus injection.

To facilitate continuous administration to critically ill patients, cimetidine can be added to hyperalimentation solutions. The delivery of 37.5 to 50 milligrams/hour results in steady-state concentrations of 0.6 to 1.0 microgram/milliliter of cimetidine in patients without renal failure.

A summary of published studies attesting to the efficacy of antacids, H2-receptor antagonists, and sucralfate (see

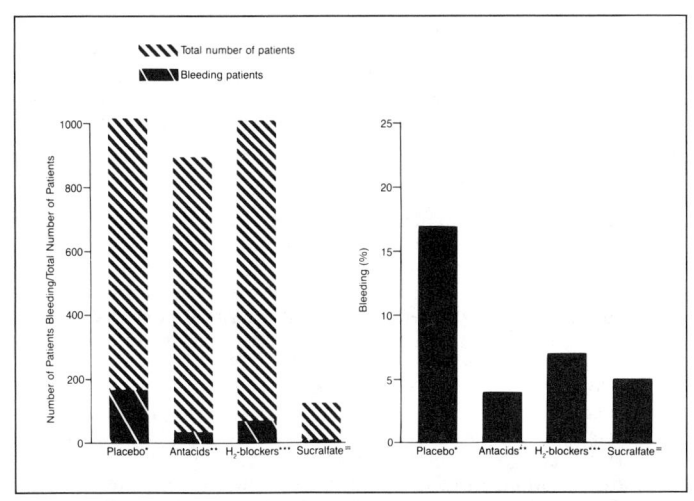

Fig. 2–3. Comparison of bleeding rates in 21 prospective studies of prophylaxis against stress ulcer bleeding in medical and surgical patients. (From GR Zuckerman, R Shuman. Therapeutic goals and treatment options for prevention of stress ulcer syndrome, Am J Med 1987; 83 (suppl 6A): 33.)

Ch. 3) in the prevention of stress-related mucosal bleeding is presented in Fig. 2–3.

The failure of either intensive antacid therapy or cimetidine to control gastric pH should alert the practitioner to the possibility of sepsis. Martin was unable to raise gastric pH above 4 in 23 of 77 patients with either antacids (initial dose 60 mls/hour increased to as high as 120 mls/hour) or cimetidine (initial dose 300 mgs every 4 hours increased to as frequently as every 3 hours). Of these 23 patients with persistent acid hypersecretion, 20 were found to be septic and five of the 20 experienced serious gastrointestinal hemorrhage.

Cimetidine has been evaluated for the treatment of gastroesophageal reflux disease. Although the drug has no effect on the lower esophageal sphincter, no effect on clearance of acid from the esophagus, and no effect on gastric emptying, Behar has demonstrated that cimetidine decreases symptoms of reflux and decreases the need for antacids compared to placebo. Even in patients with scleroderma and severe gastroesophageal reflux symptoms, cimetidine promoted healing of esophagitis. Cimetidine promotes healing of other complications of gastroesophageal reflux disease such as esophageal stenoses. In patients with Barrett's esophagus, Mulholland has shown that concurrent use of cimetidine and methscopolamine decreases gastrin-stimulated acid secretion and the number of reflux episodes per 24 hours. Interestingly, Lieberman has demonstrated that intensive short-term therapy (300 mg cimetidine 4 times a day and 10 mg metoclopramide 4 times a day) for gastroesophageal disease not associated with decreased lower esophageal sphincter pressure (< 5 mm Hg) may suffice to allow for gradual tapering and ultimate discontinuation of cimetidine and metoclopramide.

SIDE EFFECTS

It is likely that no drug in use today in gastroenterology has been scrutinized for the development of side effects as closely as has cimetidine. Given the drug's astonishingly widespread use and the number of organ systems with H2-receptors, the frequency of hepatic, central nervous system, renal, cardiovascular, and endocrine side effects is surprisingly low.

Hepatotoxicity was one of the first side effects noted after introduction of cimetidine. Villeneuve published a case report of an 83-year-old female who developed a hypersensitivity-type reaction to cimetidine. She had begun cimetidine, 300 milligrams orally 4 times a day, in October, 1977, for iron-deficiency anemia associated with Barrett's esophagus. In February, 1978, her liver-associated enzymes showed a serum glutamic oxaloacetate transferase (SGOT) of 935 U/liter, an alkaline phosphatase of 160 U/liter, and a bilirubin of 15 milligram/deciliter. Cimetidine was discontinued, and the liver-associated enzymes normalized. One month after resumption of cimetidine, the serum glutamic oxaloacetate transferase was noted to be elevated to 189 U/liter, the alkaline phosphatase was 171 U/liter, and the bilirubin was 6.5 milligrams/deciliter. There was no evidence of hemolysis.

This type of reaction is rare. In a retrospective analysis of 8553 recipients of cimetidine, Porter found only one possible case of cimetidine-induced hepatitis (Table 2–5). The liver test abnormalities normalized over 6 months after discontinuation of the drug.

Low levels of transaminase elevation are not uncommon with intravenous cimetidine. Cohen prospectively evaluated 100 normal volunteers receiving intravenous bolus injection and infusion of cimetidine and ranitidine 4 times a day for 7 to 10 days. Transaminase values less than 100 U/liter were noted in 19 percent of cimetidine and 24 percent of ranitidine recipients, typically after 5 to 7 days of therapy. No functional abnormalities were noted (i.e., elevation of prothrombin time, decreased albumin level, or elevation of serum bilirubin).

The incidence and severity of mental status changes associated with cimetidine are almost invariably increased in patients with renal or hepatic failure. It is postulated that disruption of the so-called blood–brain barrier facilitates passage of cimetidine into the central nervous system, with disorientation and confusion occurring at drug levels lower than expected. Except in the renal failure and liver failure patient, serum trough concentrations of cimetidine greater than 1.25 micrograms/milliliter are rarely associated with

Table 2–5. Intravenous cimetidine use in 1189 hospitalized patients: Adverse reactions ranked by investigator's impression

Adverse reaction	Definite or probable	Possible	Total
Neuropsychiatric	11	8	19
Blood disorders	5	3	8
Rash	2	1	3
Increased creatinine	2	1	3
Drug fever	1	2	3
Drowsiness		1	1
Nausea		1	1
Convulsions	1		1
Abnormal coagulation	1		1
Alterred liver tests		1	1
Totals (%)	23(1.9%)	17(1.4%)	41(3.5%)

Reproduced with permission from Porter JB, et al. Intensive hospital monitoring study of intravenous cimetidine. Arch Int Med 1986; 146: 2237–2239. Copyright 1986 American Medical Association.

central nervous system abnormalities. To minimize the possibility of these untoward side effects, cimetidine dosages should be reduced in renal and hepatic failure patients.

Renal disease is rare as a consequence of cimetidine therapy. Rudnick has described two cases of acute, partially reversible interstitial nephritis from cimetidine use. Symptoms of fatigue, fever, and anorexia developed 1 month after initiation of therapy. Serum creatinine levels of 6.7 and 8.1 milligrams/deciliter were seen in conjunction with moderately severe azotemia (blood urea nitrogen of 32 and 88 mg/dl) were noted. Cellular invasion of the interstitium with preserved glomerular and vascular architecture were seen on kidney biopsy. Near normalization of renal function occurred within 1 month of cessation of therapy.

Cimetidine and ranitidine have been associated with the development of sinus bradycardia after oral and intravenous administration. In one case of cimetidine-associated bradycardia Jefferys noted that the heart rate increased from 44 beats per minute to 64 beats per minute over 10 hours after cessation of cimetidine. With an intravenous rechallenge of 200 milligrams of cimetidine the patient's heart rate fell from 70 beats per minute to 44 beats per minute and returned to normal within 3 hours.

Tanner (Ann Intern Med 1988; 109:434) reviewed a total of 39 spontaneous domestic reports to the Food and Drug Administration of bradycardia associated with cimetidine and ranitidine use (24 cases with cimetidine, 15 with ranitidine). At the time of this 1988 report, about 144 million prescriptions for cimetidine (1.6 cases of bradycardia per 10 million prescriptions), 41.5 million prescriptions for ranitidine (3.6 cases of bradycardia per 10 million prescriptions), and 1.5 million prescriptions for famotidine (no reports received) were noted.

The anti-androgenic effects of cimetidine were published as early as 1979, when decreased rat and dog seminal vesicles and prostate weights were noted. Jensen reported anti-androgenic effects in Zollinger-Ellison patients. A total of 50 percent of the 22 men with Zollinger-Ellison syndrome and gastric hypersecretion taking a mean daily cimetidine dose of 5.3 grams experienced either impotence, tender gynecomastia, or both. Gynecomastia is not observed more frequently in patients on cimetidine than on placebo who are not treated for Zollinger-Ellison. With discontinuation of cimetidine, the impotence and tenderness disappeared over a month. Resolution of gynecomastia took as long as 3 months.

A potential benefit of the anti-androgenic activity of cimetidine is Terruzzi's observation that high-density lipoprotein (HDL) levels increase an average of 14 percent with cimetidine, 800 milligrams daily (Table 2–6). The clinical applicability of this observation remains unknown.

Cimetidine is known to bind reversibly the cytochrome P-450 system and to alter levels of drugs metabolized by this system. Theophylline, warfarin, diazepam, and dilantin serum concentrations are increased approximately 30 percent by concurrent cimetidine therapy. Increases in theophylline levels can be minimized by nocturnal cimetidine administration. Compared to a rise in theophylline concentration in young adults from a baseline of 7 micrograms/milliliter to 10 micrograms/milliliter with the administration of cimetidine, 300 milligrams 4 times a day, nocturnal dosing of 800 milligrams of cimetidine only increased theophylline levels from a baseline of 7 micrograms/milliliter to 8 micrograms/milliliter (Fig. 2–4).

Table 2–6. Factors affecting HDL cholesterol

Increased levels	Decreased levels
Female sex	Male sex
Physical activity	Smoking
Lean body	Obesity
Estrogens	Androgens
Nicotinic acid	Hypertriglyceridemia
Alcohol	High-carbohydrate diet
Heparin	Diabetes
Familial hyperalphalipoproteinemia	Tangier disease

Reproduced with permission from Sabesin SM, Weidman SW. Histamine H2-receptor antagonists and high-density lipoproteins. Pharm 1987; 7: 116S–119S.

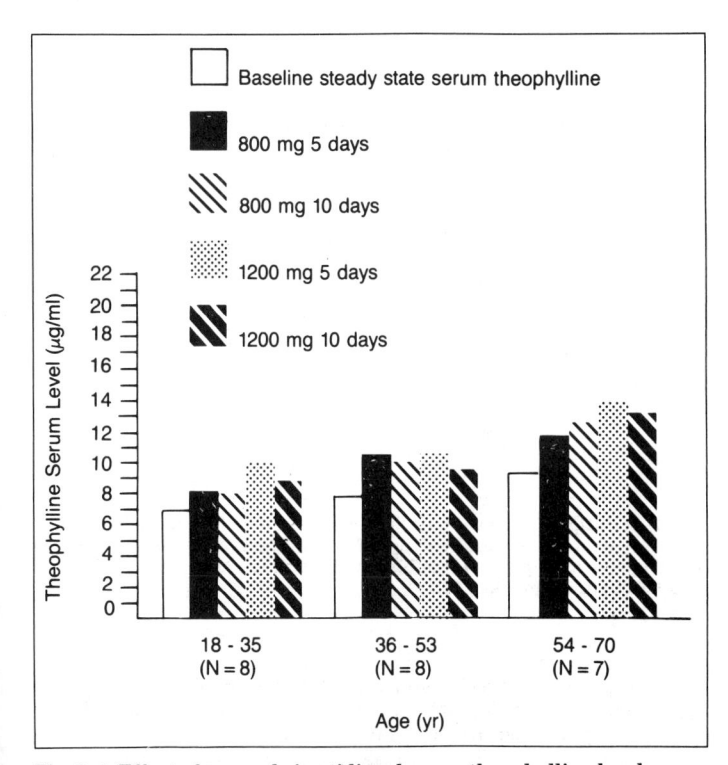

Fig. 2–4. Effect of age and cimetidine dose on theophylline level. (From C De Angelis, et al. Effect of low-dose cimetidine on theophylline metabolism. Clin Pharm 1983; 2:563–567.)

Although the addition of cimetidine to the drug regimen of a patient taking warfarin increases serum warfarin levels, little change is noted in serum prothrombin time. The reason is that the R(−) enantiomer of warfarin is the more potent anticoagulant but only the R(+) enantiomer serum concentration is increased by cimetidine.

Cimetidine's affinity for the cytochrome P-450 system is potentially beneficial in acetaminophen overdose. Mitchell has shown that pre- and post-treatment with cimetidine of rats given toxic doses of acetaminophen decreases both the magnitude of the rise and mortality rates. As depicted in Fig. 2–5, Black postulates that the benefit from cimetidine occurs by inhibition of production of the postulated acetaminophen toxic metabolite (N-acetyl-p-benzoquinone imine). Cimetidine, 37.5 milligrams/hour intravenously, serves only as an adjunct to the primary medical therapy of N-acetyl cysteine (Mucomyst, 140 mg/kg loading dose orally as soon as possible after the ingestion of acetaminophen, then 70 mg/kg orally every 4 hours for 17 doses).

Ingested cimetidine can cause a false-positive Hemoccult

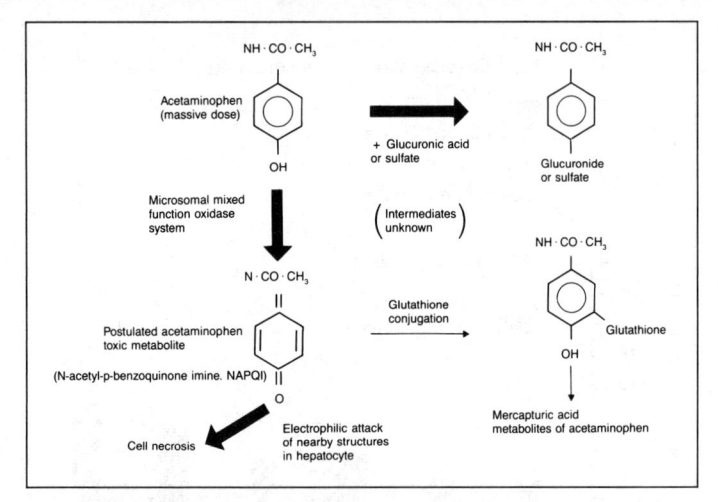

Fig. 2–5. Pathways of acetaminophen metabolism following ingestion of massive quantities of the drug. (From M Black. Hepatotoxic and hepatoprotective potential of histamine (H2)-receptor antagonists. Am J Med; 83 (suppl 6A): 71.)

reaction on gastric aspirates. Because the false-positive reaction is concentration dependent, any positive stool Hemoccult test requires full investigation.

ADMINISTRATION

The oral and parenteral doses and dosage intervals are presented in Table 2–3. Chronic renal failure patients with creatinine clearances less than 20 to 35 milliliters/minute should be dosed every 12 hours instead of every 6 hours.

Continuous infusions of cimetidine should be given as a primed infusion with a 150 milligram loading dose followed by a constant infusion. The infusion solution is made by adding 900 milligrams of cimetidine to 250 milliliters of 5 percent dextrose in water (final cimetidine concentration, 3.6 mgs/ml 5% D/W). The initial infusion rate is 10 milliliters/hour (36 mgs/hour). If gastric pH by nasogastric aspirate is less than 4, the infusion rate can be increased to 14 milliliters/hour (50 mgs/hour).

PEARLS AND PITFALLS

1. Rapid intravenous administration of cimetidine and ranitidine can cause bradycardia.
2. The introduction of cimetidine to patients receiving either theophylline, warfarin, dilantin, diazepam, lidocaine, propranolol, or procainamide may require downward adjustment of the dosages of these medications.

3. Antacids modestly inhibit the oral absorption of cimetidine.
4. Failure to neutralize the gastric pH of a seriously ill patient receiving cimetidine for prophylaxis against stress-related mucosal bleeding should raise the possibility of sepsis.
5. Gynecomastia from high-dose cimetidine therapy may require 3 months to resolve.

Ranitidine

Ranitidine was introduced into clinical practice in July, 1983. Potent, effective, and safe, it has broadened the utility of H2-receptor antagonists in the treatment of acid-peptic diseases.

MECHANISM OF ACTION

Ranitidine is a potent competitive inhibitor of the binding of histamine to parietal cell H2-receptors. As depicted in Fig. 2–1, it has a furan ring instead of the imidazole ring of cimetidine. Ranitidine binds minimally to androgen receptors, the cytochrome P-450 system, and peripheral lymphocytes. Brogden has shown that on a molar basis, ranitidine is about 12 times more potent at inhibiting pentagastrin-stimulated acid output in humans than is cimetidine. As with cimetidine, pepsin secretion is reduced by virtue of the overall decrease in gastric acid secretion, although the concentration of pepsin is not substantially reduced.

PHARMACOKINETICS

Absorption of an oral dose of ranitidine, 150 milligrams, is rapid, occurs in the upper digestive tract, and is not inhibited by food. Although peak drug levels occur about 2 hours after ingestion, significant inhibition of acid secretion continues for 8 to 10 hours. Peak serum concentration after a 150 milligram dose range from 200 to 600 micrograms/milliliter and correlate with the percent reduction in acid output ($r = 0.81$, according to Lebert). The mean inhibition of 24-hour acid secretion in duodenal ulcer patients receiving 150 milligrams of ranitidine twice a day is 70 percent.

Chronic liver disease can alter ranitidine pharmacokinetics. In normal patients and patients with compensated cirrhosis (albumin $>$ 3 g/dL, no ascites), bioavailability of ranitidine is approximately 50 percent, half-life is about 2.5 hours, and the volume of distribution is 1.2 liters. However, in cirrhotic patients with prolonged prothrombin times (twice normal), ranitidine serum concentrations tended to be higher, bioavailability tended to be higher, and half-life was longer, effects felt to be secondary to decreased hepatic metabolism and a slight decrease in glomerular filtration rate. Only in patients with severe renal and hepatic disease is dose reduction necessary.

The pharmacokinetic properties of intravenous ranitidine are presented in Table 2–2.

INDICATIONS

As outlined in Table 2–3, ranitidine is indicated for treatment of active duodenal ulcer disease, short-term maintenance against recurrence of duodenal ulcer disease, active gastric ulcer disease, gastroesophageal reflux disease, and Zollinger-Ellison syndrome and other gastric acid hypersecretory states.

Numerous studies have demonstrated the effectiveness of ranitidine in the short-term treatment of uncomplicated duodenal ulcer disease. Ulcer healing by endoscopic criteria has been documented in about 70 percent of patients after 4 weeks of ranitidine therapy, 150 milligrams twice a day, and in about 90 percent after a total of 8 weeks of drug. These figures are comparable to published studies on the effectiveness of cimetidine in the short-term therapy of duodenal ulcer disease.

Nocturnal administration of ranitidine, 300 milligrams, was studied in an effort to improve patient compliance. Colin-Jones reported the results of a trial of 102 patients treated with either 150 milligrams of ranitidine twice a day or 300 milligrams of ranitidine at bedtime. Healing rates for the patients receiving ranitidine twice a day were 84 percent (48 of 57), compared to 96 percent (43 of 45) for the patients receiving the single bedtime dose. Pain relief was comparable between the two treatment groups. Untoward side effects were rare (one patient receiving ranitidine, 150 mgs twice a day, developed cholestatic jaundice that resolved and did not necessitate drug withdrawal).

Maintenance of remission of duodenal ulcer disease is a desired effect of any treatment regimen. The cumulative remission rate for symptomatic recurrences in 367 duodenal ulcer patients treated with ranitidine and reported by Penston and Wormsley was 95 percent at 1 year, 88 percent at 3 years, and 86 percent at 5 years. Significantly, recurrent duodenal ulcer bleeding was rare (1.1%) in patients receiving continuous therapy. These figures are considerably better than those reported by Gough, who found that the cumulative relapse rate by a life-table method of analysis for patients receiving ranitidine, 150 milligrams orally at bedtime, was 23 percent. This relapse rate compared favorably to that seen with cimetidine, 400 milligrams orally at bedtime (37%, $p < 0.05$). Silvis also found ranitidine more efficacious in the prevention of duodenal ulcer relapse than was cimetidine. In a multicenter study of 126 patients, the recurrence rate for the cohort receiving ranitidine, 150 milligrams at bedtime, was 16 percent, compared to a relapse rate of 43 percent for the cohort receiving cimetidine, 400 milligrams at bedtime.

Ranitidine is effective in the treatment of acute gastric ulcers. Wright reported that ranitidine, 150 milligrams twice a day, healed 58 percent of benign gastric ulcers after

4 weeks. After 8 weeks of continued therapy, 77 percent of the gastric ulcers were healed. These results are similar to Bardham's, who found 68 to 85 gastric ulcers healed after 8 weeks of ranitidine therapy (150 mgs orally twice a day). Cessation of smoking, long duration of therapy (up to 12 weeks), and cessation of agents injurious to the gastric mucosa appear to be factors that correlate with successful healing of gastric ulcers.

Ranitidine is useful in the treatment of patients with gastroesophageal reflux disease. Compared to placebo, ranitidine clearly improves symptoms of heartburn. In addition, in a trial reported by Zimmerman of 64 patients (older than 60 years) with gastroesophageal reflux disease treated with either ranitidine, 150 milligrams twice a day, or placebo, endoscopic evidence of healing was observed in 52 percent of the ranitidine patients, compared to only 33 percent of the placebo patients.

Patients with severe gastroesophageal reflux disease complicated by nonallergic asthma or cough may also benefit from ranitidine therapy. The best predictor of benefit in this situation was found by di Stefano to be a positive pulmonary aspiration test (egg labelled with 4.5 µCi of 99 mTc-DTPA).

Berenson found that cessation of smoking does not appear to be an independent variable for treatment success in gastroesophageal reflux disease. In a study of 232 gastroesophageal reflux disease patients, age of onset, duration, complications, heartburn frequency and severity, dysphagia, antacid consumption, endoscopic findings, and histopathology were no different between the 85 smokers and 147 nonsmokers.

Like cimetidine, ranitidine is approved for use in patients with Zollinger-Ellison syndrome and other gastric acid hypersecretory states. Collen gave patients sufficient ranitidine to suppress basal acid secretion to less than 10 milliequivalents/hour. Four patients were maintained on 1.2 grams of ranitidine/day, whereas six required 3.2 grams/day. On therapy, no patient developed peptic ulcers according to endoscopic criteria. The follow-up period was at least 6 months long. Unlike cimetidine, no adverse effects like impotence or tender gynecomastia were noted.

Like cimetidine, ranitidine is used in several clinical situations in which suppression of gastric acid is desirable. Dawson studied 158 consecutive patients with acute upper gastrointestinal hemorrhage comparing ranitidine, 150 milligrams orally 3 times a day, to placebo in ability to decrease the incidence of recurrent hemorrhage. Among patients with duodenal ulcer as the etiology of their upper gastrointestinal hemorrhage, the rate of rebleeding with ranitidine treatment, 3 of 27, was significantly lower than among patients treated with placebo, 11 of 26 ($p < 0.05$).

Ranitidine is also effective in raising gastric pH in critically ill patients with respiratory failure. In a prospective evaluation, Rigaud gave a 35 milligram loading dose and 17.5 milligrams/hour by continuous intravenous infusion and found that gastric pH was maintained above 4 65 percent of the time.

Ranitidine can decrease the incidence of stress-related mucosal bleeding in critically ill patients. Reid found that only two of 33 patients in a group receiving a primed infusion of ranitidine (50 mg loading dose with 12.5 mg/hour) had clinical evidence of upper gastrointestinal hemorrhage. Other authors question the need for prophylaxis against stress-related mucosal damage and bleeding. Reusser found no benefit to ranitidine and antacids compared to placebo in a 7-day study of 40 severe head injury patients in the prevention of mucosal damage and bleeding. The study found that endoscopic evidence of any mucosal abnormalities was rare. These results are at variance with those of Peura and others who found mucosal abnormalities in 80 percent or more of severely ill patients. Most authors remain convinced that patients at risk for stress-related mucosal damage benefit from the use of agents that decrease gastric acid secretion and increase mucosal defensive factors. For example, Siepler found that ranitidine, 50 milligram bolus with an 8 milligram/hour infusion, was equivalent to cimetidine, 300 milligram bolus with a 50 milligram/hour infusion, in elevating gastric pH above 5, preventing upper gastrointestinal hemorrhage, and decreasing transfusion requirements in 227 intensive care unit patients.

Ranitidine has proven effective in suppression of gastric acid hypersecretion resistant to cimetidine therapy. Three cases were reported by Danilewitz in 1982. All three patients were treated with intravenous cimetidine (one received a total of 1.2 g/day, two received a total of 2.4 g/day, all intravenously) and experienced persistent high-volume gastric outputs and basal acid secretion (pH of gastric aspirate 1, acid output 15 mEq/hour). With initiation of ranitidine, 300 milligrams/day in divided doses, acid secretion was controlled.

Ranitidine is effective in controlling the high acid outputs characteristic of many patients with Barrett's esophagus. Collen found that the mean basal acid output was 8.3 mEq/hour in the Barrett's patients, compared to a mean basal acid output of 3.2 mEq/hour in normal controls (p = 0.001). He also noted that ranitidine dosages correlated with the basal acid output in these patients. Using the formula, daily ranitidine dose equals 100 times the BAO minus 407, 15 of the Barrett's patients in the study required a mean of 890 milligrams/day for complete control of symptoms and healing of esophagitis. No untoward side effects were noted from use of these higher doses of ranitidine.

Ranitidine can also prevent the development of duodenal ulcers in patients receiving nonsteroidal anti-inflammatory agents. Lanza studied 119 patients receiving nonsteroidal anti-inflammatory agents for rheumatologic conditions and found that ranitidine, 150 milligrams orally twice a day, prevented the development of duodenal ulcers in 62 patients, compared to the development of duodenal ulcers in 4 of 57 patients on placebo (p<0.01).

SIDE EFFECTS

Ranitidine is a remarkably safe agent with rare side effects limited primarily to drug-induced hepatitis and headache.

In an analysis of the short- and long-term untoward effects of oral ranitidine, Simon found some elevations in the liver-associated enzymes of ranitidine-treated patients. The elevations were small, of little clinical significance, and infrequent. The incidence of drug-induced hepatitis from ranitidine was estimated by Dobbs to be 0.06 to 0.08 percent.

Ranitidine is not known to possess antiandrogenic properties, is not known to change serum concentrations of high-density lipoproteins, and is not thought to be useful in the treatment of acetaminophen overdose. In fact, Bredfeldt speculates that ranitidine may compete with acetaminophen for available hepatic glutathione thereby inhibiting acetaminophen metabolism and potentiating toxicity.

The incidence of hepatitis has been reported sporadically but appears to be as high or higher with ranitidine than cimetidine. In an analysis of the short- and long-term untoward effects of oral ranitidine, Simon found some elevations in the liver-associated enzymes of ranitidine-treated patients. The elevations were small, of little clinical significance, and infrequent. The incidence of drug-induced hepatitis was estimated by Dobbs to be 0.06 to 0.08 percent.

The incidence of drug-induced hepatitis is higher with intravenous administration. Cohen conducted a prospective evaluation of 100 normal volunteers and found transaminase values of less than 100 Units/liter in 9 percent of the subjects receiving 50 milligrams of ranitidine every 6 hours for 5 days, and in 28 percent receiving 100 milligrams of ranitidine every 6 hours for 5 days.

Headache and other central nervous system effects may complicate ranitidine therapy (Table 2–7). In Cohen's study, four of the 51 patients receiving ranitidine developed headache, compared to no headache in the seven subjects receiving saline injections and three in the group of 43 receiving intravenous cimetidine.

As with cimetidine, bradycardia from both oral and intravenous ranitidine use is well-described but rare (see Tanner letter, page 25).

A recent study showed that gastric emptying, as measured by nuclear medicine emptying times, is impaired in duodenal ulcer patients treated with ranitidine.

Clinically significant interactions with theophylline have also been well documented. A study of hospitalized patients found the frequency of this interaction roughly comparable to the experience with cimetidine. Ranitidine also causes a slight decrease in warfarin clearance, but this has not been clinically significant.

ADMINISTRATION

The oral and parenteral doses and dosage intervals are presented in Table 2–3. The dosage of ranitidine should be re-

Table 2-7. Central nervous system toxicities following rantidine administration: Case reports

Author, year	Number of patients	Symptoms	Dose	Recurrence on rechallenge
Billings, 1986	3	Depression	150 mg bid	yes
Epstein, 1985	5	Headache	150 mg bid	yes
Silverstone, 1984	1	Confusion	150 mg bid	no
Hughes, 1983	1	Confusion	150 mg bid	no
Mandal, 1986	1	Confusion	150 mg bid	no
Mani, 1984	1	Confusion	150 mg bid	no
Price, 1985	1	Hallucinations	150 mg bid	yes
Sonnenblick, 1986	1	Hallucinations	150 mg bid	no

Reproduced with permission from Freston JW. Safety perspectives on parenteral H2-receptor antagonists. Am J Med 1987; 83 (suppl 6A): 60.

duced to 150 milligrams every 24 hours for renal failure patients with creatinine clearances less than 50 milliliters/minute.

Continuous infusion ranitidine should be given as a primed infusion with a 50 milligram loading dose followed by a constant infusion. The infusion solution is made by adding 300 milligrams of ranitidine to 250 milliliters of five percent dextrose in water (final ranitidine concentration, 1.2 mgs/mL 5% D/W). The initial infusion rate is ten milliliters/hour (12 mgs/hour).

PEARLS AND PITFALLS

1. Ranitidine is the only H2-receptor antagonist currently approved by the Food and Drug Administration for treatment of gastroesophageal reflux disease.
2. Ranitidine contains a furan ring and has no known antiandrogenic activity.
3. Ranitidine is 5 to 10 times more potent on a molar basis than is cimetidine.
4. Intravenous ranitidine is associated with rises in liver-associated enzymes (usually < 100 U/l) without demonstrable changes in synthetic function (albumin, bilirubin, or coagulation parameters).
5. Ranitidine has no role in the treatment of acute acetaminophen overdose.
6. Ranitidine bioavailability is not changed in patients with chronic liver disease unless severe hepatic decompensation occurs.

Famotidine

Famotidine is a newer, more potent, competitive histamine H2-receptor antagonist effective in the treatment of duodenal ulcer disease, benign gastric ulcer, and Zollinger-Ellison syndrome. At this time, after careful study and intense scrutiny, famotidine appears to be relatively free of untoward side effects.

MECHANISM OF ACTION, PHARMACOKINETICS, AND PHARMACODYNAMICS

Famotidine is based on a thiazole ring, compared to an imidazole ring for cimetidine and a furan ring for ranitidine (see Fig. 2–1). Like these agents, it is a competitive antagonist for the histamine H2-receptor. It is estimated to be 30 to 40 times more potent than cimetidine and 7 to 10 times more potent than ranitidine. Famotidine inhibits basal and pentagastrin-stimulated parietal cell acid output but has no effect on nonparietal cell (bicarbonate) gastric secretion. Reductions in pepsin output parallel reductions in volume of secretion, not changes in pepsin concentration. The half-life of famotidine is longer than those of cimetidine or ranitidine (Table 2–2) such that significant inhibition of pentagastrin-stimulated acid secretion (50% of control) persists even 12 hours after a 20 milligram oral dose.

Famotidine does not influence serum concentrations of medications metabolized by the cytochrome P-450 mixed-function oxidase system. Unlike cimetidine, an agent known to have the property of impairing hepatic microsomal drug oxidizing capacity, famotidine does not increase serum concentrations of diazepam. The effect of famotidine administration on serum concentrations of other agents metabolized by this system—theophyllin, warfarin, lidocaine, acetaminophen, azothymidine (AZT)—has not been studied but is likely to be similar.

The effect of famotidine on renal tubular secretory mechanisms was studied by Klotz. Because renal clearance of famotidine exceeds the creatinine clearance, one can assume that famotidine, like many drugs, is secreted by the renal proximal tubule. With respect to procainamide, Klotz found that famotidine does not interfere with the clearance, half-life, or plasma concentration of procainamide or its metabolite N-acetyl procainamide.

INDICATIONS

As depicted in Table 2–3, famotidine is indicated for the short-term treatment of duodenal ulcer, prophylaxis against recurrence of duodenal ulcer, short-term treatment of benign gastric ulcer, and long-term treatment of the Zollinger-Ellison syndrome. Other uses not yet FDA-approved are under study and include prophylaxis against stress-related mucosal damage, ulceration and bleeding, and gastroesophageal reflux disease.

Famotidine is indicated for the short-term treatment of duodenal ulcer in a dose of either 20 milligrams twice a day or 40 milligrams at bedtime. Although more potent on a milligram per milligram basis than either cimetidine or ranitidine, famotidine is no more efficacious. After 4 weeks of therapy with famotidine, 20 milligrams twice a day, Simon showed that 35 of 42 patients (83%) were healed according to endoscopic criteria. Pain relief was prompt, with 70 percent of patients pain-free after 2 weeks of therapy. These figures are comparable to healing and pain relief rates seen with cimetidine and ranitidine. In Simon's study, one patient in the famotidine group was withdrawn from therapy because of skin rash. In another study of famotidine, Lyon found that the most common side effect from oral famotidine therapy was headache, reported in 2 percent of patients.

Of patients treated with famotidine, Reynolds found four risk factors associated with nonhealing of duodenal ulcer. Alcohol use, prior documented duodenal ulcer, a history of upper gastrointestinal bleeding, and a duodenal ulcer greater than 10 millimeters in diameter were independently associated with nonhealing after 4 weeks of therapy. Because Collen has shown that bleeding duodenal ulcers are associated with idiopathic gastric acid hypersecretion, one could justify gastric analysis and increased drug dosages (i.e., 40 mgs twice a day) in this subset of duodenal ulcer patients at risk for nonhealing. Extension of Collen's recommendations to other patients at risk for nonhealing awaits further research but is logical from the results of currently available studies.

Famotidine is currently indicated for the treatment of benign gastric ulcer. Like the other H2-receptor antagonists, treatment success is more a function of duration of drug therapy than of drug selection or dosage. Eight to 12 weeks are often required for complete healing of benign gastric ulcer: Healing rate of benign gastric ulcer is 2 to 3 millimeters/week regardless of ulcer size or drug therapy. Cessation of smoking and use of nonsteroidal anti-inflammatory agents is necessary for optimal ulcer healing.

Although omeprazole is the drug of choice for the treatment of Zollinger-Ellison syndrome, famotidine may be useful as a second-line agent. In areas of the country where omeprazole is unavailable or the patient is reluctant to travel to national referral centers like the National Institute of Health (phone, (301) 496 4201), famotidine is the agent of choice for Zollinger-Ellison syndrome. In previous studies by Collen and Jensen, 25 percent of patients required more than 7 grams of cimetidine or more than 3 grams of ranitidine to control gastric acid secretion. Howard found that famotidine (mean daily dose 240 mgs, range 80–480 mgs) was effective in controlling symptoms and gastric acid output. It was free of significant side effects, had a duration of action approximately 30 percent longer than either cimetidine or ranitidine, and was more potent (32 times more potent than cimetidine, 9 times more potent than ranitidine). Despite this increased potency, Corleto has demonstrated a loss of efficacy of famotidine in the control of gastric acid secretion in patients with Zollinger-Ellison syndrome. In nine Zollinger-Ellison syndrome patients, control of basal acid output to levels less than 10 mEq/hour was lost in six of the nine within 7 to 15 months after initiation of therapy. The authors do not offer an explanation for the loss of control of acid output but comment that no significant increase in parietal cell mass occurred to cause the loss of efficacy of famotidine. In this study, omeprazole (a hydrogen ion-potassium ATPase inhibitor) did suppress acid completely in these six patients.

Unlike cimetidine, there is no known increase in serum HDL cholesterol during famotidine therapy.

The use of famotidine to prevent stress-related mucosal damage, ulceration, and bleeding was the subject of an abstract by Welage et al. In a study of 42 critically ill intensive care unit patients, better control of gastric pH (pH > 4) was achieved with famotidine, 20 milligrams intravenously every 12 hours, compared to cimetidine, 300 milligrams intravenously every 6 hours. Gastric pH readings were greater than 4 in 81 percent of measurements among the famotidine-treated patients, compared to only 31 percent of the time among the cimetidine-treated patients. Gross gastrointestinal bleeding, length of intensive care unit stay, transfusion requirements, and cost of hospitalization were not commented on in this study.

ADMINISTRATION

The dosages for famotidine are listed in Table 2–3. The use of one-time-a-day dosing for acute duodenal ulcer disease and benign gastric ulcer improves patient compliance. The drug is best given at dinnertime instead of at bedtime in order to suppress more completely the evening and nighttime surge of gastric acid secretion.

We prefer to give famotidine as a continuous infusion for the prevention of stress-related mucosal damage and as an adjunct to the treatment of upper gastrointestinal hemorrhage from peptic ulcer disease. Famotidine, 50 milligrams in 250 milliliters of 5 percent dextrose in water delivered at a rate of 10 milliliters/hour gives 2 milligrams of famotidine/hour. This dosage is sufficient to suppress gastric acid secretion to a pH of greater than 4 in over 85 percent of patients. It is necessary to check the gastric pH at least twice in the first 24 hours of therapy to confirm this level of acid suppression. If gastric pH is less than 4, then an increase in infusion rate to 15 milliliters/hour (3 mgs famotidine/hour) is justified. The addition of antacids should be reversed for those rare patients in whom parenteral infusion of potent H2-receptor antagonists fails to achieve adequate control of gastric acid secretion.

PEARLS AND PITFALLS

1. Famotidine is approximately 25 times more potent than cimetidine and 10 times more potent than ranitidine.
2. To date, no study has demonstrated greater efficacy of famotidine than cimetidine or ranitidine in the treatment of duodenal ulcer disease or benign gastric ulcer disease.
3. Famotidine does not bind to any appreciable degree to the cytochrome P-450 system and does not alter significantly the serum concentration of drugs known to be metabolized via this system (diazepam, dilantin, phenytoin, theophylline).
4. Famotidine has no antiandrogenic side effects.
5. The incidence of famotidine-induced headache can be as high as five percent of patients.

Nizatidine

Nizatidine is the newest competitor in the histamine H2-receptor antagonist category. Introduced in the spring of 1988, it is approved for treatment of active duodenal ulcer and maintenance therapy of healed duodenal ulcer. In controlled studies, it has been shown as effective as cimetidine, ranitidine, and famotidine in the rate of healing and relief of symptoms in duodenal ulcer disease. Its application to other acid-related conditions awaits further study.

MECHANISM OF ACTION, PHARMACODYNAMICS, AND PHARMACOKINETICS

Nizatidine, a structural analogue of histamine, contains a thiazole ring (Fig. 2–1) and is a competitive antagonist of histamine for parietal cell H2-receptors. Ninety percent of the drug is available for tissue absorption, with peak plasma concentration occurring .5 to 3 hours after ingestion (700 to 1800 µg/l for a 150 mg dose; 1400 to 3600 µg/l for a 300 mg dose). The drug is chiefly excreted in the urine via active tubular secretion (90%). About 7 percent of the drug is metabolized to N2-monodesmethylnizatidine. Sixty percent of an oral dose of the drug is found unchanged in the urine. People with normal kidney function accumulate minimal amounts of the drug. Because of its rapid clearance, the drug's half-life is only 1 to 2 hours (Table 2–2). The half-life in people with renal impairment is prolonged up to 3.5 to 11 hours.

While a 300 milligram dose of nizatidine suppresses 90 percent of nocturnal gastric acid secretion for up to 10 hours, a 150 milligram dose inhibits 98 percent of meal-stimulated gastric acid output for 4 hours. Normal doses do not have any effect on serum gastrin levels or gastric pepsin concentration. The rate of nizatidine absorption is decreased by 10 percent with concurrent use of simethicone-containing antacids, but is unaffected by ingestion of propantheline.

INDICATIONS

Nizatidine is indicated for the short-term (8 week) treatment of acute duodenal ulcer disease and for maintenance therapy of healed duodenal ulcer (Table 2–3). The recommended dosage for active therapy is 150 milligrams twice a day or 300 milligrams at bedtime. Maintenance dosage is 150 milligrams at bedtime. Patients with abnormal creatinine clearance (< 50 mls/minute but > 20 ml/minute) should receive a reduced dose of nizatidine, 150 milligrams orally every 24 hours, for treatment of acute duodenal ulcer disease, and patients with a creatinine clearance less than 20 milliliters/day should be dosed every other day.

In a double-blind, prospective, endoscopically guided study of 43 patients with duodenal ulcer receiving either nizatidine, 150 milligrams orally twice a day for 8 weeks, or placebo showed healing rates of 82 percent in the nizatidine group versus 50 percent in the placebo group. The only statistically significant laboratory event was an increase in serum creatinine from 1.05 to 1.1 milligrams/deciliter in the active therapy group. Healing correlated with symptomatic relief of ulcer pain.

Bovera reported similar healing rates of duodenal ulcers and ulcer pain relief when comparing nizatidine, 300 milligrams at bedtime, and ranitidine, 300 milligrams at bedtime, for acute duodenal ulcer disease. The nizatidine group had ulcer healing rates of 78 percent and 91 percent, respectively, at 4 and 8 weeks, while the ranitidine group showed 78 percent and 95 percent healing.

Simon's European study concluded that nizatidine and ranitidine were equally effective in duodenal ulcer healing, with 92 percent and 93 percent of ulcers healed, respectively, after 8 weeks of therapy. No serious complications were reported.

A 1-year maintenance study by Cerulli showed recurrent ulcer rates of 34 percent in the nizatidine group, as opposed to 64 percent for the placebo group—figures similar to previously published figures for cimetidine, ranitidine, and famotidine. Although treatment of gastric ulcer is not currently an approved indication in the United States, Naccarato treated 275 gastric ulcer patients in Italy with either nizatidine, 150 milligrams twice daily; nizatidine, 300 milligrams at bedtime; or ranitidine, 150 milligrams twice a day. Patients underwent routine endoscopic evaluation every 4 weeks. Healing rates after 8 weeks of therapy were: nizatidine, 150 milligrams twice a day, 90 percent; nizatidine, 300 milligrams at bedtime, 86.5 percent; and ranitidine, 150 milligrams twice a day, 86.7 percent.

SIDE EFFECTS AND UNTOWARD ACTIONS

Most frequent reported side effects include sweating (1%), urticaria (0.5%) and somnolence (0.3%), figures higher than those reported in placebo-treated groups.

ANTIANDROGENIC SIDE EFFECTS

Gynecomastia and impotence were reported at the same rate as in placebo-treated groups.

Drug-related elevations in liver-associated enzymes have been reported. One case of an elevation of the serum glutamic-pyruevate transaminase (SGPT) greater than 2000 IU/l has been seen. With discontinuation of the drug, the liver enzyme returned to normal. No abnormalities in liver function (bilirubin, albumin, or prothrombin time) were recorded.

PEARLS AND PITFALLS

1. The dose of nizatidine should be reduced to 150 milligrams/day orally for treatment of acute duodenal ulcer disease in patients with chronic renal failure.
2. Drug-induced hepatitis is rare but possible with oral nizatidine therapy.
3. Patients with severe renal disease (creatinine clearance < 20 mls/minute) should receive 150 milligrams of nizatidine orally every other day for treatment of acute duodenal ulcer disease, and 150 milligrams of nizatidine orally every third day for maintenance therapy.

References

CIMETIDINE

1. Behar J, et al. Medical and surgical management of reflux esophagitis. NEJM 1975; 293:263–268.

   Before the era of H2-receptor antagonists, surgical remedies like the Belsey Mark IV anterior fundoplication were clearly superior (73% good to excellent response) to medical therapy (19% good to excellent response).

2. Cannon LA, et al. Sucralfate versus antacids and cimetidine in preventing acute gastrointestinal bleeding in the ventilator patient [abstr]. Crit Care Med 1986; 14:358.

   A randomized study of 62 ventilator-dependent patients designed to compare the efficacy of sucralfate, antacids, and cimetidine in the prevention of upper gastrointestinal hemorrhage. Frank hemorrhage and coffee-ground nasogastric aspirate was least in the sucralfate, 1 gram every 6 hours, while cimetidine, 300 mg IV every 6 hours, was associated with coffee-ground material in 11 of 21 patients (52%).

3. Capurso L, et al. Comparison of cimetidine, 800 mgs once daily and 400 mgs twice daily, in acute duodenal ulceration. Br Med J 1984; 289:1418–1420.

   A seven-center trial of 187 acute duodenal ulcer patients entered prospectively in a double-blind fashion to receive either 800 mgs of cimetidine at night or 400 mgs of cimetidine bid. After 4 weeks of therapy, 76 of 91 (84%) patients receiving 800 mgs of cimetidine at night and 65 of 96 (68%) patients receiving 400 mgs of cimetidine twice a day were healed.

4. Choonara JA, et al. Stereoselective interaction between the R enantiomer of warfarin and cimetidine. Br J Clin Pharm 1986; 21:271–277.

   Although it is recognized that serum warfarin levels are increased with concurrent cimetidine therapy, drug interaction occurs only with the R(+) enantiomer. Because the R(−) enantiomer is a more potent anticoagulant, accumulation of the less potent R(+) enantiomer may explain the observed increase (20–40%) in warfarin blood levels without a corresponding increase in prothrombin time.

5. Cocco AE, Cocco DV. A survey of cimetidine prescribing. NEJM 1981; 304:1281.

   The authors clearly demonstrate that cimetidine is used for a number of conditions and symptoms that are beyond FDA approval but are thought related to secretion of gastric acid. No unexpected, untoward effects were noted by this practice.

6. Cohen A, Fabre L. Tolerance to repeated intravenous doses of ranitidine HCl and cimetidine HCl in normal volunteers. Cur Ther Res 1983; 34:475–482.

   A prospective evaluation of 100 normal volunteers receiving intravenous bolus injections and infusions of ranitidine and cimetidine for 7–10 days. Drug-induced hepatitis with transaminase values less than 100 U/l were noted typically after 5–7 days of therapy in 24% of the ranitidine- and 19% of the cimetidine-treated subjects.

7. Craven DE, Driks MR. Nosocomial pneumonia in the intubated patient. Sem Resp Infect 1987; 2:20–33.

The etiology of nosocomial pneumonia in intubated patients is postulated to result from gastric colonization, transgression of the lower esophageal sphincter, erosion of esophageal and oropharyngeal mucosal surfaces enhancing gram-negative bacillary adherence, and aspiration of stagnant oropharyngeal secretions. Preliminary data from 95 patients shows a 26.4% rate of pneumonia in 53 patients receiving antacids or H2-receptor antagonists, compared to a 11.9% rate in 42 patients receiving sucralfate alone.

8. De Angelis C, et al. Effect of low-dose cimetidine on theophylline metabolism. Clin Pharm 1983; 2:563–567.

Alterations of serum theophylline levels in patients receiving theophylline and cimetidine concurrently can be minimized by a one-time nocturnal dose, 800 mgs at bedtime. The one-time nocturnal dose results in only a 15–20% increase in basal levels compared to a 300 mg 4 times a day regimen, which raises basal levels up to 40%.

9. DeLattre M, Moccia P, Prinzie A. Cimetidine, 800 mg at night, in the treatment of acute duodenal ulceration. Cur Ther Res 1985; 37:677–684.

Healing rates of ulcers treated with cimetidine, 400 mgs bid, and cimetidine, 800 mgs qhs, were comparable at 4 weeks (72% versus 76%) and at 8 weeks (92% versus 94%).

10. Dobbs JH, Muir JG, Smith RN. H2-antagonists and hepatitis. AIM 1986; 103:803.

Hepatitis can be regarded as a rare (0.06%–0.08%) and idiosyncratic complication of cimetidine and ranitidine therapy.

11. Dooley CP, et al. Histological gastritis in duodenal ulcer: Relationship to *Campylobacter pylori* and effect of ulcer therapy. Am J Gastro 1988; 83:278–281.

A study of 54 patients (90% of whom had *C. pylori* on initial antral biopsy) with duodenal ulcer, randomized to treatment with either colloidal bismuth subcitrate (CBS), 5 mls po qid for 6 weeks, or cimetidine, 400 mgs po bid. After 6 weeks of therapy, 24 of 28 patients (86%) on CBS and 20 of 26 patients (77%) on cimetidine had healed duodenal ulcers. However, after treatment with CBS, the prevalence of *C. pylori* decreased from 90%–53%, whereas no change in prevalence of *C. pylori* was noted in the cimetidine-treated group.

12. Driks MR, et al. Nosocomial pneumonia in intubated patients given sucralfate compared with antacids or histamine type-2 blockers: The role of gastric colonization. NEJM 1987; 317:1376–1382.

A study of 130 intubated patients receiving sucralfate, antacids, H2-receptor antagonists, or both antacids and H2-receptor antagonists for stress-related mucosal defense, which showed that pneumonia developed in 7 of the 61 patients (11.5%) treated with sucralfate, in 9 of the 39 patients (23%) treated with antacids, in 1 of the 17 patients

(5.9%) treated with H2-receptor antagonists, and in 6 of the 13 patients (46%) treated with a combination of antacids and H2-receptor antagonists.

13. Evreux M, et al. Endoscopic and clinical evaluation of cisapride and cimetidine in reflux esophagitis. Gastroenterology 1988; 94:A120.

    Cisapride, 10 mgs qid, and cimetidine, 400 mgs qid, were equivalent in the treatment of patients with GERD in terms of symptoms and ulceration healing.

14. Fedeli G, et al. A controlled study comparing cimetidine treatment to an intensive antacid regimen in the therapy of uncomplicated duodenal ulcer. Dig Dis Sci 1979; 24:758–762.

    A prospective, randomized, endoscopically controlled study of 51 uncomplicated duodenal ulcer patients demonstrating equal efficacy of cimetidine, 200 mgs tid and 400 mgs qhs, and antacids, 30 mls 1 and 3 hours after meals and at bedtime, in healing rates after 4 weeks of therapy (78% versus 75% healed). Eleven of the 24 patients in the antacid group developed diarrhea.

15. Finkelstein W, Isselbacher KJ. Cimetidine. NEJM 1978; 299:992–996.

    Black synthesized the first H2-receptor antagonist, burimamide, in 1972. It was not absorbed orally. Metiamide, the second H2-receptor antagonist, was active orally, but it caused agranulocytosis. These facts are typical of those found in this landmark review of the mechanism of action (antagonism of the effects of histamine at the parietal cell H2-receptor), pharmacokinetics (a weak imidazole base with a 2-hour half-life), clinical effectiveness (duodenal ulcer, gastric ulcer, Zollinger-Ellison syndrome, gastroesophageal reflux disease), and side effects.

16. Fitzpatrick W, Blackwood WS, Northfield TC. Bedtime cimetidine maintenance treatment: Optimum dose and effect on subsequent natural history of duodenal ulcer. Gut 1982; 23:239–242.

    A prospective double-blind comparison of cimetidine and placebo as prophylaxis against duodenal ulcer recurrence. Equal numbers, 12 of 19 (63%) and 10 of 17 (59%) of cimetidine, 400 mgs qhs, and placebo-treated patients relapsed within 6 weeks. The authors contend that cimetidine does not alter the natural history of duodenal ulcer disease.

17. Frank WO, et al. Continuous cimetidine infusion regimens—effects on intragastric pH in ulcer patients [abstr]. Gastroenterology 1988; 94:A134.

    Primed, continuous infusion regimens of cimetidine, 37.5 mg/hr (900 mg/24 hours), maintained gastric pH greater than 4 for more time than 300 mgs of cimetidine IV bolus every 6 hours.

18. Freston JW. Cimetidine II. Adverse reactions and patterns of use. AIM 1982; 97:728–734.

    The author reviews the reported adverse effects of this agent 5 years after its introduction. Given the "astonishingly widespread use of the drug," the frequency of side effects is "surprisingly low." Central nervous system, hematologic, renal, endocrine, cardiovascular, hepatotoxic, and immunologic reactions are reviewed. Drug interactions are summarized. The author concludes that the favorable safety record of the drug is likely to be maintained if its use is reversed for those conditions for which evidence exists as to its efficacy.

19. Gledhill T, et al. Single nocturnal dose of an H2-receptor antagonist for the treatment of duodenal ulcer. Gut 1983; 24:904–908.

    The mean 24-hour acid output and nocturnal (100–600) acid output in 12 duodenal ulcer patients were compared before and after cimetidine, 400 mgs bid, cimetidine, 800 mgs qhs, ranitidine, 150 mgs bid, and ranitidine, 300 mgs qhs. Nighttime cimetidine and the two ranitidine regimens resulted in significant reductions in nocturnal acid output compared to cimetidine, 400 mgs bid.

20. Gollapudi P, Sontag S, Miller T. Surgery for complications of peptic ulcer before and after availability of cimetidine. Gastroenterology 1988; 94:A150.

    The mean number of surgical procedures per year at the reporting institution was 21 for the 5 years preceding cimetidine availability, 7 for the 3 years after its introduction in 1978, and 17 for the subsequent 3 years. Almost two-thirds of the surgical patients required surgery for bleeding or perforation, of whom half were completely asymptomatic at the time of presentation.

21. Greenblatt DJ, et al. Clinical importance of the interaction of diazepam and cimetidine. NEJM 1984; 310:1639–1643.

    Plasma concentrations of diazepam rise an average of 57 percent with the addition of cimetidine, 300 mgs qid. Despite this increase, there is little subjective or objective evidence of clinically significant changes in sedation levels, antianxiety effect, or test tracking.

22. Halloran LG, et al. Prevention of acute gastrointestinal complications after severe head injury: A controlled trial of cimetidine prophylaxis. Am J Surg 1980; 139:44–48.

    A prospective, randomized study of 50 patients with severe head injury from 1977–1979 who received corticosteroids, a prophylactic anticonvulsant, and either cimetidine, 300 mgs every 4 hours, or placebo for stress ulcer prophylaxis. Only 2 of the 26 cimetidine-treated group required blood transfusion for acute upper gastrointestinal hemorrhage, whereas 8 of 24 placebo-treated patients required 2 or more units of PRBCs to maintain a stable hematocrit.

23. Hansky J, et al. Effects of long-term cimetidine on serum gastrin in duodenal ulcer. Dig Dis Sci 1979; 24:468–470.

    A modest but statistically significant increase in basal and food-stimulated gastrin levels were noted in 16 duodenal ulcer patients with cimetidine therapy. Before treatment (400 mgs bid), the mean basal gastrin level was 27.5 pMs/l and the mean food-stimulated gastrin level was 1.67 nMs/l. After 6 months of cimetidine, the mean basal gastrin level was 38.5 pMs/l, and the mean food-stimulated gastrin level was 4.36 nMs/l.

24. Hasan M, Sircus W. The factors determining success or fail-

ure of cimetidine treatment of peptic ulcer. J Clin Gastro 1981; 3:225–229.

A retrospective study of 80 cimetidine-treatment failures showing that early age of onset, smoking, continued nonsteroidal anti-inflammatory agent use, and heavy alcohol intake ($>$ 5 pints of beer a day) correlated with treatment failure. When compared to a control group, the percent reduction in maximal acid output by cimetidine was equivalent between the two groups.

25. Hauser A, et al. More on false-positive Hemoccult reaction with cimetidine. NEJM 1981; 304:847–848.

    The authors demonstrate that all forms of oral cimetidine can cause a false-positive Hemoccult reaction.

26. Hentschel E, et al. Effect of cimetidine treatment in the prevention of gastric ulcer relapse: A 1-year double-blind, multicenter study. Gut 1983; 24:853–856.

    Of 130 patients with benign gastric ulcer, 112 (86%) were healed after 8 weeks of cimetidine therapy, 200 mgs tid with 400 mgs qhs. Of the 112, 84 were followed for 1 year, half on cimetidine, 400 mgs qhs, and half on placebo. On maintenance therapy, 86% of the cimetidine group remained in remission by endoscopic criteria, compared to 45% on placebo.

27. Jefferys DB, Vale JA. Cimetidine and bradycardia. *Lancet* 1978; i:828.

    A letter detailing a putative role of oral cimetidine in the development of symptomatic bradycardia in a 39-year-old male and a 62-year-old male.

28. Jensen RT, et al. Cimetidine-induced impotence and breast changes in patients with gastric hypersecretory states. NEJM 1983; 308:883–887.

    A total of 11 of 22 men (50%) with Zollinger-Ellison syndrome or idiopathic hypersecretion taking a mean daily cimetidine dose of 5.3 g/day had reversible impotence, breast changes (gynecomastia or breast tenderness), or both. Gynecomastia may take longer than 3 months to resolve after cessation of drug. These problems were not encountered during ranitidine usage.

29. Katz LB, Fernandez JA, Shriver DA. Rioprostil, but not cimetidine, heals preexisting aspirin-induced gastric lesions in dogs during daily aspirin administration. Gastroenterology 1988; 94:A218.

    Rioprostil, 100 mcgs/kg, an antisecretory dose, healed preexisting aspirin-induced gastric lesions in 80% of dogs after 11 days of therapy despite daily administration of 975 mgs of aspirin. No healing of the gastric lesions was noted on once-a-day cimetidine therapy, 30 mgs/kg.

30. Kingsley AN. Prophylaxis for acute stress ulcers: Antacids or cimetidine. Am Surg 1985; 51:545–547.

    A prospective study of stress-induced gastric mucosal ulceration in 249 critically ill patients, randomized to receive either bolus antacids, cimetidine, or continuous infusion antacids or cimetidine. With a regimen of 50 mgs/hour of cimetidine, the author found the lowest frequency of bleeding (1 of 59 or 1.7%).

31. Krag E. Cimetidine treatment of protein-losing gastropathy (Menetrier's disease). Scan J Gastro 1978; 13:635–639.

    The use of cimetidine in this case of Menetrier's disease was associated with an increase in serum albumin, a decrease in gastric protein loss, and a decrease in gastric hyperrugosity.

32. La Brooy SJ, et al. Controlled trial of cimetidine in upper gastrointestinal hemorrhage. Gut 1979; 20:892–895.

    A prospective trial, under the aegis of P. Cotton, of 101 patients presenting with acute upper gastrointestinal hemorrhage, comparing the rate of continued or recurrent bleeding in patients receiving cimetidine to the rate of continued or recurrent bleeding in patients receiving placebo. All patients received the antacid magnesium trisilicate BPC, 10 mls every two hours. The bleeding continued or recurred in 11 of 51 (21.5%) of patients on cimetidine and antacid and in 12 of 50 (24%) of patients on placebo and antacid. Analysis of subgroups, i.e., patients with duodenal ulcer over the age of 60 presenting with severe hemorrhage or nonpeptic etiologies, showed no trend toward benefit from treatment.

33. Lieberman DA. Medical therapy for chronic reflux esophagitis. Long-term follow-up. Arch Int Med 1987; 147:1717–1720.

    A series of 20 patients with a 13-year mean duration of symptoms, followed prospectively for a mean of 26 months, after remission induced by 1.2 g of cimetidine and 40 mgs metoclopramide daily, showed that both drugs were able to be gradually tapered and then discontinued after an average of 8 weeks of full-dose therapy. Early relapse was associated with a low LES pressure. Intensive short-term therapy may be adequate treatment for patients without decreased LES pressures.

34. Martin LF, Max MH, Polk HC. Failure of gastric pH control by antacids or cimetidine in the critically ill: A valid sign of sepsis. Surgery 1980; 88:59.

    The authors found that 20 of 28 patients whose gastric pH could not be raised above 4 were septic, compared to 8 of 47 patients whose gastric pH could be raised above 4. They propose inability to raise gastric pH above 4 as a sign of sepsis.

35. Mitchell MC, et al. Cimetidine protects against acetaminophen hepatotoxicity in rats. Gastroenterology 1981; 81:1052–1060.

    Cimetidine given to rats 4 and 10 hours after intraperitoneal installation of toxic doses of acetaminophen was compared to placebo controls. Cimetidine resulted in significant improvement in survival (75% versus 40%) and decreased transaminase elevation (mean SGOT 3800 U/l versus 7200 U/l in placebo-treated rats). The postulated mechanism is cimetidine binding of the cytochrome P-450 system with inhibition of production of toxic acetaminophen metabolites.

36. Moore RA, et al. Cimetidine and parenteral nutrition. J Parent Ent Nut 1981; 5:61–63.

A study of four patients demonstrating the feasibility of adding cimetidine to TPN solutions. Patients received 38–56 mgs of cimetidine/hour with serum concentrations ranging from 0.6–1.0 mcg/ml.

37. Ostensen H, et al. Smoking, alcohol, coffee, and familial factors: Any associations with peptic ulcer disease? Scand J Gastro 1985; 20:1227–1235.

    An epidemiologic study showing that cigarette smoking and a positive family history correlated in a positive manner with the development of both gastric and duodenal ulcers. Coffee drinking and moderate intake of alcohol were of no importance in this regard.

38. Ostro MJ, et al. Control of gastric pH with cimetidine: Boluses versus primed infusions. Gastroenterology 1985; 89: 532–537.

    A study of 23 acutely ill patients receiving cimetidine for stress mucosal ulceration prophylaxis. The gastric pH was maintained continuously above 4 in only 5 patients given 300 mgs IV every 6 hrs, whereas 14 of the 23 maintained a gastric pH greater than 4 on 37.5 mgs of cimetidine/hr. An additional 6 patients achieved pH values greater than 4 when the infusion was increased to 50 mgs/hr. Thus, 20 of 23 patients (87%) achieved continuous gastric pH values greater than 4 with cimetidine infusions of 50 mgs/hr or less. No patient bled during the study period.

39. Peterson WL, et al. Reduction of 24-hour gastric acidity with combination drug therapy in patients with duodenal ulcer. Gastroenterology 1979; 77:1015–1020.

    Cimetidine administration alone at bedtime results in a more sustained rise in intragastric pH than concurrent cimetidine and antacid ingestion.

40. Peura DA, Johnson LF. Cimetidine for prevention and treatment of gastroduodenal mucosal lesions in patients in an intensive care unit. AIM 1985; 103:173–177.

    A randomized, double-blind, placebo-controlled study with serial endoscopic examinations to evaluate the efficacy of cimetidine in the prevention and treatment of stress-induced gastroduodenal lesions in 39 patients admitted to a medical intensive care unit. Cimetidine, 300 mgs every 6 hours intravenously, was compared to placebo. Endoscopic changes in the mucosa remained normal, became normal, or improved in 14 of 21 patients in the cimetidine group, compared to only 5 of 18 in the control group. Bleeding persisted or developed in only 1 of 21 patients in the cimetidine group, compared to 7 of 18 patients in the placebo group.

41. Porter JB, et al. Intensive hospital monitoring study of intravenous cimetidine. Arch Int Med 1986; 146:2237–2239.

    A review of definite or probable and possible adverse reactions to cimetidine in a hospitalized cohort of 1189 patients. A total of 23 (1.9%) definite or probable and 17 (1.4%) possible were noted.

42. Porter JB, et al. Long-term follow-up study of cimetidine. Pharmacother 1984; 4:381–384.

    A retrospective analysis of 8553 recipients of cimetidine found one possible case of cimetidine-induced hepatitis, which reversed over 6 months when cimetidine was discontinued.

43. Priebe HJ, et al. Antacid versus cimetidine in preventing acute gastrointestinal bleeding. NEJM 1980; 302:426–430.

   A randomized, prospective study of 75 patients admitted to an ICU at risk for acute gastrointestinal bleeding, comparing the rates of upper gastrointestinal bleeding in cimetidine-treated patients with that of antacid-treated patients. In the cimetidine treatment group, initial dose 300 mg IV every 6 hours and increased as high as 400 mg IV every 4 hours for pH greater than 3.5, the rate of upper gastrointestinal hemorrhage was 18% (7 of 38). In the antacid treatment group, initial dose 30 mls of Mylanta II every hour and increased as high as 120 mls of Mylanta II every hour for pH greater than 3.5, the rate of upper gastrointestinal hemorrhage was zero (0 of 37).

44. Richter JE, Castell DO. Drugs, foods, and other substances in the cause and treatment of reflux esophagitis. Med Clin N Am 1981; 65:1223–1235.

   A thorough review of alginic acid, antacids, bethanechol, metoclopramide, and cimetidine in the treatment of GERD.

45. Rudnick MR, et al. Cimetidine-induced renal failure. AIM 1982; 96:180–182.

   Two cases of acute, partially reversible interstitial nephritis developed after cimetidine use. In case A, rechallenge with cimetidine caused fever, chills, azotemia, pyuria, and eosinophiluria. Cessation of cimetidine was associated with a prompt reversal of azotemia. In case B, renal biopsy showed interstitial plasma cells, macrophages, lymphocytes, and polymorphonuclear leukocytes with focal fibrosis.

46. Saeed ZA, et al. Management of gastric hypersecretion with intravenous antisecretory medication in patients with Zollinger-Ellison Syndrome (ZES) [abstr]. Gastroenterology 1988; 94:A393.

   A study of 47 ZES patients demonstrating a clear correlation (r = 0.94) between the total daily oral dose and the continuous IV dose of cimetidine required to decrease basal acid output to less than 10 mEq/hr. This degree of acid suppression was necessary to allow an uncomplicated perioperative clinical course.

47. Schentag JJ, et al. Pharmacokinetic and clinical studies in patients with cimetidine-associated mental confusion. *Lancet* 1979; i:177–181.

   The severity of mental status changes associated with cimetidine correlated with the presence of hepatic and renal failure and serum trough cimetidine concentrations > 1.25 mcg/ml. Reduced doses of cimetidine should be given to this type of patient to avoid this type of problem.

48. Siepler J, et al. Prophylaxis of stress ulceration in the ICU: A comparison of cimetidine and ranitidine constant infusion [abstr]. Gastroenterology 1987; 92:1639.

   A nonrandomized, prospective study of 227 patients receiving continuous infusion cimetidine (N = 77), 300 mg bolus with 50 mgs/hr, or ranitidine (N = 150), 50 mg bolus with 8 mgs/hr. The amount of time with pH greater than 5

(66% versus 71%), the amount of time with pH greater than 6 (32% versus 34%), the number and percentage of upper GI bleeds (2, 2.5% versus 1, 1.6%), and transfusion requirements (3 versus 2 units PRBCs) were comparable.

49. Siepler J, Trudeau W. Treatment of UGIH by constant versus intermittent infusion of cimetidine in the intensive care unit [abstr]. Gastroenterology 1984; 86:1251.

    A prospective study of 46 indigent patients admitted for UGIH to an ICU. One-third received 50 mgs of cimetidine/hr intravenously, while two-thirds received 300 mgs of cimetidine every six hours intravenously. All patients received 30 mls of antacids every 2 hours. Rebleeding (17 of 30 versus 3 of 15) and mortality (23.8% versus 6.6%) were significantly higher in the intermittent bolus group compared to the constant infusion group.

50. Simpson CJ, et al. Effect of cimetidine on prognosis after simple closure of perforated duodenal ulcer. Br J Surg 1987; 74:104–105.

    A randomized, prospective study of the benefits of cimetidine on the postoperative course of 60 patients with perforated duodenal ulcer. Although cimetidine had no effect on the 12-month mortality rate, re-operation (second perforation or rebleeding) and symptoms were significantly more common in the control group.

51. Sontag S, et al. Cimetidine, cigarette smoking, and recurrence of duodenal ulcer. NEJM 1984; 311:689–693.

    Given that up to 90% of patients with duodenal ulcer have a recurrence after short-term therapy regardless of the agent employed for treatment (cimetidine, ranitidine, sucralfate, or antacids), this study was carried out to determine treatment regimens capable of preventing recurrences. Symptomatic ulcer recurrence occurred in 13% of the nonsmokers receiving placebo, 4% of the nonsmokers receiving cimetidine, 51% of the smokers receiving placebo, and 22% of the smokers receiving cimetidine. If all recurrences were grouped together (symptomatic and asymptomatic), nonsmokers receiving placebo had a lower recurrence rate than did smokers receiving cimetidine (21% versus 34%).

52. Steinberg WM, Lewis JH, Katz DM. Antacids inhibit absorption of cimetidine. NEJM 1982; 307:400–404.

    The concurrent administration of antacids (Mylanta II, Maalox, Alterna GEL, MOM) and cimetidine inhibits absorption of cimetidine in both the fed and fasting state. Peak serum concentrations and total cimetidine absorption were reduced in normal and duodenal ulcer patients by approximately one-third.

53. Takeuchi K, Furukawa O, Okabe S. Induction of duodenal ulcers in rats under water-immersion stress conditions. Gastroenterology 1986; 91:554–563.

    Reduction of duodenal bicarbonate secretion in rats by stress increases the mucosal susceptibility to ulceration in the presence of acid hypersecretion.

54. Terruzzi V, et al. The influence of cimetidine and ranitidine on the plasma lipid pattern. Br J Clin Pharm 1985; 19:846–848.

    A potential benefit of the antiandrogenic activity of cimetidine is the observed increase (14%) in serum HDL cholesterol after 5 weeks of cimetidine, 800 mg/day, an effect not observed with ranitidine.

55. Villeneuve JP, Warner HA. Cimetidine hepatitis. Gastroenterology 1979; 77:143–144.

    A case report of a hypersensitivity type of allergic reaction to cimetidine in an 83-year-old white female.

56. Yokoya H, et al. Functional study on "resistant ulcer" to treatment with cimetidine. Gastroenterology 1988; 94: A510.

    A study of 18 gastric ulcer patients resistant to cimetidine after 12 weeks of therapy (800 mgs/day) and 13 duodenal ulcer patients resistant to cimetidine after 8 weeks of therapy (800 mgs/day), demonstrating that resistance to gastric ulcer healing results from an increased ID50 (the cimetidine dose required for 50% inhibition of pentagastrin-induced MAO), whereas resistance to duodenal ulcer healing results from elevated BAO and MAO compared to nonresistant duodenal ulcer patients.

RANITIDINE

1. Bardham KD, et al. Gastric ulcer healing: A comparison of rioprostil versus ranitidine [abstr]. Gastroenterology 1988; 94:A22.

    A study of 48 patients with gastric ulcer comparing the healing rates of rioprostil, a methyl-substituted prostaglandin E1, 300 mcgs/day, with ranitidine, 150 mgs bid. After 8 weeks of therapy, 96% and 85%, respectively, were healed.

2. Bardham KD, Walker RR, Miller JP. A comparison of enprostil versus ranitidine in the treatment of gastric ulcer [abstr]. Gastroenterology 1988; 94:A22.

    A study of 156 patients with gastric ulcer treated for 8 weeks with either enprostil, a prostaglandin E2 analog, 35 mcgs bid, or ranitidine, 150 mgs bid. Healing rates at 8 weeks were 72% and 80%, respectively. Diarrhea occurred in 10% and 6%, respectively.

3. Berenson MM, et al. Ranitidine treatment of gastroesophageal reflux disease: Smokers versus nonsmokers [abstr]. Am J Gastro 1985; 80:832.

    A prospective analysis of 232 gastroesophageal reflux disease patients demonstrating no difference in response to therapy with ranitidine between smokers and nonsmokers.

4. Bredfeldt JE, et al. Ranitidine, acetaminophen, and hepatotoxicity. AIM 1984; 101:719.

    A letter to the editor presenting a case of cholestatic liver disease associated with concurrent ranitidine and acetaminophen usage. One possible explanation is that both drugs compete for hepatic glutathione.

5. Cohen A, Fabre L. Tolerance to repeated intravenous doses of ranitidine HCl and cimetidine HCl in normal volunteers. Cur Ther Res 1983; 34:475–482.

    A prospective evaluation of 100 normal volunteers receiving intravenous bolus infusions of ranitidine and cimetidine 4 times a day for 7 to 10 days. Drug-induced hepatitis with transaminase values less than 100 IU/liter were noted, typically after 5 to 7 days of therapy, in 24% of the ranitidine- and 19% of the cimetidine-treated subjects.

6. Collen MJ, et al. Long-term medical therapy with ranitidine in patients with Zollinger-Ellison syndrome [abstr]. Gastroenterology 1983; 84:1127.

No adverse effects were noted in 10 ZES patients during 12 months of therapy with ranitidine in doses as high as 6 g/day.

7. Collen MJ, et al. Correlation between basal acid output and daily ranitidine dose in Barrett's esophagus [abstr]. Gastroenterology 1988; 94:A73.

A study of 36 Barrett's esophagus patients showing that ranitidine suppresses effectively the excessively high quantities of acid secreted by these patients (BAO mean, 8.3 mEq/hr). The mean daily dose of ranitidine equalled 100 times the BAO minus 407.

8. Colin-Jones DG, et al. Reducing overnight secretion of acid to heal duodenal ulcers. Am J Med 1984; 77 (suppl 5B): 116–122.

A prospective double-blind, double-placebo trial of 102 patients treated with either 150 mgs of ranitidine twice a day or 300 mgs of ranitidine at bedtime. Healing rates were 48 of 57 (84%) and 43 of 45 (96%), respectively.

9. Danilewitz M, Tim LO, Hirschowitz B. Ranitidine suppression of gastric hypersecretion resistant to cimetidine. NEJM 1982; 306:20–22.

Three cases of idiopathic gastric acid hypersecretion unresponsive to intravenous cimetidine (1200–2400 mgs/day) are presented. All three patients (aged 59, 76, and 83 years) were given intravenous ranitidine, 300 mgs/day, with adequate control of acid output. Two patients developed pneumonia, one of whom died with pseudomonas pneumonia and septicemia.

10. Dawson J, Cockel R. Ranitidine in acute upper gastrointestinal hemorrhage. BMJ 1982; 285:476–477.

A double-blind study of 158 consecutive patients with acute upper gastrointestinal hemorrhage comparing ranitidine, 150 mgs po tid, to placebo in ability to decrease the incidence of recurrent hemorrhage. Although the overall results were comparable for the two treatment groups, 14 of 76 ranitidine-treated and 21 of 75 placebo-treated patients rebled. Among patients with duodenal ulcer, the rate of rebleeding with ranitidine treatment, 3 of 27, was significantly lower than the rate of rebleeding with placebo, 11 of 26.

11. di Stefano R, et al. A positive pulmonary aspiration test predicts a favorable response to ranitidine in patients with nonallergic asthma or chronic cough [abstr]. Gastroenterology 1988; 94:A101.

A positive pulmonary aspiration test (egg labelled with 4.5 µCi of 99 mTc-DTPA) was a better predictor of a favorable clinical response in patients with nonallergic asthma or cough to ranitidine, 150 mgs orally daily, than 24-hour esophageal pH probe testing.

12. Dobbs JH, Muir JG, Smith RN. H2-antagonists and hepatitis. AIM 1986; 103:803.

    Hepatitis can be regarded as a rare (0.06–0.08%) and idiosyncratic complication of cimetidine and ranitidine therapy.

13. Gough KR, et al. Ranitidine and cimetidine in prevention of duodenal ulcer relapse. *Lancet* 1984; i:659–662.

    A prospective, randomized, double-dummy-technique study of 484 patients receiving either cimetidine, 400 mgs orally at bedtime, or ranitidine, 150 mgs orally at bedtime, showing a life-table method of analysis relapse rate at 1 year of 37% and 23%, respectively ($p < 0.05$).

14. Jensen RT, et al. Cimetidine-induced impotence and breast changes in patients with gastric hypersecretory states. NEJM 1983; 308:883–887.

    A total of 50% (11 of 22 men) of Zollinger-Ellison patients or idiopathic gastric hypersecretory patients taking a mean daily cimetidine dose of 5.3 g/day had reversible impotence, breast changes (gynecomastia or breast tenderness), or both. Gynecomastia may take longer than 3 months to resolve after cessation of drug. These problems were not encountered during ranitidine usage.

15. Karachalios GN. Ranitidine and hepatitis. AIM 1985; 103:634–635.

    A case report of a 65-year-old male admitted for an upper GI bleed secondary to a duodenal ulcer. Admission SGOT and SGPT were normal. Ranitidine, 300 mg/day, was begun. Renal function was normal. Three weeks later SGPT was 920 U/l, and the bilirubin level was 11.9 mg/dl. Liver biopsy showed cholestasis. All abnormalities resolved with discontinuation of ranitidine.

16. Koch-Weser J. Ranitidine: A new H2-receptor antagonist. NEJM 1983; 309:1367–1373.

    A review of the pharmacology and clinical use of ranitidine, with a limited and selective bibliography. The structure, mechanism of action, potency, pharmacokinetics, and clinical effectiveness in acute peptic ulcer disease, acute gastric ulcer, prophylaxis against recurrence of duodenal and gastric ulcer, acute gastrointestinal bleeding from duodenal ulcers, reflux esophagitis, Zollinger-Ellison syndrome, and cimetidine-resistant acid secretory states are detailed. Side effects were limited to headache in 1.8%. The controversial issue of the long-term effects of gastric achlorhydria and the production of N-nitroso derivatives of ranitidine are reviewed.

17. Lanza F, et al. A multicenter double-blind comparison of ranitidine versus placebo in the prophylaxis of nonsteroidal anti-inflammatory drug–induced lesion in gastric and duodenal mucosa [abstr]. Gastroenterology 1988; 94:A250.

    A prospective, endoscopically controlled study of patients receiving NSAIAs for rheumatologic conditions showing that ranitidine, 150 mgs orally twice a day, was effective in the prevention of duodenal ulcer compared to placebo (0 of 62 patients on ranitidine versus 4 of 57 patients on placebo had evidence of duodenal ulceration, $p < 0.01$).

18. Lebert PA, et al. Ranitidine kinetics and dynamics: Oral dose studies. Clin Pharm Ther 1981; 30:539–544.

    Pentagastrin-stimulated acid output in 12 normal volunteers was inhibited 70% by an oral dose of ranitidine, 80 mgs. Peak serum concentration of ranitidine correlated positively with the percent reduction in acid output (r = 0.81).

19. Morichau-Beauchant M, et al. Pharmacokinetics and bioavailability of ranitidine in normal subjects and cirrhotic patients. Dig Dis Sci 1986; 31:113–118.

    Half-life, total plasma clearance, and bioavailability of ranitidine in cirrhotic patients was comparable to those values in normal controls. Although patients (N = 5) with prolonged prothrombin times tended to have higher ranitidine serum concentrations than normals (N = 8), the differences were not significant statistically.

20. Offit K, Sojka DA. Possible ranitidine-induced granulomatous hepatitis. NEJM 1984; 310:1603–1604.

    A case report of a 66-year-old male on ranitidine, 150 mgs/qhs for 4 weeks, who presented with fever and malaise. Liver test values were SGOT 128 U/l, SGPT 145 U/l, AP 466 U/l, and gamma-glutamyl transpeptidase 535 U/l. Biopsy showed granulomatous inflammation with eosinophilia. Fever and liver test abnormalities abated 1 week after discontinuation of the drug.

21. Okolicsanyi L, et al. Oral and intravenous pharmacokinetics of ranitidine in patients with liver cirrhosis. Int J Clin Pharm Ther Tox 1984; 22:329–332.

    Bioavailability of ranitidine in normals and compensated cirrhotic patients (albumin > 3 gm/dl, no ascites) was equivalent.

22. Penston JG, Wormsley KG. Long-term treatment of duodenal ulcers. Gastroenterology 1988; 94:A349.

    Long-term treatment of patients with previously documented duodenal ulcers with either ranitidine or cimetidine was associated with symptomatic recurrences in only 16% at 3 years (12% for ranitidine, 27% for cimetidine). Although 82 of the 432 patients (19%) presented with an upper gastrointestinal hemorrhage, only 5 of the 432 patients (1.1%) on maintenance therapy had a recurrent DU with hemorrhage.

23. Reid SR, Baycliff CD. The comparative efficacy of cimetidine and ranitidine in controlling gastric pH in critically ill patients. Can Anaesth Soc J 1986; 33:287–293.

    A randomized, prospective study of 71 patients admitted to an ICU, designed to evaluate the effectiveness of a primed infusion of cimetidine, 300 mg bolus with a 50 mgs/hr infusion, compared to a primed infusion of ranitidine, 50 mg bolus with a 12.5 mgs/hr infusion. Thirteen of the 38 patients in the cimetidine group (31.6%) and three of the 33 patients in the ranitidine group (9.1%) were "poorly" controlled (pH < 5 on more than 25% of the readings). One cimetidine and two ranitidine patients had clinical evidence of bleeding. No significant adverse effects attributable to the drugs occurred. Both agents effectively prevent stress-induced UGI hemorrhage.

24. Reusser P, et al. A randomized, controlled, endoscopic study

of ranitidine and antacids for the prevention of gastroduodenal stress lesions and bleeding in critically ill patients [abstr]. Gastroenterology 1988; 94:A373.

A 7-day study of 40 ventilator-dependent patients with severe head lesions admitted to an intensive care unit, who received either ranitidine, 150–200 mgs daily, plus antacids (dosage not specified), or no specific treatment. Gastric pH was > 4 in the treatment group significantly more often than in the control group (77% versus 33%). Endoscopic evidence of mucosal damage (1 GU, 1 DU) and clinical evidence of upper gastrointestinal tract bleeding was rare in both groups. The authors question the value of stress-related mucosal damage prophylaxis.

25. Rigaud D, et al. Intragastric pH profile during acute respiratory failure in patients with chronic obstructive pulmonary disease. Chest 1986; 90:58–62.

    A prospective evaluation of the ability of ranitidine, 35 mg loading dose and 17.5 mgs/hr continuous infusion, to elevate gastric pH in 12 COPD patients with respiratory failure. Gastric pH was maintained above 4 for 65% of the time.

26. Siepler J, et al. Prophylaxis of stress ulceration in the ICU: A comparison of cimetidine and ranitidine constant infusion [abstr]. Gastroenterology 1987; 93:1639.

    A nonrandomized, prospective study of 227 patients receiving continuous infusion cimetidine (N = 77), 300 mg bolus with 50 mgs/hr, ranitidine (N = 150), 50 mg bolus with 8 mgs/hr. The amount of time with pH greater than 5 (66–71%), the amount of time with pH greater than 6 (32–34%), the number and percentage of upper GI bleeds (2/2.5% and 1/1.6%), and transfusion requirements (3 and 2) were equivalent.

27. Silvis SE, et al. Final report on the United States multicenter trial comparing ranitidine to cimetidine as maintenance therapy following healing of duodenal ulcer. J Clin Gastro 1985; 7:482–487.

    The authors found an ulcer relapse rate at 1 year of 43% for cimetidine, 400 mgs at bedtime, and an ulcer relapse rate at 1 year of 16% for ranitidine, 150 mgs at bedtime (p < 0.01).

28. Simon B, Muller P, Dammonn H-G. Safety profile of ranitidine. In Riley AJ (ed), Ranitidine, Seventh World Congress Gastroenterology. Stockholm, 1982.

    An analysis of short- and long-term untoward consequences of ranitidine. With regard to liver enzymes, some elevations were noted in the ranitidine-exposed group of 4532 (12.9%) and in the placebo-treated group (9.24%). However, the elevations were small, isolated, and rarely of clinical significance.

29. Smith IL, et al. Ranitidine disposition and systemic availability in hepatic cirrhosis. Clin Pharm Ther 1984; 35:487–494.

    A study of 10 cirrhotic patients demonstrating that half-life (2.7 hours), plasma clearance (470 mls/min), and volume of distribution (1.2 l/kg) are not significantly different than for those of normal subjects. Renal dysfunction and

advanced years appear to be the known factors to prolong ranitidine half-life.
30. Strum WB. Ranitidine. JAMA 1983; 250:1894–1896.

A review of ranitidine emphasizing that its chemical structure is a substituted furan ring, that its relative potency is 5 to 12 times that of cimetidine, that it is useful in acute duodenal and gastric ulcer disease, and that it is not associated with antiandrogenic side effects.
31. Zeldis JB, Friedman LS, Isselbacher KJ. Ranitidine: A new H2-receptor antagonist. NEJM 1983; 309:1368–1373.

A comprehensive review of the mechanism of action, pharmacokinetics, efficacy, and side effects of ranitidine.
32. Zimmerman TW, et al. Ranitidine treatment of gastroesophageal reflux disease in the elderly. Gastroenterology 1985; 88:1644.

A retrospective analysis of the response of 64 patients 60 years old or older to ranitidine or placebo treatment of gastroesophageal reflux disease. Symptom improvement and endoscopic healing of esophageal abnormalities were significantly more likely to occur in the ranitidine (150 mgs po bid) group than in the placebo group. No significant untoward effects were seen.

FAMOTIDINE

1. Aono M, et al. Effect of famotidine and cimetidine on high density lipoprotein cholesterol levels in peptic ulcer patients [abstr]. Dig Dis Sci 1986; 31:493S.

There is no known associated increase in serum HDL cholesterol with famotidine.
2. Chiverton SG, Hunt RH. Pharmacokinetics and pharmacodynamics of treatment for peptic ulcer disease in the elderly. Am J Gastro 1988; 83:211–215.

A review of the drug therapy of peptic ulcer disease in the elderly. The authors emphasize:

If a patient is taking warfarin, phenytoin, or theophylline, and is stable, the addition of cimetidine requires dose reduction of warfarin, phenytoin, and theophylline and measurement of prothrombin time and serum drug levels.

Decreased renal tubular excretion of procainamide by concurrent cimetidine administration has an especially noteworthy propensity for toxicity.

Decreased acid secretion may inhibit iron and ketoconazole absorption.

Famotidine does not influence drugs eliminated by the P-450 mixed-function oxidase system.

Long-term treatment of elderly patients with impaired renal function with the basic aluminum salt sucralfate raises the specter of aluminum and dialysis dementia, even though long-term treatment of patients with normal renal function was *not* associated with elevation of plasma aluminum levels.

Colloidal bismuth compliance may be limited by its ammoniacal taste, blackening of the stool, and darkening of the tongue. Theoretical concern about increased plasma bismuth levels (toxic > 100 mcgs/l) in renal failure patients has not been observed.

3. Corleto V, et al. Loss of efficacy of famotidine in the control of gastric acid secretion in patients with Zollinger-Ellison syndrome, reversed by omeprazole [abstr]. Gastroenterology 1988; 94:A79.

The authors studied nine ZES patients and found that BAO increased to > 10 mEq/hr, despite initial control with 80–400 mgs/day of famotidine, in six of the nine within 7 to 15 months of starting the drug. Complete acid suppression was achieved with omeprazole, 20–60 mgs/day.

4. Klotz U, Arvela P, Rosenkranz B. Famotidine, a new H2-receptor antagonist, does not affect hepatic elimination of diazepam or tubular secretion of procainamide. Eur J Clin Pharm 1985; 28:671–675.

In contrast to cimetidine, an agent known to delay hepatic clearance of diazepam and renal tubular secretion of procainamide, famotidine did not alter significantly the half-life of diazepam (t ½ 45.6 hours pre- and 39.0 hours post-famotidine) or procainamide (t ½ 2.9 hours pre- and 3.0 hours post-famotidine) in eight healthy male volunteers.

5. Locniskar A, et al. Interaction of diazepam with famotidine and cimetidine, two H2-receptor antagonists. J Clin Pharm 1986; 26:299–303.

Eleven volunteers received diazepam concurrently with either famotidine, 40 mgs bid, or cimetidine, 300 mgs qid. Cimetidine increased significantly the elimination half-life of diazepam (55–72 hrs). Famotidine did not alter diazepam pharmacokinetics. In this article, no comments were made about clinically significant changes in subject performance.

6. Lyon DT. Efficacy and safety of famotidine in the management of benign gastric ulcers. Am J Med 1986; suppl 4B: 33–41.

The most common side effect of famotidine is headache, reported in 2 percent of these patients treated for gastric ulcer.

7. McCallum RW, et al. MK-208, a novel histamine H2-receptor inhibitor with prolonged antisecretory effect. Dig Dis Sci 1985; 30:1139–1144.

MK-208 (famotidine, Pepcid) is a guanidinothiazole derivative that is a potent H2 blocker devoid of antiandrogenic activity with a longer duration of action than cimetidine (up to 7 hours). Five mgs of MK-208 was equipotent to 300 mgs of cimetidine in suppressing pentagastrin-stimulated acid output.

8. Reynolds, JC. Four independent variables predict duodenal ulcer healing by famotidine in a relatively unselected patient population: A multivariate analysis of a prospective, multicenter study [abstr]. Gastroenterology 1988; 94:A374.

A prospective evaluation of 135 patients that identified four risk factors associated with nonhealing of duodenal ulcer at 4 weeks: (1) alcohol use (3.9-fold increased risk over normal of not being healed); (2) prior DU (2.7-fold increased risk over normal of not being healed); (3) history of bleeding (1.9-fold increased risk over normal of not being healed); and (4) ulcer size greater than 10 mm (6.2-fold increased risk over normal of not being healed). Use of NSAID or ASA prior to entry increased the odds of healing.

9. Simon B, et al. Famotidine versus ranitidine for the short-term treatment of duodenal ulcer. Digestion 1985; 32 (suppl 1):32–37.

    A prospective, randomized trial of three famotidine regimens compared to ranitidine. Famotidine was given 40 mgs at bedtime, 20 mgs twice a day, and 40 mgs twice a day. Ranitidine was given 150 mgs twice a day. At 4 weeks, the healing rates for the four treatment regimens were 91%, 83%, 90%, and 93%. At 8 weeks, the healing rates for the four treatment regimens were 98%, 95%, 100%, and 93%.

10. Smith, JL, et al. Famotidine, a new H2-receptor antagonist. Dig Dis Sci 1985; 30:308–312.

    Famotidine decreases dramatically acid output from parietal cells with parallel decrements in pepsin production. Nonparietal cell secretion (bicarbonate) is not decreased significantly. Pentagastrin-stimulated acid secretion remained decreased (50% of control) 12 hours after a 20 mg oral dose of famotidine.

11. Welage LS, et al. An evaluation of intravenous famotidine versus cimetidine therapy in the critically ill [abstr]. Gastroenterology 1988; 94:A491.

    In this study of 42 critically ill ICU patients, famotidine-induced acid suppression (20 mg IV q12h) was greater than cimetidine-induced acid suppression (300 mg IV q6h). Among the famotidine-treated patients, 81% of the gastric pH readings were > 4, whereas among the cimetidine-treated cohort, only 31% of the gastric pH measurements were > 4.

NIZATIDINE

1. Bovera E, et al. Nizatidine in the short-term treatment of duodenal ulcer—An Italian multicenter study. Hepatogastroent 1987; 34:269–271.

    A double-blind study comparing nizatidine, 300 mgs at bedtime, to ranitidine, 300 mgs at bedtime, for treatment of active duodenal ulcer disease showed them similar in healing response.

2. Cerulli, MA, et al. Nizatidine as maintenance therapy of duodenal ulcer disease in remission. Scand J Gastro Suppl 1987; 136:79–83.

    Nizatidine, 150 mgs, versus placebo was superior in prevention of duodenal ulcer disease in a 1-year study.

3. Cloud, ML. Safety of nizatidine in clinical trials conducted in the USA and Europe. Scand J Gastro Suppl 1987; 136:29–36.

    No significant adverse reactions were found in 3800 nizatidine-treated patients.

4. Dyck WP, et al. Treatment of duodenal ulceration in the United States. Scand J Gastro Suppl 1987; 136:37–55.

A dose-response study showing equivalent healing rates of nizatidine, 300 mgs at bedtime, and 150 mgs twice a day, significantly better than nizatidine, 25 mgs twice a day and placebo.

5. Hentschel E, et al. Nizatidine versus ranitidine in the prevention of duodenal ulcer relapse. Six-month interim results of a European multicenter study. Scand J Gastro Suppl 1987; 136:84–88.

   Statistically similar recurrence rates of duodenal ulcer were seen when comparing nizatidine, 150 mgs at bedtime, and ranitidine 150 mgs at bedtime.

6. Levendoglu H, Mehl B, Wait C. Nizatidine, a new histamine blocker in the treatment of active duodenal ulcers. Am J Gastro 1986; 12:1167–1170.

   Nizatidine, 150 mgs twice a day, compared with placebo was more effective in healing duodenal ulcer (82%–50% respectively) after 8 weeks of treatment.

7. Naccaratto R, et al. Nizatidine versus ranitidine in gastric ulcer disease: A European multicenter trial. Scand J Gastro Suppl 1987; 136:71–78.

   Benign gastric ulcer healing rates were similar when comparing nizatidine, 150 mgs daily, nizatidine, 300 mgs at bedtime, and ranitidine, 150 mgs twice daily (90%, 86.5% respectively) at 8 weeks.

8. Simon B, et al. 300 milligrams nizatidine at night versus 300 milligrams ranitidine at night in patients with duodenal ulcer: A multicenter trial in Europe. Scand J Gastro Suppl 1987; 136:61–70.

   A large (859-patient), six-center trial of duodenal ulcer patients showing equivalent rates of healing (92%–93%) and nocturnal pain relief (> 90% in both) in patients treated with either nizatidine or ranitidine (both 300 mgs at bedtime).

Cytoprotective Agents

Thomas Dorsey

Sucralfate

Sucralfate (Carafate-Marion) was introduced in Japan by the Chugai Pharmaceutical Company in 1968 for therapy of peptic ulcer disease. The drug was approved for use in the United States in 1981.

Sulfated saccharides such as Heparin and chondroitin sulfate have been known since early in this century to inhibit peptic activity, and in 1932 the concept that chondroitin sulfate in the gastric mucus was the major factor protecting the stomach from autodigestion was advanced. In 1954, Levy demonstrated that chondroitin sulfate inhibited pepsin activity and protected against experimental gastric ulceration in an animal model. Other agents such as amylopectin sulfate were developed. This drug also showed evidence of activity in animal studies but was limited by side effects common to this group of compounds, including anticoagulation and the induction of colonic ulceration. Subsequent efforts to produce a compound with the same activity but without the side effects led to the development of sucralfate.

PHARMACOLOGY

The base compound of sucralfate is sucrose, which has its eight alcohol groups sulfated forming sucrose octasulfate. This substance is then complexed with polyaluminum hydroxide [Al(OH)]+ to form sucralfate. The compound is a white amorphous powder insoluble in water and alcohol. It is poorly absorbed from the gut because of its high polarity, low solubility, and propensity for binding protein and bile acids. Ninety-five to 97 percent is excreted in the stool. Three to 5 percent of a dose is dissociated into sucrose octasulfate and aluminum base, which are absorbed. Sucrose octasulfate cannot be metabolized by the human and is excreted unchanged in the urine, as is the aluminum salt.

MECHANISM OF ACTION

Sucralfate mechanism of action is multifactorial and differs from those of the antisecretory and acid-neutralizing drugs.

Upon entering the acid environment of the stomach (pH < 3-4), some of the aluminum ions are dissociated and the compound becomes negatively charged. Polymerization occurs via intra- and intermolecular bridging, forming a viscous adhesive gel that retains its form even if the pH is subsequently raised (i.e., on entering the duodenum).

Sucralfate binds to normal mucosa, erosions, and ulcers. Binding to damaged areas of epithelium is more avid by a factor of 6-7 times than binding to normal mucosa. In addition, binding is better to duodenal than to gastric ulcers.

Sucralfate binds strongly to albumin, fibrinogen, and other proteins found in the ulcer base. Most of these proteins are positively charged at an acidic pH. Pepsin is negatively charged at this pH, as is sucralfate; thus, the binding of sucralfate proteins in the ulcer base prevents the binding of pepsin and subsequent digestion. In addition, it forms a physical barrier preventing diffusion of hydrogen ions from the gastric lumen to the gastric mucosa and acts as an antacid in the local microenvironment by slowly dissociating aluminum ions. The barrier also prevents bile acids from contacting the ulcer base.

Macroscopically, sucralfate binds for at least 6 hours. Although food removes sucralfate from normal mucosa, it does not affect sucralfate binding to damaged tissue other than by attaching to the luminal surface of the sucralfate patch. All traces of sucralfate are gone from the mucosa by 24 hours after a single dose.

Newer studies have shown that sucralfate-binding is less acid-dependent than previously thought. Aside from the barrier effect, sucralfate has a variety of luminal effects. Sucralfate absorbs pepsin. One gram of sucralfate decreases pepsin activity by 32–55 percent. Bile acids are also absorbed and sucralfate is as effective as cholestyramine in this regard. Aluminum ions also form an insoluble complex with bile acids.

Despite these luminal effects, there is no significant alteration in the volume or pH of gastric secretions and no change in the pepsin concentration. Thus, the barrier of gastric acid is maintained, preventing infection or colonization, as can occur with therapy using antacids or H2-antagonists. In addition, there is evidence that sucralfate may have a direct antibacterial effect against Escherichia coli and Pseudomonas.

The final mechanism of actions falls under the concept of cytoprotection, which refers to enhancement of mucosal defense mechanisms (mucus, bicarbonate secretion, epithelial cell renewal, and microcirculatory effects) by prostaglandin dependent or independent mechanisms without alterations of gastric secretion. An example of the prostaglandin independent mechanisms includes increases in both gastric and duodenal mucosal bicarbonate production. Two nonprostaglandin-mediated effects are (1) an increased secretion of soluble mucus and (2) binding of epidermal growth factor that is then carried to the ulcer base and kept in contact with the underlying mucosa for a prolonged period of time.

INDICATIONS

1. Peptic ulcer disease. In duodenal ulcer disease, sucralfate is significantly better than placebo and equivalent to cimetidine in short-term duodenal ulcer healing. It decreases the severity and frequency of symptoms, both during the day and nocturnally, and decreases antacid use. It has been shown that a dose of 2 grams twice a day

is effective in healing duodenal ulcers. In maintenance therapy of duodenal ulcer, it is superior to placebo in decreasing relapse rates. Remissions last longer in patients maintained on sucralfate when compared to cimetidine, but at 1 year the total percentages are not significantly different. Lam recently presented evidence that sucralfate is superior to cimetidine in the rate of healing and duration of remission in duodenal ulcer disease in smokers. In gastric ulcer, sucralfate is superior to placebo and equivalent to cimetidine in short-term ulcer healing. It is less effective in gastric ulcer than in duodenal ulcer. It is effective for pain relief and is as effective as cimetidine in maintaining remission.

2. Nonulcer dyspepsia. Several studies have reported that sucralfate is superior to placebo in relief of symptoms in nonulcer dyspepsia.

3. Drug-induced gastritis. Sucralfate has been shown to decrease the mucosal injury associated with the use of aspirin and nonsteroidal anti-inflammatory drugs, both long and short term, in animal and human studies via a prostaglandin dependent mechanism. In addition, sucralfate appears more effective than cimetidine in protection of the gastric mucosa from alcohol-induced injury.

4. Stress-related mucosal damage. Sucralfate is superior to placebo and equivalent to antacids and cimetidine in the prevention of stress ulceration. In addition, it has been suggested that by preservation of the gastric acid barrier and perhaps by direct antibacterial action, sucralfate decreases gastric colonization and subsequent nosocomial pneumonia. Driks has demonstrated this in ventilator patients.

5. Bile reflux gastritis. The bile-absorbing action and barrier effects of sucralfate make it an attractive option in the therapy of bile reflux gastritis. One study has shown significant improvement in histology without significant endoscopic or symptomatic improvement. More studies are needed.

6. Gastroesophageal reflux disease. Sucralfate suspension has shown efficacy equal to antacids, cimetidine, and ranitidine and symptomatic relief and endoscopic appearance in patients with reflux esophagitis. Its use in sclerotherapy-induced ulcerations and radiation esophagitis need to be studied further.

7. Miscellaneous uses. Sucralfate after meals has been used with success in a small number of patients with chemotherapy-induced oral stomatitis. Several articles, including one by Pera, have investigated the use of Technitium-99m–labeled sucralfate in the localization of peptic ulcers; however, it seems unlikely that this method would supplant currently existing diagnostic modalities. Several authors have shown that sucralfate is effective in lowering the serum phosphate level in renal failure patients. However, like other phosphate binders, sucralfate caused an elevation in the serum aluminum levels. Finally, in a preliminary study by Carling, sucralfate was shown to adhere to colitic mucosa and, when labeled with

Technitium-99m, may be useful in the determination of the extent of disease. A small number of patients were treated with a 10 percent sucralfate enema, 100 cc per rectum twice a day for 6 weeks. A large percentage of these patients had symptomatic improvement. These findings are preliminary and must be further investigated before sucralfate can be recommended in this setting.

SIDE EFFECTS

Side effects are uncommon, occurring in less than 5 percent of patients in most series, and are usually transient and seldom require discontinuation of the drug. The most common side effect is constipation, which occurs in 2 to 4 percent of patients. Other side effects, which occur in less than 1 to 2 percent of patients, are not significantly different from those reported while on placebo and include dry mouth, nausea, dyspepsia, headache, rash, dizziness, drowsiness, diarrhea, back pain, and vertigo. There has been one reported case of bezoar formation. In animals, there has been no evidence of mutogenicity, carcinogenicity, and lethal overdosage (LD-50) could not be induced.

LABORATORY ABNORMALITIES

There have been no changes noted in coagulation parameters, hematologic, renal, or liver biochemical values. There are no electrocardiographic changes or changes in fecal occult blood positivity. As noted, in renal failure patients, aluminum levels may increase and phosphate levels may normalize. There are rare reports of hypophosphatemia in otherwise normal patients.

DRUG INTERACTIONS

Sucralfate decreases the bioavailability of tetracycline, cimetidine, dilantin, digoxin, and coumadin by binding these agents in the gut and decreasing their absorption. Sucralfate should not be given within 2 hours of other drugs.

PREGNANCY

Sucralfate did not decrease fertility in animal studies. Chronic high doses of sucralfate did not cause birth defects in the mouse, rat, or rabbit models. There are no human studies, but sucralfate is probably safe for use in pregnancy. There are no studies available in nursing women, but significant levels are unlikely in breast milk. There are no data on the use of sucralfate in children.

DOSAGE AND ADMINISTRATION

Sucralfate is available as a one gram tablet. The suspension is not currently available commercially. Schneider has described a method of preparing individual doses by placing a 1-gram tablet in a 20-cc syringe (by removing and subsequently replacing the plunger) and drawing up to 20 cc of water and letting it stand for 5 minutes with occasional shaking.

There are no known contraindications to the use of sucralfate. In the adult, recommended dosage is 1 gram postorally 4 times a day given 1 hour before meals and at bedtime, or 2 hours after meals and at bedtime. Two grams twice a day have been shown effective in short-term healing of duodenal ulcer. Antacid should not be given within 30 minutes of sucralfate.

PEARLS AND PITFALLS

1. Sucralfate is a nonsystemic drug with few side effects aside from constipation, which is seen in 2 to 4 percent of patients.
2. It is as effective as cimetidine in the healing of duodenal ulcer and gastric ulcer and maintenance of duodenal ulcer healing. Some practitioners use sucralfate for maintenance therapy of gastric ulcers.
3. Particular settings for sucralfate that may offer advantages over the H2 blockers include chronic renal failure patients, smokers, and pregnant patients.
4. Sucralfate has shown efficacy in gastroesophageal reflux disease, drug-induced gastritis, stress-related mucosal damage, and nonulcer dyspepsia.
5. The usual dose is 1 gram postorally 4 times a day 1 hour before meals and at bedtime. Two grams twice a day have been shown as effective as the traditional dose in healing duodenal ulcer. Antacids should not be given within 30 minutes of a dose. Sucralfate can also interfere with the absorption of other drugs; administration of sucralfate and another agent should be separated by 2 hours.

Misoprostol

Prostaglandins are naturally occurring 20-carbon oxygenated fatty acids found in a wide variety of mammalian tissues. These compounds have widely varying biological activities; for example, prostaglandins of the E and F2 types stimulate contraction of uterine smooth muscle, prostaglandins of the A, E, and I type are potent vasodilators, and prostaglandins of the E type are bronchodilators. Naturally occurring E2 and prostacyclin I2 are found in gastric mucosa and regulate gastric mucosal blood flow and acid secretion, and exhibit cytoprotective properties (as defined by Roberts), including stimulation of mucous and bicarbonate secretion.

Synthesized prostaglandin E1, misoprostol, has these cytoprotective properties as well as gastric acid antisecretory effects. It has been shown to protect the mucosa of the stomach from inflammatory and noxious stimuli. It has been released for use in 12 foreign countries and holds promise as a treatment for preventing gastric ulceration, for treatment of gastric and duodenal ulcers, and for treatment of refractory peptic ulcer disease.

MECHANISM OF ACTION

Misoprostol is a synthetic prostaglandin E1 methyl ester analog with gastric cytoprotective activity at low doses, gastric antisecretory activity at higher doses, and few systemic actions.

PHARMACODYNAMICS AND PHARMACOKINETICS

When given orally, misoprostol blocks histamine-, pentagastrin-, and meal-stimulated gastric acid output. Misoprostol does not interfere with gastrin release nor alter serum gastrin levels. The primary acid-inhibiting effect is to lower the concentration of acid with little effect on the volume of gastric output. Misoprostol binds to the E-type prostaglandin receptors, which number approximately 8000 per parietal cell.

In rat ulcer models, the dose of misoprostol that prevented gastric ulceration (10-150) µgs/kg) was well below the dose (1000 µgs/kg) required to inhibit gastric acid secretion. Aspirin- and ethanol-induced ulcerations in dog and rat models were reduced by low-dose misoprostol administration.

Oral misoprostol has no significant effects on blood pressure, heart rate, or electrocardiogram measurements. Transient hypotension can accompany intravenous bolus administration.

Misoprostol does not inhibit platelet aggregation in a muscarinic receptor–binding assay.

Misoprostol has no anti-estrogenic, progestational, or androgenic activity.

Peak concentrations of misoprostol are reached one-half hour after dosing, with an elimination half-life of one and a half hours. The tissue-to-plasma ratio for misoprostol for the stomach was about 70.

Savarino has shown that misoprostol, 400 micrograms twice a day, was inferior to ranitidine, 150 milligrams twice a day, in decreasing gastric acid output. Utilizing 24-hour pH probes, the area under the curve was no different for misoprostol and placebo, whereas the area under the curve for the ranitidine-treated group was significantly less than either misoprostol or placebo.

INDICATIONS

Although now currently approved by the FDA for use in the United States for the prevention of aspirin- and NSAID-induced gastric ulcers in patients at high risk of complications from a gastric ulcer, it is often necessary to reduce the dose from 200 µg to 100 µg 4 times a day.

In a randomized, single-blind study of the palliative effect of misoprostol, sucralfate, and placebo on the acute effects of aspirin-induced gastric and duodenal mucosal damage, Lanza showed that misoprostol, 200 micrograms orally 4 times a day, was more efficacious than either placebo or sucralfate in preventing lesions induced by eight 325 milligram tablets of nonenteric coated aspirin in 30 healthy volunteers. A significant degree of protection of gastric mucosa was provided by the antisecretory dose of misoprostol (10 of 10 subjects showed no aspirin-induced gastric mucosal damage) compared to sucralfate (2 of 10 subjects were normal) or placebo (0 of 10 subjects were normal). There was only a trend in favor of misoprostol in terms of duodenal mucosal protection. Long-term benefits of this type of therapy were not addressed in this study.

Gonvers has shown that misoprostol, 800 micrograms a day, was comparable to ranitidine, 300 milligrams a day, in the treatment of benign gastric ulcer. In this endoscopically guided, randomized, double-blind study, 21 of 37 ranitidine-treated patients (56%) and 16 of 42 misoprostol-treated patients (38%) were healed after 4 weeks of therapy. After 8 weeks of therapy, 86 percent of the ranitidine group and 74 percent of the misoprostol group were healed. Interestingly, in smokers, ranitidine was superior to misoprostol, with a higher healing rate at 4 weeks (73% versus 20%). This fact counters the argument that misoprostol is cytoprotective at these antisecretory doses and can overcome the negative effects of cigarette smoking on ulcer healing.

Misoprostol at a cytoprotective dose of 50 micrograms orally every 6 hours healed only 42 percent of ulcers in a study by Brand. Given what is known about the pathogenesis of duodenal ulcers, i.e., relative gastric acid hypersecretion, it is not surprising that an antisecretory dose of the drug, 200 micrograms 4 times a day, is required for duodenal ulcer healing.

In a multicenter, European, endoscopically controlled, double-dummy, double-blinded study of 731 patients, Nicholson has shown that misoprostol, 200 micrograms 4 times a day, is as efficacious as cimetidine, 300 milligrams 4 times a day, in the treatment of uncomplicated duodenal ulcer disease. At this antisecretory dose, and analyzed utilizing the intent-to-treat rule, misoprostol healed 63 percent of duodenal ulcers, compared to a cimetidine healing rate of 70 percent ($p = 0.098$).

In patients with refractory duodenal ulcer disease—defined by persistance of a duodenal ulcer crater after 4 weeks of conventional doses of cimetidine or ranitidine—misoprostol, 200 micrograms 4 times a day, was associated with healing in about 40 percent of cases, compared to a placebo healing rate of about 20 percent ($p = 0.02$). Comparison of misoprostol to continued or adjusted doses of H2-receptor antagonists or to omeprazole was not performed.

In a review of the humanitarian use of misoprostol for severe, life-threatening, upper gastrointestinal hemorrhage refractory to cimetidine, ranitidine, antacids, and sucralfate, Corboy has shown a "favorable" clinical outcome in 52 of 83 treatment courses (63%). Analyzing the outcome by diagnosis, he found favorable outcomes in 20 of 28 duodenal ulcer patients (17%), 24 of 41 gastric ulcer patients (58%), 14 of 23 reflux esophagitis patients (61%), and 39 of 63 hemorrhagic gastritis patients (62%).

PEARLS AND PITFALLS

1. In low doses, misoprostol has only cytoprotective action (increased mucous and bicarbonate secretion), while at high doses the drug has gastric acid and pepsin antisecretory effects.
2. In patients with refractory duodenal ulcer disease, misoprostol has been shown to heal 40 percent of ulcers.
3. In a short-term study of the effect of aspirin on the gastric mucosa, misoprostol has been shown to be more efficacious than sucralfate in the prevention of gastric erosions.
4. Extragastric side effects of misoprostol are uncommon except for diarrhea (10% incidence). Cardiovascular, hematologic, and hormonal side effects are very rare.

References

SUCRALFATE

1. Aarimaa M, et al. Mucosal defense in ulcer disease. Scand J Gastro 1987; 23:1.

    A current review of actions of sucralfate and its use in peptic ulcer disease (symposium).

2. Brooks WS. Sucralfate: Non-ulcer uses. Am J Gastro 1985; 80:206.

    Reviews use of sucralfate in esophagitis, drug-induced gastritis, bile reflux gastritis, and miscellaneous other uses.

3. Cannon LA, et al. Prophylaxis of upper gastrointestinal tract bleeding in mechanically ventilated patients. Arch Intern Med 1987; 147:2101.

    Sucralfate as efficacious as antacids or cimetidine.

4. Carling L, Kageri I, and Borvall E. Sucralfate enema: Effective in inflammatory bowel disease. Endoscopy 1986; 18:115.

    A preliminary report of a potential new use for sucralfate.

5. Driks MR, Craven DE, Bartolome MD. Nosocomial pneumonia in intubated patients given sucralfate as compared with antacid or histamine type-2 blockers. NEJM 1987; 317:1376.

    The sucralfate group suffered less nosocomial pneumonia in intubated patients.

6. Hameeteman W, et al. Sucralfate versus cimetidine in reflux esophagitis. J Clin Gastro 1987; 9:390.

    Sucralfate is equivalent to cimetidine in therapy of reflux esophagitis.

7. Lam SK, et al. Sucralfate overcomes adverse effects of cigarette smoking on duodenal ulcer healing and prolongs subsequent remission. Gastroenterology 1987; 92:1193.

   Sucralfate superior to cimetidine in duodenal ulcer in smokers.

8. Leung ACT, et al. Aluminum hydroxide versus sucralfate as a phosphate binder in uraemia. BMJ 1983; 286:1379.

   Sucralfate as effective as Al(OH) in decreasing serum phosphate, but both cause elevated serum aluminum levels.

9. Marks, IN, et al. Second International Sucralfate Symposium. Scand J Gastro 1983; 18:1.

   Symposium on sucralfate mechanism of action and use in ulcer healing and maintenance therapy.

10. Marks, IN, Samloff IM. Third International Sucralfate Symposium. Am J Med 1985; 79:1.

    Symposium on use of sucralfate in peptic ulcer disease, reflux gastritis, and stress bleeding.

11. Pera, A, et al. Gastric ulceration localization by direct in vivo labelling of sucralfate. Radiology 1985; 156:783.

    Early work on using sucralfate to image ulcers.

12. Sabesin, SM, Lam SK. International Sucralfate Research Conference. Am J Med 1987; 83:1.

    Symposium stressing cytoprotection activities of sucralfate and its use in reflux esophagitis, nonulcer dyspepsia, and drug-induced mucosal damage.

13. Samloff IM. Gastritis, duodenitis, and peptic ulcer disease. J Clin Gastro 1983; 3:103.

    Development, pharmacology, mechanism, and safety of sucralfate in peptic ulcer disease.

14. Schneider JS, Ovellette SM. Sucralfate administration via nasogastric tube. NEJM 1984; 310:990.

    A method of preparing sucralfate suspension.

MISOPROSTOL

1. Agrawal NM, et al. Healing of benign gastric ulcer: A placebo-controlled comparison of two dosage regimens of misoprostol, a synthetic analog of prostaglandin E1. Dig Dis Sci 1985; 30:164S.

   A multicenter, randomized double-blind, parallel-group comparison of two doses of misoprostol and placebo showed 8-week healing rates in the intent-to-treat cohort of misoprostol, 100 μgs 4 times a day (62%), 25 μgs 4 times a day (50%), and placebo (45%). Diarrhea was experienced by 10 percent of patients.

2. Brand DL, et al. Misoprostol, a synthetic PGE1 analog, in the treatment of duodenal ulcers: A multicenter double-blind study. Dig Dis Sci 1985; 30:147S.

   After 4 weeks of therapy, 77 percent of patients taking misoprostol, 200 μgs 4 times a day, 43 percent of patients taking misoprostol, 50 μgs 4 times a day, and 51 percent of patients taking placebo were healed.

3. Bright-Asare P, Sontag SJ, et al. Efficacy of misoprostol (twice-daily dosage) in acute healing of duodenal ulcer. A

multicenter, double-blind controlled trial. Dig Dis Sci 1986; 31:63S.

Three hundred-thirty patients with duodenal ulcer received either placebo, misoprostol, 200 µgs, or misoprostol 400 µgs 2 times a day for 4 weeks. Healing rates at 4 weeks for a total of 280 evaluable patients were: misoprostol, 400 µgs bid, 65%; misoprostol, 200 µgs bid, 53%; and placebo 42%. Interestingly, the percentage of nonsmokers who healed at 4 weeks was higher than that of smokers in both misoprostol-treatment groups.

4. Corboy ED, et al. Humanitarian use of misoprostol in severe refractory upper gastrointestinal disease. Am J Med 1987; 83:49.

In humanitarian clinical trials, misoprostol was frequently associated with symptomatic relief and improvement in upper gastrointestinal hemorrhage from a variety of causes, including peptic ulcer disease, esophagitis, and hemorrhagic gastritis.

5. Dajani EZ. Overview of the mucosal protective effects of misoprostol in man. Prostaglandins 1987; 33:117.

Beneficial effects of misoprostol include reducing aspirin-induced gastric bleeding, aspirin-induced fecal occult blood loss, and ethanol-induced gastric damage. In the ethanol study, the mucosal protective effect was greater than that given by cimetidine.

6. Fich A, et al. Effect of misoprostol and cimetidine on gastric cell labelling index. Gastroenterology 1985; 89:57.

The number of antral and fundic labelled cells was significantly lower after misoprostol as compared to pretreatment, whereas the number of antral and fundic labelled cells was significantly higher after cimetidine than before therapy. The authors conclude that the decreased gastric cell turnover induced by misoprostol indicates that the trophic effect of prostanoids on gastric mucosa is not due to an increase in cellular kinetics.

7. Fich A, et al. Effect of misoprostol and cimetidine on gastric cell turnover. Dig Dis Sci 1985; 30:133S.

Misoprostol significantly decreased the number of labelled cells in antral and fundic gastric pits. Cimetidine significantly increased the number of labelled cells. The authors conclude that the decreased cell turnover induced by misoprostol does not appear to be a mechanism responsible for its mucosal protective and healing activity.

8. Gonvers JJ, et al. Gastric ulcer: A double-blind comparison of 800 micrograms misoprostol versus 300 milligrams ranitidine. Hepatogastroenterology 1987; 34:233.

In 79 gastric ulcer patients receiving either ranitidine or misoprostol, the 8-week healing rates were 86 percent for ranitidine and 74 percent for misoprostol. In smokers, ranitidine was superior to misoprostol, leading to a higher 4-week healing rate (73% versus 20%). There is no evidence that misoprostol overcomes the negative effect of smoking on gastric ulcer healing.

9. Herting RL, Clay GA. Overview of clinical safety of misoprostol. Dig Dis Sci 1986; 31:47S.

Misoprostol has a dose-related antisecretory effect that lasts 3-5 hours. Use of the drug does not result in rebound ulcer recurrence in the first 12 months after therapy. There is a tropic effect on the pregnant uterus. No significant effects on blood pressure, pulse, platelets, the immune system, pulmonary vasculature, or endocrine system were found.

10. Lam SK, et al. Prostaglandin E1 (misoprostol) overcomes the adverse effect of chronic cigarette smoking on duodenal ulcer healing. Dig Dis Sci 1986; 31:68S.

   A double-blind, randomized trial of 229 patients with duodenal ulcer receiving either placebo, misoprostol, 200 µgs 4 times a day, or misoprostol, 300 µgs 4 times a day, showing 4-week ulcer healing rates for the misoprostol groups of 61% and 71%, respectively. The time-healing curves for smokers and nonsmokers overlapped, implying that smoking is not a factor in the rate of healing of duodenal ulcers of patients treated with misoprostol.

11. Lanza F, et al. A blinded, endoscopic comparative study of misoprostol versus sucralfate and placebo in the prevention of aspirin-induced gastric and duodenal ulceration. Am J Gastro 1988; 83:143.

   Thirty healthy volunteers were randomized into three equal groups receiving either misoprostol, 200 µgs, sucralfate, 1 gm, or placebo, co-administered with 650 mgs of aspirin, 4 times a day for 7 days. A clinically significant degree of protection of the gastric mucosa was achieved with misoprostol (10/10, 100%) compared to sucralfate (2/10, 20%) or placebo (0/10, 0%). In the duodenum, nine of 10 subjects taking misoprostol showed no damage, compared to only five of 10 taking sucralfate, and three of 10 taking placebo.

12. Londong W. Anti-ulcer drugs in antisecretory doses for "cytoprotection" in arthritic patients? Klinische Wochenschrift 1986; 64:32.

   No study reviewed by the author of cytoprotective use of misoprostol, pirenzapine, or H2-receptor antagonists corresponds to Robert's definition of cytoprotection because all are being given in antisecretory doses in clinical trials.

13. Mazure PA. Comparative efficacy of misoprostol and cimetidine in the treatment of acute duodenal ulcer: Results of major studies. Am J Med 1987; 83:22.

   Misoprostol has potent antisecretory activity in addition to a mucosal protective action at low doses. In one study reviewed by the author the rate of disappearance of mucosal erosions was significantly greater for misoprostol than for cimetidine.

14. McGuigan JE, Chang Y, Dajani EZ. Effect of misoprostol, an anti-ulcer prostaglandin, on serum gastrin in patients with duodenal ulcer. Dig Dis Sci 1986; 31:120S.

   There was no significant difference in fasting serum gastrin or in integrated gastrin responses in duodenal ulcer patients after treatment with placebo or misoprostol, 50, 100, or 200 µgs 4 times a day for 4 weeks.

15. Monk JP, Clissold SP. Misoprostol: A preliminary review of

its pharmacodynamic and pharmacokinetic properties, and therapeutic efficacy in the treatment of peptic ulcer disease. Drugs 1987; 33:1.

In this large review, the author notes that duodenal ulcer pain relief from misoprostol therapy is less than pain relief resulting from cimetidine therapy. There are no studies to date on the use of misoprostol for maintenance therapy after documented ulcer healing.

16. Newman RD, et al. Misoprostol in the treatment of duodenal ulcer refractory to H2-blocker therapy: A placebo-controlled multicenter, double-blind, randomized trial. Am J Med 1987; 83:27.

    A study of 225 patients with duodenal ulcer persisting after at least 4 weeks of adequate, conventional therapy with cimetidine or ranitidine. Misoprostol, 200 μgs 4 times a day, was significantly superior to placebo in healing duodenal ulcers (37% versus 20%, respectively).

17. Ogawa M, et al. Inhibitory effects of prostaglandin E1 on T-cell mediated cytotoxicity against isolated mouse liver cells. Gastroenterology 1988; 94:1024.

    The cytotoxicity of mouse T-cells for mouse hepatocytes in a model for chronic auto-immune liver disease was significantly decreased in vitro by the addition of prostaglandin E1 at concentrations $>10-7$ M. This study suggests a possible new and exciting role for prostaglandin E1 in the treatment and modulation of "lupoid" hepatitis.

18. Quimby QF, et al. Active smoking depresses prostaglandin synthesis inhuman gastric mucosa. Ann Int Med 1986; 104:616.

    The accumulation in culture medium of prostaglandin E2 and F1a from fundic, antral, and duodenal mucosa was significantly depressed by active smoking. This depression may help explain slower ulcer healing and predisposition to ulcer recurrence in smokers.

19. Rachmilewitz D, Chapman JW, Nicholson PA. A multicenter, international, controlled comparison of two dosage regimens of misoprostol with cimetidine in treatment of gastric ulcer in outpatients. Dig Dis Sci 1986; 31:75S.

    On an intent-to-treat basis, ulcer healing rates for misoprostol, 50 and 200 μgs 4 times a day, and cimetidine, 300 mgs 4 times a day, were 39 percent, 51 percent, and 58 percent, respectively. Cimetidine, 300 mgs 4 times a day relieved global pain significantly better than misoprostol, 200 μgs, at 2 weeks but not at 4 weeks.

20. Robert A. Cytoprotection by prostaglandins. Gastroenterology 1979; 77:761.

    Hypothetical mechanisms by which cytoprotection occurs are: (1) mucus secretion, (2) restoration of the sodium pump, (3) activation of the enzyme adenyl cyclase, (4) alteration of gastric blood flow, and (5) protection of the gastric mucosal barrier by decreased transmucosal fluxes of sodium, potassium, and hydrogen ion.

21. Savarino V, et al. Evaluation of antisecretory activity of misoprostol in duodenal ulcer patients using long-term intragastric pH monitoring. Dig Dis Sci 1988; 33:293.

Ranitidine, 150 mgs bid, was significantly more effective in decreasing gastric acidity than was misoprostol, 400 μgs bid.

22. Wildeman RA. Focus on misoprostol: Review of worldwide safety data. Clin and Invest Med 1987; 10:243.

Misoprostol has been released for use in 12 countries and reports from over 100,000 patients reveal only mild adverse side effects, including a 7-percent incidence of diarrhea and a 13-percent incidence of abdominal pain, only rarely (<1%) so severe as to warrant discontinuation of the drug.

4

Bismuth

Margaret Andrea, James King,
and Michael M. Van Ness

For years bismuth preparations have been recognized to have antidiarrheal and antipeptic properties, but more recently selective antibacterial actions have been recognized. Although the literature contains few clinical trials and much is unknown about potential mechanisms of action, renewed interest in the potential benefits of bismuth compounds has sparked further research in its application to the problem of refractory and recurrent peptic ulcer disease.

MECHANISM OF ACTION AND PHARMACOKINETICS

Bismuth salts have numerous and varied actions in the gastrointestinal tract.

All salts of bismuth are fluid-absorptive.

Bismuth oxide, precipitated from bismuth salts by acid present in the digestive system, forms a tenacious layer on the digestive mucosa. Bismuth oxide has particular affinity for granulation tissue (i.e., ulcer base).

Bismuth salts fix chloride ion with the formation of insoluble bismuth oxychloride.

Bismuth compounds inhibit the growth of enterococci, staphylococci, and pseudomonas species.

Bismuth decreases gastric and intestinal motility, reduces intestinal spasticity, and prolongs intestinal transit time.

Bismuth ion increases directly the secretion of mucous in both the stomach and the intestine.

Bismuth ion attenuates the role of pepsin by chelation of the protein and protein precursor.

Although bismuth is not systemically absorbed after an oral dose, the amount of salicylate absorbed when one 8-ounce bottle is taken over 3.5 hours (the recommended dose) is equivalent to taking eight 325-milligram aspirin tablets.

The mean inhibitory concentration of colloidal bismuth subcitrate for *C. pylori* is less than 25 milligrams/liter.

INDICATIONS

Bismuth subsalicylate (Pepto-Bismol) is approved by the Food and Drug Administration for the symptomatic treatment of indigestion, nausea, and diarrhea.

Hamilton treated 80 duodenal ulcer patients with either tripotassium dicitrato bismuthate (TDB), one tablet 4 times a day, or cimetidine, 200 milligrams 3 times a day with 400 milligrams at bedtime. After 6 weeks of therapy, ulcers were healed in 75 percent of both treatment groups. However, duodenal ulcers recurred in 43 percent of patients in the 12 months after treatment with TDB and in 78 percent of patients after cimetidine treatment.

Martin has shown ulcer relapse rates similar to those reported by Hamilton. In a study of 55 patients treated with either TDB or cimetidine and followed for a year after documented healing of duodenal ulcers, 23 of 27 cimetidine-treated patients relapsed, compared to 11 of 28 placebo-treated patients. The mechanism of this difference is unknown, although it is known that ultrastructural abnormalities of the duodenal epithelial cell found in ulcer patients return to normal more often with TDB than with cimetidine.

Boyes treated 20 gastric ulcer patients with either TDB, 5 milliliters 4 times a day, or placebo for 4 weeks. Endoscopic healing of the ulcer was documented in nine of 10 patients receiving bismuth, compared to only three of 10 receiving placebo.

Goldenberg has shown that tripotassium dinitrato bismuthate (De-Nol) prevents stress-, alcohol- and aspirin-induced mucosal damage.

The use of bismuth-containing compounds for the treatment of gastritis (nonimmune, type B) with or without concurrent or sequential antibiotic therapy is controversial. Although Bizzozero (1893), Salomon (1896), and Doenges (1939) described spiral bacteria in the stomachs of animals and humans in the late-nineteenth and early-twentieth centuries, it was not until the reports of Marshall and Warren in 1983 and 1984 that renewed interest developed in this area. An etiologic relationship between spiral-shaped organisms *(C. pylori)* and gastritis was suggested by their results. Likewise, Buck found a strong correlation between the presence of gastritis (27 of 39 or 67%) and curved or spiral gram-negative bacilli. One proposed mechanism of injury caused by *C. pylori* is the rapid hydrolysis of urea at intercellular junctions with back-diffusion of hydrogen ion.

Some authors are skeptical of an etiologic relationship between *C. pylori* and gastritis, gastric ulcer, or duodenal ulcer. Dooley and Hornick are not yet prepared to label peptic ulcer disease a bacterial infection.

ADMINISTRATION

Each tablespoon (15 mls) of Pepto-Bismol liquid contains 262 milligrams of bismuth subsalicylate.

Each tablet of Pepto-Bismol contains 300 milligrams of bismuth subsalicylate. The tablets have none of the ammonical taste or smell characteristic of the liquid.

For symptomatic treatment of indigestion, nausea, and diarrhea, the usual dosage is 2 tablespoons or two tablets every one-half to one hour, not to exceed eight doses per day. Children are dosed according to age: 3 to 6 years, 1 teaspoon or one-half tablet; 6 to 10 years, 2 teaspoons or one tablet; 10 to 14 years, 4 teaspoons or one-and-a-half tablets. Tablets may be chewed or allowed to dissolve in the mouth.

For prevention of traveler's diarrhea, bismuth subsalicylate (Pepto-Bismol), 60 milliliters (2 ounces) 4 times a day is indicated.

For treatment of duodenal ulcer disease, De-Nol (colloidal bismuth, tripotassium dicitrato bismuthate, TDB) in doses ranging from 15 to 60 milliliters a day (5-10 mls orally 3-6 times a day) can be justified based on the results of studies done by Shreeve, Salmon, Hamilton, and VanTrappen.

For treatment of gastric ulcer disease, TDB, 5 milliliters diluted in 15 milliliters of water, is justifiable based on the results of work by Boyes, Sutton, and Tanner.

Despite some reservation, the use of combination antibiotic and bismuth therapy is justifiable for the treatment of gastritis. The highest published rates of clearance of *C. pylori* in gastritis patients were put forward by Borsch. He used bismuth subsalicylate, 600 milligrams 3 times a day, amoxicillin suspension, 500 milligrams 3 times a day, and metronidazole, 500-milligram tablets 3 times a day, for 2 weeks and achieved 100 percent (23 of 23) clearance after 2 weeks of therapy, with 90 percent remaining clear after an additional 2 weeks of observation.

SIDE EFFECTS

Side effects of bismuth subsalicylate include blackening of the stool; salicylate-induced tinnitus from rapid ingestion, prolonged use, or concurrent aspirin use; and bleeding due to salicylate-induced platelet inhibition.

There are no known drug interactions or inhibition of drug absorption from bismuth compounds. As a practical matter, it is prudent to avoid concurrent drug and bismuth administration.

There are no known acute or chronic toxic effects of bismuth salts. There is no established LD50 for bismuth subsalicylate.

Long-term use of the bismuth congeners, bismuth subnitrate, and bismuth subgallate is associated with neurotoxicity.

PEARLS AND PITFALLS

1. Bismuth is considered to act at a pH of 1 to 6, with optimum pH of 4 or less, requiring dosing at least an hour before or after meals.
2. Given the systemic absorption of aspirin with Pepto-Bismol, the use of Pepto-Bismol (bismuth subsalicylate) in children 12 years of age or younger for viral syndromes such as influenza and varicella may risk the development of Reye's syndrome.

References

1. Borsch G, Mai U, Opferkuch W. Oral triple therapy may effectively eradicate *Campylobacter pylori* in man: A pilot study [abstr.]. Gastroenterology 1988; 94:A44.

    An aggressive and intensive antibiotic regimen cleared *C. pylori* from 100 percent of patients as judged by CLOtest and culture.

2. Boyes BE, et al. Treatment of gastric ulceration with a bismuth preparation. Postgrad Med J 1975; 51(S5):29–33.

   Twenty patients with gastric ulcer were selected to receive either placebo or a bismuth preparation (TDB). The mean percentage reduction in the cross-sectional area of the ulcer by radiographic criteria was 91% in the TDB treatment group and 36% in the control group. Ninety percent of the ulcers were healed at endoscopy, compared to only 30% healing in the control group.

3. Buck GE, et al. Relation of *Campylobacter pyloris* to gastritis and peptic ulcer. J Infect Dis. 1986; 153:664–669.

   Of 39 biopsies of the gastric mucosa of patients with gastritis, 27 showed spiral gram-negative bacilli compatible with *C. pylori*.

4. Dooley CP, Cohen H. The clinical significance of *Campylobacter pylori*. AIM 1988; 108:70–79.

   Although eradication of the organism is associated with healing of gastritis and a lower relapse rate in duodenal ulcer disease, the authors conclude that a role for the organism in other upper gastrointestinal diseases is unproven.

5. Goldenberg MM, et al. Protective effect of Pepto-Bismol liquid on the gastric mucosa of rats. Gastroenterology 1975; 69:636.

   Bismuth subsalicylate may prove useful, like sucralfate and H2-receptor antagonists, in the prevention of stress-, alcohol-, and aspirin-induced gastric mucosal damage.

6. Hamilton I, et al. Healing and recurrence of duodenal ulcer after treatment with tripotassium dicitrato bismuthate (TDB) tablets or cimetidine. Gut 1986; 27:106–110.

   Eighty duodenal ulcer patients were randomized to receive either TDB or cimetidine. Healing occurred in 78% and 74% of the two treatment groups. The percentage of recurrences in the 12 months after treatment in the patient groups were 78% in the cimetidine group but only 43% in the bismuth group.

7. Hazell SL, Lee A. *Campylobacter pyloris,* urease, hydrogen ion back-diffusion, and gastric ulcers. *Lancet* 1986; i:15–17.

   The authors speculate as to the etiology and mechanism of *C. pylori*–induced gastritis.

8. Hornick RB. Peptic ulcer disease: A bacterial infection? NEJM 1987; 316:1598–1599.

   The prospects in this area of research are exciting, intriguing, and promising, but unproven.

9. Marshall BJ, Warren JR. Unidentified curved bacilli in the stomach of patients with gastritis and peptic ulceration. *Lancet* 1984; ii:1311–1314.

   An association between the presence of spiral-shaped bacilli and chronic gastritis, duodenal ulcer, or gastric ulcer is postulated by the author.

10. Martin DF, et al. Difference in relapse rates of duodenal ulcer after healing with cimetidine or tripotassium dicitrato bismuthate. *Lancet* 1981; i:7–10.

    Although no difference was noted in ulcer healing rates after 1 and 2 months of therapy between cimetidine and TDB, the relapse rate was higher in the cimetidine-treated group (23:27) compared to the bismuth group (11:28).

11. Salmon PR, et al. Evaluation of colloidal bismuth (De-Nol) in the treatment of duodenal ulcer employing endoscopic selection and follow-up. Gut 1974; 15:189–193.

    A greater number (9:10) of patients treated with colloidal bismuth showed endoscopic and symptomatic improvement than did those receiving placebo (6:10).

12. Shreeve DR. A double-blind study of tripotassium dicitrato bismuthate in duodenal ulcer. Postgrad Med J 1975; 51(S5), 33–36.

    A double-blind study of duodenal ulcer patients treated with either TDB or placebo. The healing rate after 4 weeks of therapy by endoscopy was 14 of 19 in the TDB group and 4 of 19 ($p < 0.005$) in the placebo group.

13. Shreeve DR, Klass HJ, Jones PE. Comparison of cimetidine and tripotassium dicitrato bismuthate in healing and relapse of duodenal ulcers. Digestion 1983; 28:96–101.

    In a comparison of healing and relapse rates of cimetidine-treated and bismuth-treated patients with duodenal ulcers, the rate of healing at 4 weeks was 75% in the bismuth-treated patients and 54% in the cimetidine-treated patients. The relapse rate at 1 year was 47% for the bismuth group and 60% for the cimetidine group.

14. Sutton DR. Gastric ulcer healing with tripotassium dicitrato bismuthate and subsequent relapse. Gut 1982; 23: 621–624.

    Gastric ulcer healing occurred in 18 of the 25 (72%) patients given TDB and in nine (36%) of the patients given placebo. During a follow-up period of 44 months, relapse occurred in 13 (45%).

15. Tanner AR, et al. Efficacy of cimetidine and tripotassium dicitrato bismuthate (De-Nol) in chronic gastric ulceration: A comparative study. Med J Austral 1979; 1:1–2.

    Of 57 gastric ulcer patients evaluated endoscopically after 6 weeks of bismuth therapy, 20 (67%) were healed, compared to 17 of 27 patients (63%) treated with cimetidine.

16. VanTrappen G, et al. Randomized, open-controlled trial of colloidal bismuth subcitrate tablets and cimetidine in the treatment of duodenal ulcer. Gut 1980; 21:329–333.

    For the treatment of acute duodenal ulcer disease, colloidal bismuth and cimetidine were equivalent in terms of pain relief and ulcer healing.

17. Wilson TR. The pharmacology of tripotassium dicitrato bismuthate (TDB). Postgrad Med J 1975; 51 (S5):18–21.

    TDB is a colloidal bismuth preparation that is free from toxicity and capable of facilitating the healing of gastric ulcers in both humans and experimental animals.

5
Metoclopramide
David G. Litaker

Since its initial approval by the FDA in 1981 for diabetic gastroparesis, the prokinetic agent metoclopramide has been applied to a variety of clinical situations, leading to broader usage. This drug is a prototype of a class of medications including Cisapride and Dazopride, which are likely to extend dramatically the ability of the clinician to treat patients with altered gastrointestinal motility.

MECHANISM OF ACTION

Developed in the early 1960s, metoclopramide (2-methoxy-5-chloroprocainamide) is a procainamide derivative with clinically insignificant anesthetic and antidysrhythmic effects. Although the exact mechanism of action is not understood, extensive research over the last 20 years suggests that it is a potent dopamine-receptor antagonist with cholinomimetic properties.

Stimulation of dopamine receptors in the gastrointestinal tract results in gastric relaxation and decreased forward passage of a tracer-labelled food bolus from the stomach into the proximal small bowel. This effect is vagally mediated and is abolished by vagotomy. Pharmacologic inhibition of this effect occurs with metoclopramide and can be counterantagonized by administration of levodopa. The prokinetic effect of metoclopramide is also explained by an apparent cholinomimetic effect on the gastrointestinal tract thought to be secondary to enhanced acetylcholine release resulting in increased smooth-muscle contraction. Unlike other cholinomimetic agents such as bethanecol, there has been no evidence of increased acid secretion or gastrin release.

Metoclopramide coordinates forward propulsion of esophagogastric contents in an effective manner. Use of this drug in normal human volunteers results in increased lower-esophageal sphincter pressure, increased amplitude and duration of esophageal peristalsis, increased antral peristaltic contractions, relaxation of the pyloric sphincter, and decreased proximal small-bowel transit time. Although little physiologic response in the distal small bowel or colon was documented in the early research, subsequent investigators have reported an increase in the amplitude of colonic contractions and a decrease in the transit time of the colon in both normal volunteers and patients with severe diabetic enteropathy.

Metoclopramide is rapidly absorbed into the gastrointestinal tract, with peak serum levels appearing in 1 hour. The normal half-life ranges from 3 to 6 hours and is increased to as long as 24 hours in patients with renal impairment due to almost complete renal excretion. Because of weak protein binding, drug removal can be effectively achieved by dialysis.

INDICATIONS

Current indications for metoclopramide include treatment of diabetic gastroparesis, gastroesophageal reflux, reduction of cancer chemotherapy–associated emesis, and the facilitation of small-bowel intubation and radiographic examination of the stomach and small bowel. In addition, a number of as-yet unapproved uses have been identified. The use of metoclopramide to reduce the risk of aspiration of gastric contents in the patient facing emergent surgery and to treat patients with the gastrointestinal complications of scleroderma, dystrophica myotonica, and adynamic or chemotherapy-induced ileus is justified by reports in the medical literature.

Diabetic Gastroparesis

Diabetic gastroparesis is a condition characterized by decreased gastric emptying and generalized gastric atony. The diagnosis is suspected on clinical grounds in longstanding diabetic patients with early satiety, nausea, vomiting, and weight loss but is confirmed by radiographic or scintigraphic examination. Ricci described significantly increased gastric emptying in these patients and a marked reduction of symptoms following oral administration of metoclopramide. A subsequent case report suggests responsiveness to a rectal-suppository form in a patient intolerant of oral dosages. The long-term efficacy and symptomatic benefit of metoclopramide in this setting has not been documented completely.

Gastroesophageal Reflux

Gastroesophageal reflux results from decreased lower-esophageal sphincter pressure, regurgitation of acid from the stomach to the esophagus, and inadequate clearance of regurgitated material. In a number of clinical trials, the prokinetic effects of metoclopramide have resulted in diminution of symptoms compared with placebo, but have not correlated with a decreased incidence of esophagitis on endoscopy follow-up.

Chemotherapy-induced Emesis

The etiology of emesis in the setting of cancer treatment is multifactorial. Stimulation of the chemoreceptor trigger zone, amomorphine (a dopamine agonist) release, and delayed gastric emptying have all been observed following the administration of chemotherapeutic agents. Cisplatin, one of the most emetogenic agents, has been shown to disrupt normal smooth-muscle pacemaker potentials in the stomach of dogs and to result in gastrointestinal retroperistalsis. Metoclopramide, in this model, corrects such dysmotility by peripherally enhancing forward motility and centrally inhibiting the dopamine-agonist effect at the chemoreceptor trigger zone. Similar effects have been observed in humans, but it appears that inhibition of the chemoreceptor trigger-zone activity is clinically insignificant.

Small-Bowel Radiographic Examination

Metoclopramide has long been recognized to decrease the transit time of barium or tracer-labelled meals through the small bowel. When studied in a double-blinded fashion with other prokinetic agents such as domperidone, metoclopramide shortened the radiographic examination to a greater extent, caused no difference in technical quality of the study compared with controls, and resulted in less radiation exposure to the patient.

Nonapproved Indications

The rationale for application of metoclopramide to other clinical problems or diseases is based on its ability to enhance esophagogastric motility. A beneficial effect in patients with esophageal dysmotility and delayed gastric emptying due to both progressive systemic sclerosis or dystrophica myotonica has been reported and appears to address a primary pathophysiologic defect. In addition, metoclopramide has reported efficacy in reducing the risk of aspiration in patients in whom reflux of gastric contents may be more common, such as the chronically debilitated nursing-home occupant or the patient in need of emergent surgery. The future role for this and similar prokinetic agents requires further study to determine long-term benefit, the limitations of side effects, and the extent of drug–drug interactions.

CONTRAINDICATIONS

Metoclopramide should not be used in patients with suspected or known mechanical intestinal obstruction, gastrointestinal perforation, known sensitivity or intolerance, or in known epileptic patients or patients likely to be treated with drugs causing extrapyramidal side effects. The presence of pheochromocytoma is felt to be an absolute contraindication since metoclopramide can result in increased catecholamine release from the tumor. If this situation should occur, the appropriate treatment of the resultant hypertension is an alpha-receptor blocking agent such as phentolamine. Because of inadequate controlled studies, the use of metoclopramide is relatively contraindicated in the pregnant patient.

ADMINISTRATION

Metoclopramide is dispensed in 10-milligram tablets. It is also available in syrup (5 mgs/ml) and injectable forms (5 mgs/ml). Treatment for gastroesophageal reflux is 10 to 15 milligrams 4 times a day 30 minutes before meals, and at bedtime as needed, for control of symptoms. Diabetic gastroparesis is usually treated with 10 milligrams before meals but may require parenteral administration depending on the severity of symptoms. Once gastric emptying improves, conversion to an oral regimen is usually possible.

Significant relief of symptoms may be experienced early in the course of therapy and continue to improve for up to 3 weeks. The dosage for small-bowel intubation and radiographic examination is 10 milligrams intravenously. To prevent chemotherapy-induced emesis, a loading dose of 1 to 2 milligrams/kilogram of body weight is used, with .5 to 1 milligram/kilogram given every 3 to 4 hours subsequently while receiving chemotherapy.

PEARLS AND PITFALLS

1. Because metoclopramide decreases gastric-emptying time as well as gastrointestinal transit time, insulin-dependent diabetic patients may need to increase the amount of regular insulin and decrease the amount of NPH (or other long-acting) insulin preparations used. When metoclopramide is begun, close attention must be given to blood glucose levels.
2. Drowsiness and central nervous system depression seen with metoclopramide are substantially increased in patients concomitantly receiving dopamine antagonists such as phenothiazines.
3. Dystonic reactions associated with metoclopramide should be immediately treated with 50 milligrams of diphenhydramine intravenously.

References

1. Akwari OE. The gastrointestinal tract in chemotherapy-induced emesis: A final common pathway. Drugs 1983; 25: 18–34.

   This paper summarizes the current understanding of gastrointestinal motility and the derangements in normal function thought to be induced by emetic agents. Metoclopramide is effective in preventing emesis by direct gastrointestinal as well as central effects.

2. Alphin RS, et al. Antagonism of cisplatin-induced emesis by metoclopramide and dazopride through enhancement of gastric motility. Dig Dis Sci 1986; 31:524–529.

   The authors further investigate the antiemetic effects of metoclopramide and dazopride by studying the central and peripheral sites of action in nonhuman subjects treated with cisplatin. They conclude that metoclopramide acts predominantly by enhancing gastrointestinal motility and inhibiting amomorphine-induced emesis, but has little antagonistic effect at central dopamine receptors (e.g., at the chemoreceptor trigger zone) in clinically used doses.

3. Battle WM, et al. Colonic dysfunction in diabetes mellitus. Gastroenterology 1980; 79:1217–1221.

   The authors investigate the myoelectrical and motility abnormalities seen in the colons of diabetic patients with constipation. They conclude that these patients have evidence of an autonomic enteropathy with absent postprandial gastrocolonic response which responds to the use of neostigmine and metoclopramide.

4. Beam L, Bianchi C, Crema C. Effects of metoclopramide on isolated colon: 1. Peripheral sensitization to acetylcholine. Eur J Pharmacol 1970; 12:320–331.

   The authors report the augmentation of acetylcholine release from postganglionic nerve terminals and sensitization of muscarinic receptors in gastrointestinal smooth muscle in isolated human smooth muscle and guinea pig colon. This study expands the understanding of metoclopramide as an unconventional cholinergic drug that relies on intrinsic stores of acetylcholine.

5. Gipson SL, et al. Pharmacologic reduction of the risk of aspiration. South Med J 1986; 79:1356–1358.

   Forty women undergoing gynecologic surgery received metoclopramide, cimetidine, a combination of the two, or no treatment at all. A resultant decrease in gastric volume and increase in gastric pH are documented and support the use of this drug in reducing the risk of gastric-content aspiration in the preoperative patient.

6. Horowitz M, et al. Gastric and esophageal emptying in dystrophica myotonica: Effect of metoclopramide. Gastroenterology 1987; 92:570–577.

   Dystrophica myotonica, a systemic disease characterized by myotonia and skeletal muscle-wasting, also involves smooth muscle and is associated for this reason with abnormal esophageal- and gastric-emptying. This paper documents the prokinetic effects of metoclopramide in these patients and supports its use in treating gastroparesis.

7. Johnson DA, et al. Metoclopramide response in patients with progressive systemic sclerosis: Effects on esophageal and gastric motility abnormalities. Arch Intern Med 1987; 147:1597–1601.

   Metoclopramide improved lower-esophageal pressure and gastric-emptying in 12 patients with progressive systemic sclerosis. Although use does not alter survival data, metoclopramide may improve the quality of life in patients who suffer from debilitating symptoms.

8. McCallum RW. Review of the current status of prokinetic agents in gastroenterology. Am J Gastro 1985; 80:1008–1016.

   This review article details the evolution of prokinetic agents in gastroenterology, including metoclopramide and its congeners dazopride and cisipride.

9. Morewood DJW, Whitehouse GH. A comparison of three methods for performing barium follow-through studies of the small intestine. Brit J Rad 1986; 59:971–973.

   Gastric-emptying time is decreased in patients pretreated with either domperidone or metoclopramide prior to barium examination of the stomach or small bowel, compared with rapid-transit barium. This article is representative of the literature that supports the use of metoclopramide in this setting.

10. Ricci DA, et al. Effect of metoclopramide in diabetic gastroparesis. J Clin Gastro 1985; 7:25–32.

    Gastric-emptying time by scintigraphic study showed a significant improvement in diabetic patients receiving metoclopramide compared with placebo. This paper supports continued use of metoclopramide in relieving symptoms of diabetic patients with gastroparesis.

11. Trapnell BC, et al. Metoclopramide suppositories in the treatment of diabetic gastroparesis. Arch Intern Med 1986; 146:2278–2279.

   Diabetic patients with symptoms of severe gastroparesis who are intolerant of oral dosages of metoclopramide may respond to a rectal route of administration, according to this case report. The clinical efficacy of the drug was verified by gastric-emptying studies and serum levels before and after the dose was given.

12. Valenzuela JE. Dopamine as a possible nerve transmitter in gastric relaxation. Gastroenterology 1976; 71:1019–1022.

   The author documented that dopamine receptors are found in the pyloric smooth muscle of the canine, feline, and human species. This work formed the basis of the research leading to metoclopramide's development.

13. Winnan J, et al. Double-blind trials of metoclopramide versus placebo-antacid in symptomatic gastroesophageal reflux. Gastroenterology 1980; 78:1292.

   The efficacy of metoclopramide versus placebo-antacid regimens was studied in a double-blinded fashion. Metoclopramide was significantly more effective than placebo and antacid in improving symptoms and increasing gastric-emptying, which was delayed in reflux patients, but did not result in an increased rate of healing in patients with esophagitis on endoscopy.

Omeprazole

Michael Carboni

Omeprazole is the first member of a new class of potent gastric acid inhibitors under investigation for the treatment of peptic ulcer disease, Zollinger-Ellison syndrome, and erosive reflux esophagitis. Early results indicate that omeprazole is more potent and may be more convenient than traditional H2-receptor antagonists.

MECHANISM OF ACTION, PHARMACODYNAMICS, AND PHARMACOKINETICS

Omeprazole is a substituted benzimidazole. It inhibits gastric acid secretion by noncompetitive inhibition of the $H+/K+$ ATPase proton pump. This proton pump is the final step in gastric acid secretion and lies within the secretory membrane of parietal cells. Omeprazole is not only a powerful inhibitor of basal acid output but, unlike the H2-receptor antagonists, also inhibits stimulated gastric acid output.

Omeprazole is a lipid soluble weak base. It is acid labile, necessitating formulation as enteric-coated granules in order to reach the small intestine. As omeprazole is absorbed and gastric acid secretion is inhibited, intragastric pH rises, increasing its absorption and bioavailability.

The plasma half-life of omeprazole is about 50 minutes. Because omeprazole accumulates in parietal cells, its effective half-life is considerably longer (18-24 hours). Omeprazole's inhibition of acid secretion is dose-dependent and increases over time due to increasing absorption. A single dose reaches peak inhibitory effect in 2 to 4 hours, while repeated daily doses require 3 to 5 days for maximum acid inhibition. With repeated daily doses, inhibition of acid output remains for days even with cessation of drug therapy. Eventually complete recovery of acid output occurs.

Twenty-four-hour intragastric acidity studies demonstrate that oral omeprazole in doses of 20 to 80 milligrams inhibit gastric acid secretion by 50 to 100 percent within hours of drug ingestion. Repeated dosing with 20 milligrams gradually increases the level of inhibition to nearly 100 percent. With a single morning dose, nocturnal secretion is decreased by 50 percent, as is meal-stimulated and pentagastrin-stimulated acid secretion. Intravenous dosing is under investigation and is equally effective in its inhibition of gastric output.

Other physiologic effects include elevation of serum gastrin. Hypergastrinemia from endogenous production, as seen in Zollinger-Ellison syndrome, is not aggravated by omeprazole therapy. Omeprazole does not affect gastric emptying or secretion of intrinsic factor. It does appear to increase intragastric concentrations of bile acid, the significance of which is unknown.

INDICATIONS

Zollinger-Ellison Syndrome

The primary indication for omeprazole therapy is Zollinger-Ellison syndrome (ZES). Zollinger-Ellison syndrome patients may be resistant to treatment with high doses of H2-receptor antagonists. Because of its beneficial clinical effects and pronounced, long-lasting reduction in gastric acid secretion, omeprazole is the drug of choice for treatment of ZES patients. The drug is available on a compassionate-use basis from Merke, Sharp, and Dohme (Director of Clinical Research, Merke, Sharp, and Dohme Research Laboratories, West Point, PA, 19486, (215) 834–2624, or (215) 661–5000).

Since omeprazole is such a potent gastric acid inhibitor, anticholinergic therapy is not needed, as it may be with H2-receptor antagonists. No adverse effects in humans have been noted, even with long-term therapy of Zollinger-Ellison patients. Since omeprazole has been associated with gastric carcinoids in rats, histologic monitoring of the gastric mucosa for enterochromaffinlike cell hyperplasia is recommended. If discovered, therapy with omeprazole should be discontinued. With discontinuation of treatment, the hyperplasia is reversible.

Recommended doses for the treatment of ZES are not fixed but are titrated to keep basal acid output less than 10 milliequivalents/hour. Dosages range from 20 to 80 milligrams daily.

Erosive Reflux Esophagitis

Omeprazole has been shown to be better than H2-receptor antagonists in a study of eight patients with erosive esophagitis. Seven of these patients were healed with 30 milligrams of omeprazole daily for 4 weeks. The remaining patient had a 95-percent reduction in the area of erosion.

Gastric Ulcer Disease

Omeprazole (20 mgs daily) has been found to be equal in potency and efficacy to daily ranitidine therapy (150 mgs twice a day). Healing rates are not affected by smoking.

Duodenal Ulcer Disease

With once-daily dosing, it is possible to almost completely inhibit 24-hour intragastric acidity in most duodenal ulcer patients. Direct comparative studies indicate that omeprazole is superior to H2-receptor antagonists in short-term treatment of duodenal ulcers. The majority of patients heal within 2 to 4 weeks with faster and more pronounced pain relief on omeprazole. Optimum recommended therapy is 20 to 30 milligrams for 4 weeks. Although doses up to 60 milligrams may increase the number of patients healed, the benefits of higher dosages do not outweigh the risk of enterochromaffinlike cell hyperplasia.

Intravenous therapy is also available if immediate reductions in acidity are needed. A single bolus injection of 10 milligrams of omeprazole is comparable with the inhibition by 20 milligrams of a single oral dose. Intravenous injections reach peak inhibitory effects within 2 hours.

Healing rates of duodenal ulcers treated with omeprazole are impaired by smoking. Sixty percent of the smokers studied endoscopically healed in 6 to 8 weeks.

The recurrence rate of duodenal ulcers treated with omeprazole is approximately 50 percent within 1 year, comparable to that seen with H2-receptor antagonists.

SIDE EFFECTS AND CARCINOGENICITY

Because it is specific for the H+/K+ ATPase of parietal cells, omeprazole lacks any systemic effects beyond that of gastric acid inhibition. In addition, omeprazole has been well tolerated and has no known adverse clinical effects.

Studies in rats and rabbits have shown no fetal toxicity, teratogenicity, or mutagenicity with omeprazole. Pregnancy does not appear to be an absolute contraindication. No hepatic or renal toxicity has been demonstrated. Studies done in patients with chronic renal failure indicate that omeprazole is safe, effective, and nondialyzable.

Omeprazole does not have an association with gastric carcinoids, established by 2-year oncogenicity studies in rats. Doses 10 times those used therapeutically in humans have produced low-malignant carcinoid tumors from the enterochromaffinlike (ECL) cells of rat gastric mucosa. These tumors may have arisen from direct effects of omeprazole, but they more likely arose from ECL-cell hyperplasia induced by secondary hypergastrinemia. To date, these findings have restricted human use of omeprazole to ZES patients.

References

1. Archambult AP, et al. Omeprazole (20 mg daily) versus cimetidine (1200 mg daily) in duodenal ulcer healing and pain relief. Gastroenterology 1988; 94:1130–1134.
   A study of 169 patients with acute duodenal ulcers comparing omeprazole with cimetidine.
2. Bardhan KD, et al. A comparison of two different doses of omeprazole versus ranitidine in treatment of duodenal ulcers. J Clin Gastro 1986; 8:408–413.
   A study of 105 duodenal ulcer patients treated with either omeprazole or ranitidine.
3. Bardram L, Stadil F. Omeprazole in Zollinger-Ellison syndrome. Scand J Gastro 1986; 21:374–378.
   Omeprazole treatment investigated in nine patients resistant to H2-receptor antagonists.
4. Bardram L, Thomsen P, Stadil F. Gastric endocrine cells in omeprazole-treated and untreated patients with Zollinger-Ellison syndrome. Digestion 1986; 35:116–122.
   Gastric endocrine cell hyperplasia investigated in 19 patients with ZES receiving omeprazole, H2-receptor antagonists, or no treatment.
5. Brook CW, et al. Relapse of duodenal ulceration after healing with omeprazole. Med J Austral 1987; 147:595–597.

During a 12-month period, the recurrence rate of duodenal ulcers was documented in 55 patients previously healed with omeprazole.

6. Carlsson E, et al. Pharmacology and toxicology of omeprazole, with special reference to the effects on gastric mucosa. Scand J Gastro 1986; 118:131–138.

    Studies illustrating that omeprazole causes hypergastrinemia in rats and, after long-term treatment with high doses, hyperplasia of oxyntic endocrine ECL cells with possible development of gastric carcinoids.

7. Classen M, et al. Omeprazole heals duodenal, but not gastric ulcers more rapidly than ranitidine. Hepatogastroenterology 1985; 32:243–245.

    Healing rates of omeprazole versus ranitidine studied in 334 patients with duodenal ulcers and 184 patients with gastric ulcers.

8. Dammann HG, et al. Intragastric acidity under 28-day omeprazole treatment. Hepatogastroenterology 1985; 32:191–194.

    A study done to determine the effect of 28-day treatment with oral omeprazole while measuring 24-hour intragastric H+ activity in 15 healthy subjects.

9. Delchier JC, et al. Effectiveness of omeprazole in seven patients with Zollinger-Ellison syndrome resistant to histamine H2-receptor antagonists. Dig Dis Sci 1986; 31:693–699.

    Treatment with omeprazole evaluated in seven patients with ZES resistant to H2-receptor antagonists.

10. Ekman L, et al. Toxicology studies on omeprazole. Scand J Gastro 1985; 108:53–69.

    Studies done in several species of animals looking for clinical toxicity, oncogenicity, fetal toxicity and teratogenicity, and mutagenicity.

11. Festen HP, et al. Effect of single and repeated doses of oral omeprazole on gastric acid and pepsin secretion and fasting serum gastrin and serum pepsinogen I levels. Dig Dis Sci 1986; 31:561–566.

    Twelve healthy volunteers studied to determine the effect of omeprazole on gastric acid and pepsin secretion and fasting serum gastrin and serum pepsinogen I levels.

12. Havu N. Enterochromaffinlike cells carcinoids of gastric mucosa in rats after life-long inhibition of gastric secretion. Digestion 1986; 35:42–55.

    Oncogenicity studies in rats showing an association with long-term inhibition of gastric acid secretion and compensatory rise in serum gastrin with hyperplasia of ECL cells and subsequent formation of gastric carcinoids.

13. Hetzel DJ, Shearman DJ. Omeprazole's inhibition of nocturnal gastric secretion in patients with duodenal ulcers. Brit J Clin Pharm 1984; 18:587–590.

    Overnight studies of gastric acid secretion following single morning doses of omeprazole versus placebo.

14. Horowitz M, et al. The effect of omeprazole on gastric-emptying in patients with duodenal ulcer disease. Brit J Pharm 1984; 18:791–794.

    Gastric-emptying of eight patients with history of duo-

denal ulcers assessed by dual-isotope scintigraphic technique following single oral dose of omeprazole.
15. Howden CW, et al. Effects of low-dose omeprazole on gastric secretion and plasma gastrin in patients with healed duodenal ulcers. Hepatogastroenterology 1986; 33:267-270.
  Study of six male patients with healed duodenal ulcers on 5 mg and 10 mg omeprazole and its effect versus placebo.
16. Howden CW, et al. Antisecretory effect and pharmacokinetics following low-dose omeprazole in man. Brit J Pharm 1985; 20:137-139.
  Single and repeated doses of 10 mg oral omeprazole were given to six healthy subjects to assess gastric acid activity and oral pharmacokinetics.
17. Howden CW, Forrest JA, Reid JL. Effects of single and repeated doses of omeprazole on gastric acid and pepsin secretion in man. Gut 1984; 25:707-710.
  Twelve healthy subjects studied to determine omeprazole's effect on gastric acid and pepsin secretion following single and repeated doses.
18. Howden CW, et al. Antisecretory effect and oral pharmacokinetics of omeprazole in patients with chronic renal failure. Eur J Clin Pharm 1985; 28:637-640.
  A group of patients on hemodialysis were studied to determine the effectiveness of omeprazole on gastric acid secretion.
19. Jansen JB, et al. Effect of single and repeated intravenous doses of omeprazole on pentagastrin-stimulated gastric acid secretion and pharmacokinetics in man. Gut 1988; 29:75-80.
  Healthy male volunteers studied for the effect of single and repeated IV doses of omeprazole on gastric acid secretion.
20. Kittang E, Aadland E, Schjonsby H. Effect of omeprazole on secretion of intrinsic factor, gastric acid, and pepsin in man. Gut 1985; 26:594-598.
  The effect of IV omeprazole on basal and pentagastrin-stimulated output of intrinsic factor, gastric acid, and pepsin studied in 10 healthy male adults.
21. Lamers CB. Present experiences with omeprazole in the Zollinger-Ellison syndrome. Scand J Gastro 1986; 118:123-128.
  Study of the effect of omeprazole on acid hypersecretion and acid peptic disease resulting from endogenous hypergastrinemia in ZES.
22. Lamers CB, et al. Omeprazole in Zollinger-Ellison syndrome: Effects of a single dose and of long-term treatment in patients resistant to histamine H2-receptor antagonists. NEJM 1984; 310:758-761.
  Seven patients with ZES resistant to H2-blockers treated with omeprazole in a single dose and in long-term therapy.
23. Lauritsen K, et al. Effect of omeprazole and cimetidine on duodenal ulcers: A double-blind comparative trial. NEJM 1985; 312:958-961.
  Treatment of 132 duodenal ulcer patients with omeprazole compared to cimetidine.
24. Lind T, et al. Effect of omeprazole—A gastric proton pump

inhibitor—on pentagastrin-stimulated acid secretion in man. Gut 1983; 24:270–276.

Pentagastrin-stimulated gastric acid secretion studied in 11 healthy subjects receiving varying doses of oral omeprazole.

25. Lind T, et al. Inhibition of basal and betazole- and sham-feeding-induced acid secretion by omeprazole in man. Scand J Gastro 1986; 21:1004–1010.

Healthy subjects were studied to establish the effect of omeprazole on acid secretions.

26. Londong W, et al. Dose-response study of omeprazole on meal-stimulated gastric acid secretion and gastrin release. Gastroenterology 1983; 85:1373–1378.

Eight healthy subjects receiving various doses of oral omeprazole studied to determine the effect on stimulated gastric acid secretion and gastrin release.

27. McArthur KE, et al. Omeprazole: Effective, convenient therapy for Zollinger-Ellison syndrome. Gastroenterology 1985; 88:939–944.

Eleven patients with ZES treated investigated for the acute and long-term effects of omeprazole on gastric acid secretions.

28. Meyrick-Thomas J, et al. Omeprazole in duodenal ulceration: Acid inhibition, symptom relief, endoscopic healing, and recurrence. BMJ 1984; 289:525–528.

Study comparing various doses of omeprazole on 44 patients with duodenal ulcers and its effects on acid production, symptom relief, and recurrence.

29. Naesdal J, et al. The effect of 20 mg omeprazole daily on serum gastrin, 24-hour intragastric acidity, and bile acid concentrations in duodenal ulcer patients. Scand J Gastro 1987; 22:5–12.

Serum gastrin, intragastric acidity, and bile acid concentration studied in 10 patients with duodenal ulcers receiving omeprazole treatment.

30. Naesdal J, Bodemar G, Walan A. Effect of omeprazole, a substituted benzimidazole, on 24-hour intragastric acidity in patients with peptic ulcer disease. Scand J Gastro 1984; 19:916–922.

Intragastric pH measured in patients with peptic ulcer disease treated with various doses of omeprazole.

31. Naesdal J, et al. The rate of healing of duodenal ulcers during omeprazole treatment. Scand J Gastro 1985; 20:691–695.

Healing rates of 44 duodenal ulcer patients treated with omeprazole determined.

32. Olbe L, et al. Effect of omeprazole on gastric acid secretion in man. Scand J Gastro 1986; 118:105–107.

Omeprazole's effect on basal acid secretion, vagally-stimulated and meal-stimulated acid secretion, and serum gastrin levels studied in healthy adults.

33. Sharma BK, et al. Optimal dose of oral omeprazole for maximal 24-hour decrease of intragastric acidity. Gut 1984; 25:957–964.

A series of 59 experiments in nine duodenal ulcer patients to establish optimal dosing with oral omeprazole.

34. Thompson JN, et al. Basal, sham-feed- and pentagastrin-stimulated gastric acid, pepsin, and electrolytes after omeprazole, 20 mg and 40 mg daily. Gut 1985; 26:1018–1024.

    Nine patients with duodenal ulcer studied to investigate omeprazole's effect on pepsin and gastric acid secretion, basally and following stimulation.

35. Wilson JA, Boyd EJS, Wormsley KG. Omeprazole inhibits nocturnal and pentagastrin-stimulated gastric secretion in man. Dig Dis Sci 1984; 29:797–801.

    Study of healthy male volunteers receiving oral omeprazole and its effect on overnight and pentagastrin-stimulated secretion of pepsin and gastric acid.

Inflammatory Bowel Disease Drugs

Inflammatory bowel disease, with its unknown etiology and complicated pathogenesis, is a difficult and frustrating illness to treat. Whenever physicians and their patients are faced with the task of controlling an illness for which no cure is available, the therapeutic armamentarium is limited to agents that ameliorate signs and symptoms of the disease. Such is the case with ulcerative colitis and Crohn's disease, maladies that currently affect two million Americans, inflicting pain and causing altered lifestyle, extreme financial burden, and sometimes death.

A complete review of the pathophysiologic alterations and etiologic theories of inflammatory bowel disease is clearly beyond the scope of these chapters; however, several observations should be highlighted. Various effector cells of the inflammatory response have been found in increased number within the mucosa of patients with active ulcerative colitis and Crohn's disease. These include T- and B-lymphocytes, plasma cells, macrophages, epithelioid cells, neutrophils, mast cells, and eosinophils. Inflammatory mediators secreted by these cells, such as prostaglandins, kinins, leukotrienes, chondroitin sulfate, platelet-activating factors, immunoglobulins and lymphokines, are found in high concentration in various tissues during active inflammation.

Within the gastrointestinal tract these agents cause proximate tissue injury leading to mucosal and transmural edema, vascular congestion, acute and chronic inflammatory cellular infiltration, cell death, and reactive fibrosis. While inflammatory bowel disease is not felt to be a classic autoimmune disorder, recent studies implicate an immunoregulatory defect as a major factor in its pathogenesis. As many as 50 percent of patients with early, mild Crohn's disease have been shown to have circulating T-lymphocyte populations possessing enhanced suppressor T-cell activity. In contrast, decreased suppressor T-cell activity has been demonstrated in late, severe disease. In light of evidence showing that some patients with Crohn's disease have increased B- and T-lymphocyte response to multiple mucosal and bacterial antigens, it is speculated that there is a tendency in these patients to initially mount an inappropriate immune response to one or more mucosal or microbial antigens.

Once inflammation becomes firmly entrenched, the suppressor T-cell response is incapable of turning off the immune activity. The exact role of corticosteroids in altering this process is unknown, but several of their anti-inflammatory actions have been elucidated. Corticosteroids diminish the levels of circulating leukocytes, inhibit the release of interleukin I and II, and reduce tissue levels of the inflammatory mediators and lymphokines. Both the proliferative response of T-lymphocytes to antigenic and mitogenic stimuli and their cytotoxic activity are profoundly diminished. Besides affecting cellular mediators, corticosteroids also inhibit prostaglandin and leukotriene production, by their inhibition of phospholipase A2. Prednisolone has been shown to reduce synthesis and to lower tissue levels of PGE2 in cultured rectal biopsies of patients with ulcerative colitis. The result is a reduction in vasodilation, capillary permeability, chemotaxis, and neutrophilic enzyme release within the gastrointestinal mucosa.

Ulcerative Colitis

Corticosteroids are currently recognized as the most effective agents in the treatment of ulcerative proctosigmoiditis, and mild to moderate ulcerative colitis; and frequently useful in severe colitis.

Multiple clinical trials have proven their efficacy compared to placebo. A retrospective analysis of patients with ulcerative colitis before and after the advent of steroid use, by Korelitz and Lindner in 1964, showed significant reductions in overall morbidity and mortality, a decrease in complications, and a shift from emergent to more elective surgery since these agents came into common use. Along with the clinical and gross endoscopic improvement, histologic examination of rectal biopsies of patients with active colitis shows resolution of neutrophilic infiltration of the lamina propria, an increase in mucous goblet cells, and a decrease in fragmented epithelial cells in response to steroid therapy.

Corticosteroids can be given intravenously, orally, or by rectal instillation as suppositories, rectal drip, retention enemas, and foam. They should be viewed as effective therapeutic agents for ulcerative colitis, restricted in their use to resolving new onset attacks or recurrent exacerbations, and not utilized for long-term management.

Rectally instilled steroids have been demonstrated to spread retrograde as far as the splenic flexure by scintigraphy of Technetium-99–labelled suspensions. Enemas have the most extensive spread, while foams may reach the mid–sigmoid colon. Spreading is more proximal in patients with active disease than in those with inactive colitis or controls, and there seems to be a positive correlation between the extent of disease involvement and the degree of steroid spreading. Retention enemas should be used in patients with proximal sigmoid disease, while foams are as effective and usually preferred for proctitis and distal sigmoiditis. They are especially helpful in relieving tenesmus and rectal urgency or incontinence. Most patients find foams easier to retain and more acceptable aesthetically than enemas. Steroid suppositories should be used for proctitis only. Oral agents should be used for refractory proctitis, colitis that extends to the proximal sigmoid colon, or colitis associated with systemic symptoms, significant diarrhea, or abdominal pain.

Severe colitis, necessitating hospitalization, requires parenteral corticosteroids or corticotropin (ACTH). Steroid therapy should be only one of several treatment modalities offered, and a protocol of medical management may include bedrest; correction of dehydration, electrolyte abnormalities, and anemia; nutritional supplementation; and appropriate use of sulfasalazine, antibiotics, or immunosuppressive agents.

Trials of intensive intravenous corticosteroid treatment for mild, moderate, and severe attacks of ulcerative colitis have demonstrated remission rates of 92 percent, 87 percent, and 56 percent, respectively.

The lowest remission rates occur in patients with chronic, continuous pancolitis. Truelove, using a regimen of intravenous and rectal steroids, predetermined that the absence of any improvement after 5 days of treatment constituted an absolute indication for colectomy. Further studies have shown that patients with severe colitis who receive treatment for longer than 5 days have a mean time of remission of between 8 and 10 days. Prolonging treatment for longer than 10 days or changing drugs (e.g., from hydrocortisone to ACTH) does not improve remission rates. Thus, patients failing to respond to 10 days of high-dose, intravenous steroids should have total abdominal colectomy.

A small number of patients present with or progress to fulminant colitis or toxic megacolon. There are no good, controlled trials of steroid therapy in these life-threatening cases. It is accepted practice to give at least a short trial of corticosteroids while stabilizing the patient preoperatively. There is no evidence that steroids adversely affect surgical outcome as long as they do not lead to a delay in performing an indicated colectomy. Systemic corticosteroid therapy that is successful in inducing remission of the bowel disease usually resolves flares of colitis-associated complications. Axial arthropathy and hepatic complications (pericholangitis, chronic active hepatitis, sclerosing cholangitis, and postnecrotic cirrhosis) follow an independent course, may antedate the onset of bowel disease, and do not respond to medical therapy.

In the treatment of ulcerative colitis, sulfasalazine is useful in inducing remission in mild flares of the disease and in the maintenance of remission.

Newer substituted aminosalicylic-acid compounds, 4-ASA and 5-ASA, hold promise as agents useful for treatment of mild flares of ulcerative colitis in patients intolerant of sulfasalazine. To date, these drugs appear to be as efficacious as oral sulfasalazine and rectal corticosteroids.

Crohn's Disease

Steroids were introduced as treatment for Crohn's disease in the early 1950s. Until 1979, only retrospective and uncontrolled trials evaluating efficacy were available. Most of these studies reported encouraging clinical improvement in patients treated with ACTH or corticosteroids, with greater than 50 percent of patients responding favorably. Much of the data from these early studies were conflicting, reporting progression of disease on therapy, increased complications and mortality in some treatment groups, and increased need for surgery after treatment. To answer the many questions regarding the natural history, optimal treatment, and complications of Crohn's disease, a multicenter drug study was initiated in 1971. A total of 1119 patients were entered into the study after fulfilling diagnostic criteria. The results of this National Cooperative Crohn's Disease Study (NCCDS) were published in 1979, detailing the effect of treatment with sulfasalazine, prednisone, and azathioprine compared to placebo. The conclusions drawn from this report have guided our use of steroids, anti-inflammatory agents, and immunosuppressives in Crohn's disease for the last 10 years.

The results of the NCCDS showed that in patients with active, symptomatic disease prednisone was superior to placebo in inducing and maintaining improvement. Using the Crohn's disease activity index (CDAI) to evaluate improvement, 78 percent of patients achieved at least transient remission (CDAI < 150) during 17 weeks of prednisone treatment. Response was influenced by prior drug therapy. Patients taking sulfasalazine at the time of beginning prednisone treatment responded no better than to placebo. Conversely, prior treatment with steroids precluded a significant improvement on sulfasalazine. Different responses were also noted depending on the location of active disease. Prednisone was superior to placebo only in patients with isolated ileal or ileocolonic disease. Patients with Crohn's colitis alone responded to prednisone no better than to placebo, although this group was quite small.

In a follow-up, controlled trial by Singleton in 1979, sulfasalazine was used in combination with prednisone for active and quiescent Crohn's disease to judge the former's adjunctive and steroid-sparing effect. The combination was less effective for active ileal disease than prednisone alone and exhibited no prednisone-sparing effect. Thus, the addition of sulfasalazine to steroid therapy does not appear to improve substantially the response to treatment in active Crohn's disease.

In the NCCDS, steroid therapy was administered to 274

patients in remission to assess its prophylactic effect. Steroid therapy proved to be no better than placebo in preventing relapse of active disease. Another multicenter drug trial, the European Cooperative Crohn's Disease Study (ECCDS), confirmed the effectiveness of high-dose steroids for active disease but also demonstrated beneficial results from maintenance methylprednisolone at a dose of 12.5 mgs daily. Unfortunately, no appropriate control group was used for the maintenance regimen.

Long-term corticosteroid therapy (> 6 months), high-dose corticosteroid therapy (> 15 mgs prednisone daily), or significant corticosteroid side effects (diabetes, hypertension, cataracts, or osteoporosis) justify the use of steroid-sparing agents like 6-mercaptopurine. Immunosuppressive agents like 6-mercaptopurine require careful follow-up and intensive patient counseling.

Complications of Crohn's disease like enterocutaneous fistulae often respond to use of antibacterial agents such as metronidazole, either alone or in combination with 6-mercaptopurine or 6-mercaptopurine and low-dose corticosteroids.

The use of 4-ASA and 5-ASA in the treatment of Crohn's disease is currently under intensive investigation. Initial studies suggest benefit in mild ileal or ileocolonic Crohn's disease.

Total parenteral nutrition remains a useful adjunct in the treatment of severe Crohn's disease, in the preparation of nutritionally depleted Crohn's patient for surgery, and as a life-sustaining therapy for patients with extensive Crohn's disease and nonfunctional gut.

W. Zack Taylor and Michael M. Van Ness

References

1. Elson CO, et al. An evaluation of total parenteral nutrition in the management of inflammatory bowel disease. Dig Dis Sci 1980; 25:42–48.

    Assessing the role of TPN as an adjunct in the therapy of inflammatory bowel disease.

2. Flavell Matts SG, and Gaskell KH. Retrograde colonic spread of enemata in ulcerative colitis. BMJ 1961; 2:614.

    A 40% suspension of barium in water demonstrated retrograde spread to the ascending colon when given by slow, rectal drip in U.C.

3. Haber CJ, et al. Nature and course of pancreatitis caused

by 6-mercaptopurine in the treatment of inflammatory bowel disease. Gastroenterology 1986; 91:982–986.

The authors report the clinical course of 13 cases of pancreatitis attributable to 6-MP in 400 (3.25%) patients with inflammatory bowel disease. The pancreatitis tends to occur early (within 30 days), is usually mild, and recurs with rechallenge.

4. Korelitz BI, and Lindner AE. The influence of corticotropin and adrenal steroids in the course of ulcerative colitis: A comparison with the presteroid era. Gastroenterology 1964; 46:671.

Impressive review of the positive impact of steroid therapy on the course of U.C.

5. Singleton JW. Steroids in chronic liver and inflammatory bowel diseases. Hosp Prac 1983; 12:97.

Good review of indications and regimens for steroid therapy in IBD.

6. Sutherland LR, et al. 5-aminosalicylic acid enema in the treatment of distal ulcerative colitis, proctosigmoiditis, and proctitis. Gastroenterology 1987; 92:1894–1898.

A randomized, double-blind, placebo-controlled study of 153 patients with left-sided ulcerative colitis. The 5-ASA patients had a clinical improvement rate of 63% from 4-gm nighttime enemas. The data are important in that dropouts were included in the final calculation of the intent-to-treat success rate.

7. Truelove SC, and Witts, LJ. Cortisone in ulcerative colitis. BMJ 1955; 2:1041.

Early landmark study showing favorable response of U.C. to oral cortisone.

8. Truelove, SC. Treatment of ulcerative colitis with local hydrocortisone. BMJ 1956; 2:1267.

Truelove's landmark article reporting the effectiveness of rectally instilled hydrocortisone in mild to moderately severe U.C.

9. Truelove SC. Treatment of ulcerative colitis with local hydrocortisone hemisuccinate sodium. BMJ 1958; 2:1072.

A controlled trial proving the efficacy of a water-soluble preparation of hydrocortisone for rectal instillation in U.C.

10. Truelove SC. Systemic and local corticosteroid therapy in ulcerative colitis. BMJ 1960; 1:464.

A combination of oral prednisolone, 5 mgs qid, and hydrocortisone enemas for mild to moderately severe U.C. was more effective than either agent alone.

11. Williams CN, Haber G, Aquino JA. Double-blind, placebo-controlled evaluation of 5-ASA suppositories in active distal proctitis and measurement of extent of spread using 99m Tc-labeled 5-ASA suppositories. Dig Dis Sci 1987; 32:71S–75S.

This study reiterates the utility of 5-ASA, 500-mg suppositories 3 times a day, in active proctitis. The suppositories deliver the 5-ASA to the rectum alone.

Corticosteroids

W. Zack Taylor and Michael M. Van Ness

Glucocorticoids are 21-carbon steroid molecules, structurally and functionally similar to cortisol, the principle circulating glucocorticoid in humans. Minor modifications in the structure of these compounds alter their potency, duration of action, and mineralocorticoid activity dramatically. Table 7–1 lists the most commonly used glucocorticoids by their relative potencies, dosage equivalents, and sodium-retaining potential. Two corticosteroids used to treat inflammatory bowel disease, cortisone and prednisone, lack functional activity until converted in vivo to cortisol and prednisolone, respectively. Other commercial preparations include cortisol (hydrocortisone), prednisolone, methylprednisolone, betamethasone, beclomethasone, dexamethasone, and tixocortol pivalate. In addition, corticotropin (ACTH), which is normally released from the anterior pituitary gland and regulates adrenal cortisol production, has been used with considerable success in the parenteral treatment of ulcerative colitis and Crohn's disease.

PHARMACOLOGY AND PHARMACOKINETICS

Corticosteroids are well absorbed after oral administration and clinically effective systemically when given by this route. Topical application to the skin and mucous membranes results in local activity and, in some instances, absorption and a systemic effect. Ninety percent of cortisol and its synthetic analogs is bound in plasma by two protein fractions, cortisol-binding globulin (CBG) and albumin. CBG has a high affinity for cortisol but low total binding capacity, while albumin provides for the majority of protein-bound steroid even though its affinity is less due to its considerably larger plasma pool.

The activity of glucocorticoids, as with all steroid hormones, depends on passive entry into the cell cytoplasm, binding to specific intracytosolic receptors, and ingress into the nucleus. Genomic expression is then modulated, with subsequent mRNA transcription, and translation to proteins that then govern metabolic and enzymatic pathways. Due to their intracellular location of action, the activity of glucocorticoids cannot be correlated to plasma levels. Likewise, circulating half-life and duration of action do not seem to be closely related. For example, the half-life of prednisone is 60 minutes and prednisolone 115–252 minutes; however, their relative potency and equivalent dosage is identical. Glucocorticoids clearly exert many of their actions after disappearance from plasma and not all of these effects have an equal duration. It is clear that duration of action is a function of dose, and enhanced activity can be obtained by increasing the amount administered. The protein-free, unbound fraction of circulating steroid is felt to be the active

Table 7–1. Commonly used glucocorticoids

Duration of action	Glucocorticoid potency	Equivalent glucocorticoid dose (mg)	Mineralo-corticoid activity
Short-acting			
Cortisol (hydrocortisone)	1	20	yes
Cortisone	0.8	25	yes
Prednisone	4	5	no
Prednisolone	4	5	no
Methylprednisolone	5	4	no
Intermediate-acting			
Triamcinolone	5	4	no
Long-acting			
Betamethasone	25	0.60	no
Dexamethasone	30	0.75	no

moiety. Reduced levels of albumin and steroid-binding globulin increase the levels of this active, serum-free steroid. Even though the therapeutic effect of the drug may remain unaltered, the risk of side effects will increase.

Prednisone is the most commonly used glucocorticoid and owes its activity to its metabolite, prednisolone. The conversion of prednisone to prednisolone occurs in the liver and has led to recommendations that only prednisolone be used in patients with hepatic dysfunction. Liver disease, however, prolongs prednisolone half-life and is usually accompanied by hypoalbuminemia, which increases the unbound fraction of circulating steroid. Thus, the reduced conversion and lower initial prednisolone concentration in such patients is compensated for by delayed clearance and higher levels of active steroid, preserving the effectiveness of prednisone regardless of hepatic function.

The overall steroid dose should be reduced in patients with significant liver disease who require long-term treatment, to reduce adverse side effects. Gluocorticoids are primarily metabolized in the liver and excreted in the urine as glucuronides, sulfates, and unconjugated compounds. Their elimination is not affected by alterations in renal function.

The absorption of prednisolone has been extensively studied in patients with inflammatory bowel disease. Wide absorptive variations in patients with Crohn's disease have been demonstrated. Although therapeutic serum levels with standard doses can be achieved, reduced absorption occurs in some patients with active disease. Shaffer demonstrated reduced absorption of prednisolone by isotopic measurements of drug and metabolites from plasma, urine, and feces, in patients with Crohn's disease of the ileum. Tanner, in an earlier study, found no significant difference in peak levels or total absorption of 20 milligrams prednisolone given orally, though the majority of his patients had predominantly colonic Crohn's disease. Some degree of corticosteroid malabsorption is possible in Crohn's disease, particularly when extensive small bowel inflammation is present. Mucosal integrity, surface area, and transit time of the small bowel are significant factors affecting the bioavailability of these agents. The total absorption of prednisolone does not differ between normals and patients with ulcerative colitis after oral dosing. However, there is a lower peak level and a more gradual reduction of plasma levels in patients, possibly due to delayed absorption. The overall effect of the drug does not seem to be altered.

The site of action of topically administered steroids is thought to be primarily local; however, systemic absorption occurs through the rectal mucosa with most agents. Fifty percent of administered hydrocortisone reaches the systemic circulation, and up to 90 percent absorption has been demonstrated, with retention times exceeding 8 hours. The rectally instilled steroids are classified according to this degree of absorption and concomitant adrenal suppression (Table 7–2). The largest group includes those that are highly absorbed with subsequent adrenal suppression, followed by the absorbable agents with no systemic effects, and the nonabsorbable compounds.

Several preparations have been developed that limit the systemic effects of rectal steroids. Beclomethasone dipropionate and budenoside are two compounds that are absorbed but undergo rapid first-pass hepatic metabolism. Prednisolone metasulfobenzoate is a large molecule that is poorly absorbed after rectal instillation. All of these compounds are equally or more effective than hydrocortisone and avoid adrenal suppression and steroid side effects. Tixocortol pivulate, a recently formulated, nonglucocorticoid, synthetic derivative of cortisol, is easily absorbed but has negligible systemic effects due to rapid first-pass metabolism, clearance, and elimination. It is also very effective in reducing colonic inflammation without reducing serum cortisol levels. These agents have been available for use in Europe for some time and may be approved in the United States.

MECHANISMS OF ACTION

Corticosteroids stabilize lysosomal membranes, reduce capillary permeability, function as inhibitors of chemotaxis and phagocytosis, and impair cell-mediated immunity in experimental models.

Table 7-2. Rectally administered topical steroids

Absorbable steroids	Delivery vehicle	Systemic effects/adrenal suppression
Hydrocortisone hemisuccinate (Cortenema)	Enema: 100 mgs in 60-ml aqueous solution	yes
Hydrocortisone acetate	Enema: 100 mgs in 60-ml aqueous solution	yes
	Suppository: (Cort-Dome) 15 mgs, 25 mgs	yes
	Foam: (Cortifoam) 10% in 20 gm foam	yes
	Foam: (Proctofoam-HC) 1% in 10 gm foam	yes
Prednisolone 21-phosphate	Enema: 20 mgs in 100-ml aqueous solution	yes
	Suppository: 5 mg	
Methylprednisolone acetate	Enema: 40 mgs in water	yes
Prednisolone	Enema: 100 mgs in oil	yes
Betamethasone 17-valerate	Enema: 5 mgs in aqueous solution	yes
Tixocortal pivulate	Enema: 250 mgs in 100-ml aqueous solution	no
	Suppository: 250 mgs	no
Poorly absorbable steroids		
Prednisolone metasulfobenzoate	Enema and suppository	low
Beclomethasone dipropionate	Enema and suppository	low

INDICATIONS AND ADMINISTRATION

Ulcerative Colitis

Oral

Several studies provide data on the most effective and least toxic dosage schedules. Baron compared the results of using 20, 40, and 60 milligrams of prednisone daily for attacks of mildly to moderately severe ulcerative colitis. He found the 40- and 60-milligram dose equally superior to 20 milligrams daily for remission induction.

Powell-Tuck showed that a single 40-milligram dose of prednisolone given in the morning for active proctocolitis was as effective in inducing remission as 10 milligrams taken 4 times a day, with less adrenal suppression. There is a large body of anecdotal experience favoring twice-a-day over four-times-a-day steroid dosing. For more severe cases not requiring intravenous therapy, it is prudent to split the dosage. There have been no controlled trials performed to evaluate an alternate dose regimen of steroids for acute attacks, but most reports do not support its use.

Intravenous

Resistant cases of ulcerative colitis not responding to oral steroid therapy within 10–14 days, and patients presenting with severe attacks (see Table 7–3) should receive intravenous corticosteroids. The most frequently used agents include hydrocortisone, prednisolone, methylprednisolone, and ACTH. Because of its intense mineralocorticoid effect, necessitating intravenous potassium replacement of up to 200 milligrams/day, hydrocortisone has become less popular as an intravenous agent.

Early clinical studies suggested that ACTH was superior to corticosteroids, particularly for patients with a relapse of colitis. Kaplan in 1975 and Meyer in 1982 found both agents equally effective; however, patients previously treated with steroids had a better response to hydrocortisone and those without prior treatment had significantly better improvement with ACTH. The lesser response of patients who had received prior steroid therapy to ACTH (25% improved with ACTH, compared to 53% with hydrocortisone) could not be explained by impaired adrenal responsiveness, since mean

Table 7–3. Criteria for severe colitis

1. *Diarrhea*: Six or more stools per day with macroscopic blood.
2. *Fever*: Mean evening temp. $\geq 37.5°$ C or a temp. of $\geq 37.8°$ C on at least 2 days out of 4.
3. *ESR elevation* ≥ 30 mm/hr.
4. *Anemia*: Hemoglobin level ≤ 11.5 mg/l.
5. *Tachycardia*: Mean pulse rate ≥ 90/min.

From SC Truelove, DP Jewell: Criteria for severe colitis. *Lancet* 1974; 1:1067.

serum cortisol and dehydroepiandrosterone levels were similar in both groups. Given these data, one might treat severe, initial attacks of ulcerative colitis with ACTH and recurrent, previously treated episodes with corticosteroids. In reality, both agents are usually successful.

The recommended dosages are hydrocortisone, 300–400 milligrams/day, prednisolone, 60–80 milligrams/day, methylprednisolone, 60–80 milligrams/day, and ACTH, 120 u/day. They may be administered by intermittent bolus or continuous infusion; the latter method is preferred.

Once remission is obtained, an attempt should be made to advance to equivalent oral dosages with a subsequent taper of the drug. Generally, prednisone dosage is decreased at a rate of 5 milligrams/week down to a level of 20 milligrams/day. Flares are less common above 20 milligrams daily and side effects infrequent below this dose. Subsequent weaning should proceed at a slower pace (e.g., 2.5-mg reductions every 1–2 weeks). Further tapering in 2.5-milligram weekly increments, perhaps using an alternate-day schedule, should be continued until the drug is stopped.

Alternate-day tapering once the daily dose reaches 10 to 15 milligrams may be attempted and is frequently successful. An example of this type of regimen would be converting a 15-milligram daily dose to 30 milligrams every other day, then tapering in 5-milligram increments every week to 10 days. Since adrenal suppression and systemic toxicity are negligible on alternate-day steroids, this may be a preferred regimen in patients with multiple side effects.

Topical

Proper use of rectally instilled steroids induce remission or improvement in more than 80 percent of patients with active ulcerative proctosigmoiditis. They should be administered in a single dose at bedtime. After instillation, patients should lie on the left side for at least 30 minutes, then turn to the supine and prone positions to ensure proper contact with the entire circumference of the distal colon. The solution should be retained as long as possible, preferably all night. The usual course of therapy lasts 14 to 21 days. An incomplete or partial response may dictate prolonging treatment for up to 8 weeks on a daily or alternate-day schedule, but systemic side effects and adrenal suppression should be anticipated, necessitating slow tapering.

If no response occurs after 2 weeks, twice-daily administration may be tried for up to 14 days. Lack of improvement after 1 month of treatment should prompt discontinuation of the agent and pursuance of systemic steroid or sulfasalazine treatment. If remission is achieved, treatment should be stopped or tapered off. Maintenance treatment with topical steroids is not recommended.

Crohn's Disease

Oral

A reasonable approach to the patient with Crohn's disease is to consider steroid therapy after implementing supportive care and sulfasalazine without the desired therapeutic response. For refractory patients and those with systemic symptoms such as fever, weight loss, and anorexia, steroids should be started at high doses (e.g., prednisone, 60–80 mgs daily, or the equivalent, in four divided doses). A favorable response with resolution of fever, pain, diarrhea, improvement in appetite and sense of well-being usually occurs within 10 days, at which point slow tapering of the dosage should begin. Optimally, one should make an attempt to wean off steroids completely within 4 to 6 weeks.

Many patients experience an exacerbation of symptoms with attempts to lower or discontinue steroids. Any flare should prompt reinstituting a high dose, since small incremental dosage elevations may allow the inflammatory process to become less responsive and increasingly refractory. If patients are unable to taper down to a low dose (< 10 mgs daily) of prednisone, alternate-day therapy, surgery, and use of a steroid-sparing agent should be considered. Alternate-day steroids are usually unsuccessful in Crohn's disease.

Intravenous

As with ulcerative colitis, high fever, severe diarrhea, bleeding, weight loss, anorexia, or bowel destruction necessitate continuous intravenous therapy with either ACTH (120 u daily) or corticosteroids (methylprednisolone, 48–80 mgs daily).

Topical

Topical application of steroids may be helpful in alleviating the symptoms of the colitis-related complications. Adjunctive therapy for oral ulceration includes topical application of triamcinolone acetonide dental paste (Kenalog in Orabae) 3 times a day after meals, or intralesional injections of triamcinolone acetonide, 10 milligrams/milliliter in a 0.1 to 0.5 dilutional mixture with 1 to 2 percent xylocaine hydrochloride.

Intra-articular injections of corticosteroids may give relief immediately, while waiting for the overall clinical picture to improve. The most frequently used drugs include short-acting, inexpensive agents such as hydrocortisone acetate (25 mg/ml) and the longer-acting betamethasone sodium phosphate (6 mg/ml), triamcinolone hexacetonide (20 mg/ml), or dexamethasone sodium phosphate (4 mg/ml). One may combine short- and long-acting agents or dilute them in 1 to 2 percent xylocaine HCl. Ocular steroids such as dexamethasone, 0.1 percent, or prednisone, 1 percent, are sometimes necessary in cases of severe uveitis.

CONTRAINDICATIONS

There are very few absolute contraindications to steroid therapy. Colonic perforation, peritonitis, and abscess formation are frequently listed as absolute contraindications; however, in the context of steroid use in inflammatory bowel disease, most patients are already undergoing steroid treatment when these complications occur and an increase in dosage to cover surgical stress is required. Clearly, pyogenic, viral, and systemic fungal infection are relative contraindications to beginning steroids, but steroid therapy can be given concomitantly with the appropriate antibiotic, antiviral, or antifungal agent if the clinical situation dictates.

Corticosteroids may mask the signs and symptoms of intra-abdominal or systemic sepsis, necessitating frequent, detailed evaluations of patient status. Wound healing may be delayed as a result of steroid use.

Early surgical reports indicated that preoperative steroid use increased the incidence of postoperative infection, wound dehiscence, anastomosis breakdown, and mortality. However, multiple reviews and controlled trials have proven otherwise.

All patients with latent tuberculosis or positive tuberculin reactivity should receive chemoprophylaxis during prolonged steroid therapy. Patients with previous peptic ulcer disease, diabetes mellitus, hypertension, diverticulitis, osteopenia, or myasthenia gravis may receive steroids, but close attention should be given to any flare or exacerbation of symptoms. Diuretics may be needed to offset fluid retention, and glucose homeostasis may be altered in diabetics requiring an adjustment of diet, oral agents, or insulin. There is no need to place patients on antacids or H2-antagonists for ulcer prophylaxis; however, patients with active or very recent peptic ulcers should probably receive continued acid suppression.

SIDE EFFECTS

The National Cooperative Crohn's Disease Study (NCCDS) provides the best data about steroid side effects in the treatment of inflammatory bowel disease. Prednisone, 0.25 to 0.75 milligrams/kilogram of body weight was used for up to 2 years. The most frequently occurring major side effects (peptic ulcer disease, hypertension, and psychiatric disturbances) occurred in 32 percent of patients. Only one patient in 85 suffered more than one major complication. The vast majority of complications resolved with reduction or withdrawal of treatment. The most common minor side effects were facial mooning, acne, and ecchymosis, occurring after 100 days of treatment for active disease in 50 percent, 35 percent, and 16 percent, respectively. Evident side effects occurred in roughly one-third of patients on low-dose prednisone, 0.25 milligrams/kilogram daily for prophylaxis. A total of 18 percent of steroid-treated patients had to be withdrawn from the study due to side effects.

PEARLS AND PITFALLS

1. Most studies have shown neither Crohn's disease nor ulcerative colitis to be detrimental to the outcome of pregnancy. There are some data indicating that active Crohn's

disease increases the fetal risk. If inflammatory bowel disease flares during pregnancy, corticosteroids should be used to enhance a favorable outcome. There are no perinatal or fetal adverse effects associated with corticosteroid use. Appropriate routes of administration and dosage for the disease activity present should be utilized. Fetal and newborn HPA suppression does not occur.
2. If the recommended once-daily administration of prednisone for ulcerative colitis does not result in prompt improvement, splitting the dose into a twice-a-day or 4-times-a-day regimen should be tried. A 3 to 5 day trial should be sufficient to determine whether either will be effective.
3. Patients with underlying psychiatric disease are not at increased risk to develop steroid-related psychiatric side effects. If psychiatric-emotional symptoms develop they are more than likely to resemble the primary illness. The dosage of steroid used does not affect the time of onset, duration, or severity of psychiatric symptoms. If symptoms develop, reduction or discontinuation of steroid treatment should be attempted. Neuroleptics, lithium, and electroconvulsive therapy (ECT) may also be helpful.
4. Due to the increased nonprotein-bound, active steroid in plasma, corticosteroid dosage should be reduced in patients with hypoalbuminemia to lower the incidence of side effects and toxicity.
5. If disease activity flares during corticosteroid dosage tapering in ulcerative colitis or Crohn's disease, prednisone should be increased to previous high-dose levels (e.g., 60–80 mgs daily), or intravenous treatment started. Small incremental increases in dosage usually fail to induce remission and reset the refractory-dosage level, entrenching disease activity at progressively higher doses of steroid.
6. Corticosteroids in high doses retard growth in children who have unfused epiphyses, and it is frequently recommended that steroid therapy be avoided in children under 15 years of age. It is important to remember that inflammatory bowel disease alone significantly delays linear growth, frequently prior to its diagnosis in children and adolescents. Corticosteroid treatment in doses necessary to arrest disease activity may very well be associated with accelerated growth as a result of controlling the inflammatory process. Low-dose and alternate-day schedules of treatment may suppress the disease without inhibiting growth and permit nutritional restitution and growth acceleration.

Therefore, it is prudent to withhold corticosteroids in children and adolescents with further growth potential, if alternate forms of therapy are available and equally effective. One must recognize the growth-suppressing effect of active inflammatory bowel disease and give corticosteroids as a therapeutic trial to quiet the bowel inflammation if indicated. A paradoxical acceleration of growth may follow. Long-term use of steroids should be

avoided in children, as toxicity will eventually outstrip any beneficial effect produced.
7. For those patients who require low-dose (< 15 mgs prednisone daily) steroid therapy for long periods of time, close attention should be given to the risk of developing cataracts and osteopenia. This is particularly important in older patients. Yearly ophthalmologic examination should be performed, and adequate calcium intake ensured. Low-dose vitamin D administration is advisable in most patients, to counter the inhibitory effect of steroids on calcium absorption and the increased bone resorption that occurs. Hip or knee pain should alert the physician to the possibility of aseptic necrosis of the femoral head.

References

1. Alcena V, Alexopoulos GS. Ulcerative colitis in association with chronic paranoid schizophrenia: A review of steroid-induced psychiatric disorders. J Clin Gastro 1985; 7:400.

    A good review of psychiatric side effects of steroid use.

2. Axelrod L. Glucocorticoid therapy. Medicine 1976; 55:39.

    An extensive review of glucocorticoid pharmacology and a guide to steroid therapy.

3. Baiocco P, Korelitz BI. The influence of inflammatory bowel disease and its treatment on pregnancy and fetal outcome. J Clin Gastro 1984; 6:211.

    Steroids should be administered to pregnant patients with active IBD if indicated.

4. Baron JH, et al. Outpatient treatment of ulcerative colitis. BMJ 1962; 2:441.

    Comparison of three doses of prednisone for UC reveals 40 mgs daily to be the safest and most effective regimen.

5. Elliot PR, et al. Prednisolone absorption in acute colitis. Gut 1980; 21:49.

    Total absorption of prednisolone in UC patients is equal to that seen in normals.

6. Farthing MJG, et al. Retrograde spread of hydrocortisone-containing foam given intrarectally in ulcerative colitis. BMJ 1979; 2:822.

    Technetium-99m-labeled hydrocortisone foam spread as far as the proximal sigmoid colon in active UC.

7. Flavell Matts SG. Intrarectal treatment of 100 cases of ulcerative colitis with prednisolone-21-phosphate enemata. BMJ 1961; 1:165.

    Treatment resulted in improvement in 88% patients with UC in this uncontrolled trial.

8. Friedman G. Clinical challenges in inflammatory bowel disease: Tixocortal pivulate. National Foundation for Illeitis and Colitis 1988: 8.

    A brief review of the existing data regarding tixocortal pivulate.

9. Hawkey CJ, Truelove SC. Effect of prednisolone on prostaglandin synthesis by rectal mucosa in ulcerative colitis: Investigation by laminar flow bioassay and radioimmunoassay. Gut 1981; 22:190.

Prednisolone decreases PGE2 synthesis in cultured rectal biopsies of patients with UC.

10. Jalan KN, et al. Influence of corticosteroids on the results of surgical treatment of ulcerative colitis. NEJM 1970; 282:588.

    No difference in operative results, complications, or mortality between UC patients treated and not treated with steroids.

11. Janowitz H. *Inflammatory Bowel Disease—A Personal View* Yearbook, Chicago 1985; pp 68, 73.

    A practical review with many clinical "pearls" regarding steroid therapy for ulcerative colitis and Crohn's disease.

12. Jarnerot G, et al. Intensive intravenous treatment of ulcerative colitis. Gastroenterology 1985; 89:1005.

    Results of the use of Truelove's intensive IV steroid regimen in mild, moderate, and severe UC.

13. Jay M, et al. Retrograde spreading of hydrocortisone enema in inflammatory bowel disease. Dig Dis Sci 1986; 31:139.

    Technetium-labelled hydrocortisone enema migrated to the transverse colon and spreading paralleled the extent of disease involvement in UC.

14. Jeffries WM. Low-dosage corticosteroid therapy. Arch Intern Med 1967; 119:265.

    Low-dose steroid treatment (60 mgs or less hydrocortisone daily) is safe over a long period of time.

15. Kaplan HP, et al. A controlled evaluation of intravenous adrenocorticotropic hormone and hydrocortisone in the treatment of active colitis. Gastroenterology 1975; 69:91.

    ACTH and hydrocortisone are equally effective in acute UC.

16. Kirschner BS, et al. Growth retardation in inflammatory bowel disease. Gastroenterology 1978; 75:504.

    Growth retardation, seen in 20% of children with Crohn's disease, may improve with appropriate treatment of the bowel disease.

17. Korelitz BI, Sommers SC. Response to drug therapy of ulcerative colitis. Dig Dis 1976; 21:441.

    Prednisone treatment is associated with decreased inflammatory infiltrate of the lamina propria in rectal biopsies of UC patients.

18. Kozarek R. Extracolonic manifestations of inflammatory bowel disease. Amer Fam Phys 1987; Feb, p 205.

    An excellent review.

19. Lee DAH, et al. Plasma prednisolone levels and adrenocortical responsiveness after administration of prednisolone-21-phosphate as a retention enema. Gut 1979; 20:349.

    The amount of prenisolone absorbed from a 20 mg retention enema was 44% of that absorbed from an equivalent oral dose.

20. Lennard-Jones JE. Toward optimal use of corticosteroids in ulcerative colitis and Crohn's disease. Gut 1983; 24:177.

    Excellent review of steroid therapy for IBD.

21. Lennard-Jones JE, et al. Prednisone as maintenance treatment for ulcerative colitis in remission. Lancet 1965; 1:188.

    Prednisone, 5 mg tid, was not superior to placebo in remission maintenance of UC.

22. Malchow H, et al. European cooperative Crohn's disease study (ECCDS): Results of drug treatment. Gastroenterology 1984; 86:249.

    Steroids demonstrated to be effective in achieving and maintaining remission in active Crohn's disease.

23. Meltzer RM. Steroids. In B Korelitz and N Sohn (eds.), Inflammatory bowel disease, experience and controversy. Orlando, Fla.: Grune, 1985.

    Broad review of steroid therapy in IBD.

24. Meyers S. The role of corticosteroids. Mt Sinai J Med 1983; 50:141.

    A review of the controlled trials of steroids and ACTH versus hydrocortisone for ulcerative colitis.

25. Meyers S, Janowitz H. The place of steroids in the therapy of toxic megacolon. Gastroenterology 1978; 75:729.

    Steroid treatment does not worsen the prognosis of toxic megacolon.

26. Meyers S, Janowitz H. Systemic corticosteroid therapy of ulcerative colitis. Gastroenterology 1985; 89:1189.

    An editorial review of parenteral corticosteroid use in severe UC.

27. Meyers S, et al. Corticotropin versus hydrocortisone in the intravenous treatment of ulcerative colitis. Gastroenterology 1983; 85:351.

    Confirmed the superior effect of ACTH in previously untreated patients and hydrocortisone for treated patients with UC.

28. Meyers S, et al. Predicting the outcome of corticoid therapy for acute ulcerative colitis. J Clin Gastro 1987; 9:50.

    An assessment of prognostic variables in 66 patients with UC treated with parenteral ACTH or hydrocortisone.

29. Mogadam M, et al. Pregnancy in inflammatory bowel disease: Effect of sulfasalazine and corticosteroids on fetal outcome. Gastroenterology 1981; 80:72.

    Corticosteroid treatment of IBD in pregnancy does not adversely affect fetal morbidity or mortality.

30. Pickup ME. Clinical pharmacokinetics of prednisone and prednisolone. Clin Pharm 1979; 4:111.

    Excellent review of prednisone–prednisolone bioavailability and alterations in liver disease.

31. Powell-Tuck J, Buckell NA, Lennard-Jones JE. A controlled comparison of corticotropin and hydrocortisone in the treatment of severe proctocolitis. Scand J Gastro 1977; 12:971.

    ACTH is not superior to hydrocortisone in the treatment of severe proctocolitis.

32. Powell-Tuck J, Lennard-Jones JE. A comparison of oral prednisolone given as single or multiple daily doses for active protocolitis. Scand J Gastro 1978; 13:833.

    A single, morning 40-mg dose of prednisolone for UC is as effective as 10 mgs qid.

33. Powell-Tuck J, et al. A controlled trial of alternate-day prednisolone as a maintenance treatment for ulcerative colitis in remission. Digestion 1981; 22:263.

    Prednisolone, 40 mgs orally every other day, was superior to placebo in remission maintenance for UC.

34. Routes J, Claman HN. Corticosteroids in inflammatory bowel disease. J Clin Gastro 1987; 9:529.

    A review of the immunopathogenesis of inflammatory bowel disease and the role of corticosteroids in altering inflammation.

35. Ruddell W, et al. Treatment of distal ulcerative colitis (proctosigmoiditis) in relapse: Comparison of hydrocortisone enemas and rectal hydrocortisone foam. Gut 1980; 21:885.

    Steroid enemas and foams are equally effective for proctosigmoiditis. Foam was preferred over enema by patients.

36. Shaffer JA, et al. Absorption of prednisolone with Crohn's disease. Gut 1983; 24:182.

    Patients with Crohn's disease have impaired prednisolone absorption.

37. Singleton JW, et al. National cooperative Crohn's disease study (NCCDS): Adverse reactions to study drugs. Gastroenterology 1979; 77:870.

    A review of the drug side effects from NCCDS.

38. Smith RC, et al. Low-dose steroids and clinical relapse in Crohn's disease: A controlled trial. Gut 1978; 19:606.

    Prednisone did not improve the relapse rate, nor affect recurrence or extension of disease.

39. Somerville KW, et al. Effect of treatment on symptoms and quality of life in patients with ulcerative colitis: Comparative trial of hydrocortisone acetate foam and prednisolone-21-phosphate enemas. BMJ 1985; 2:866.

    Quality of life is altered less by foams than by enemas in the treatment of distal UC.

40. Sparberg M, Kirshner J. Long-term corticosteroid therapy for regional enteritis: An analysis of 58 courses in 54 patients. Amer J Dig Dis 1966; 11:865.

    Steroid treatment for 6 months induced remission in 50% patients with Crohn's disease.

41. Summers RW, et al. National cooperative Crohn's disease study (NCCDS): Results of drug treatment. Gastroenterology 1979; 77:847.

    The best prospective study of steroid use in Crohn's disease, showing response superior to placebo in ileal and ileocolonic disease.

42. Tanner AR, et al. Serum prednisolone levels in Crohn's disease and coeliac disease following oral prednisolone administration. Digestion 1981; 21:310.

    Patients with Crohn's disease achieve therapeutic serum prednisolone levels.

43. Truelove SC, et al. Further experience in the treatment of severe attacks of ulcerative colitis. Lancet 1978; 1:1086.

    Results of intensive intravenous steroid treatment for severe UC, including indications for colectomy.

8
Sulfasalazine
Michael Canty

Sulfasalazine is the most widely used drug in the treatment of inflammatory bowel disease. It was discovered by a Swedish physician, Nana Svartz, who was looking for a drug for "rheumatic polyarthritis," in the late 1930s. She noted that her patients with ulcerative colitis experienced marked improvement in their symptoms. Multiple trials over the 4 decades since then have confirmed the efficacy of the drug in the treatment of inflammatory bowel disease.

ABSORPTION, METABOLISM, AND DISTRIBUTION

Sulfasalazine is a conjugate of (5)-aminosalicylic acid, a salicylate analogue, and sulfapyridine, a sulfonamide. They are linked by an azo bond. Approximately 20 to 30 percent of the ingested drug is absorbed from the upper gastrointestinal tract, with blood levels detectable within 1 to 2 hours of oral intake and steady-state serum levels achieved in 24 hours. Ninety percent of the absorbed drug is excreted unchanged in the bile; 10 percent is excreted unchanged in the urine. Sixty to 70 percent of the ingested drug passes directly into the colon without being absorbed.

Intestinal bacteria possessing an intracellular reductase that is inhibitable by oxygen reduce the azo bond and release sulfapyridine and (5)-aminosalicylic acid. After azo bond reduction, most of the sulfapyridine is absorbed from the colon, partially metabolized, and excreted in the urine as the free sulfonamide or its acetyl or glucuronide metabolite. Sulfapyridine is subject to polymorphic acetylation. Slow acetylators tend to have higher serum levels of total sulfapyridine. (5)-aminosalicylate remains primarily in the lumen of the colon. Only a small portion of this metabolite is absorbed and excreted in the urine as the acetylated derivative. Most (5)-aminosalicylate is recovered unchanged in the feces, although small amounts are present in an acetylated form.

MECHANISM OF ACTION

The mechanism of action of sulfasalazine is unclear. Early speculation focused on studies of histologic changes in the connective tissue associated with ulcerative colitis, as well as experimental observations that the drug and its (5)-aminosalicylate metabolite have strong affinity for connective tissue. A possible antibacterial action has been suggested because of the sulfonamide component. Recent studies have shown a diminution in the population of certain clostridial organisms, nonsporing anerobes, and enterobacteria in response to sulfasalazine. However, this antibacterial action did not correlate with an improvement in disease activity. Neither sulfasalazine nor its metabolites appears to significantly affect the immune system in vivo. Sulfasalazine was once thought to work via decreasing prostaglandin levels by inhibition of cyclooxygenase. However, more potent cyclooxygenase inhibitors (indomethacin and flubiprofen) not only show no benefit in the treatment of inflammatory bowel disease but often cause an exacerbation of the disease.

Recent interest has focused on the possible effects of sulfasalazine and its metabolites on polymorphonuclear leukocytes.. Sulfasalazine and sulfapyridine inhibit polymorphonuclear leukocyte random migration and superoxide production. (5)-aminosalicylate and sulfapyridine inhibit myeloperoxidase-mediated iodination and cytotoxicity. These effects have been proposed to occur through inhibition of the lipoxygenase pathway. The major products of this pathway are the leukotrienes and certain hydroxy-fatty acids, potent chemotactic agents that recruit inflammatory cells into sites of inflammation. Sulfasalazine and (5)-aminosalicylate block the synthesis of these products. Inhibition of the synthesis of these agents may account for some of the anti-inflammatory effects of sulfasalazine in inflammatory bowel disease. The ability of sulfasalazine and (5)-aminosalicylate to scavenge reactive oxygen (free radicals) may also play a role in their therapeutic effects in inflammatory bowel disease. (5)-aminosalicylate has been shown to be the active moiety of sulfasalazine.

INDICATIONS

Ulcerative Colitis

Controlled trials have established the value of sulfasalazine compared with placebo in the treatment of mild to moderate active disease. Topical sulfasalazine enemas are effective for distal disease. Sulfasalazine is not recommended for the initial treatment of acute, severe ulcerative colitis. It is effective in preventing relapses of inactive ulcerative colitis. The optimal duration of maintenance therapy has never been determined.

Sulfasalazine is safe during pregnancy and nursing, despite its crossing the placenta and being present in breast milk.

Crohn's Disease

Controlled trials have shown sulfasalazine to be effective in the treatment of mild to moderate ileocolic or colonic Crohn's disease. It can be used with steroids in acutely ill patients, although the added benefit is small. It has not been shown to be effective in the treatment of Crohn's disease of the small bowel or in the prevention of relapses of inactive Crohn's disease.

Maintenance therapy is not indicated in Crohn's disease.

DOSAGE

The suggested dosage in acute inflammatory bowel disease is 1 gram/15 kilograms body weight/day in divided doses.

The usual dosage is 3 to 4 grams/day. The risk of side effects or toxic reactions increases with dosages of 4 grams/day or more. To avoid side effects, the initial sulfasalazine dose should be low, 1 gram/day, with gradual daily increases of 500 milligrams/day until the therapeutic range is reached. A therapeutic response is usually apparent by 1 month.

Once remission has been achieved in ulcerative colitis, the sulfasalazine should be gradually tapered to a maintenance dose of 2 grams/day.

After remission has been induced in Crohn's disease, therapy, 500 milligrams/week, should be continued for several more months or more before slowly tapering the sulfasalazine.

SIDE EFFECTS

The overall reported incidence of side effects of sulfasalazine therapy varies from 10 to 45 percent. The most common side effects include nausea, vomiting, anorexia, headache, heartburn, epigastric distress, and diarrhea. These side effects have been directly related to the level of sulfapyridine in the serum. Accordingly, slow acetylators on high-dose therapy are most commonly affected. The side effects are usually relieved by discontinuing the drug temporarily, then resuming therapy at a lower dosage.

Dermatological manifestations include drug rashes, photosensitivity, exfoliative dermatitis, and rarely, toxic epidermal necrolysis.

Hematological side effects include neutropenia and agranulocytosis, megaloblastic anemia secondary to an effective folate deficiency, red cell aplasia, thrombocytopenia, hemolytic anemia, reticulocytosis, methemoglobinemia, and sulfhemoglobinemia. The occurrence of hemolysis appears to be directly related to sulfapyridine levels and to acetylator status.

Some patients have experienced a generalized allergic reaction, with fever, skin rash, arthralgias, and lymphadenopathy.

Recently, reversible male infertility has been described.

Cyanosis unrelated to methemoglobinemia, sulfhemoglobinemia, and oxygen desaturation has been reported.

Extremely rare side effects include neurotoxicity, pancreatitis, hair loss, hepatotoxicity, pulmonary fibrosis, a lupuslike syndrome, and hemorrhagic colitis.

DESENSITIZATION

Patients who are intolerant of or allergic to sulfasalazine may be desensitized. Desensitization should not be attempted in patients who have previously experienced agranulocytosis, frank hemolysis, hepatotoxicity, pulmonary toxicity, or toxic epidermal necrolysis.

Patients who have generalized side effects such as nausea, vomiting, headache, and malaise should have the medication stopped for 2 weeks. Sulfasalazine should then be restarted at 0.25 to 0.5 grams/day for a week, and gradually increased by 0.25 grams at weekly intervals until a dose of 2 grams/day is reached. Doses above 3 grams/day are not recommended.

Patients who have hypersensitivity or idiosyncratic reactions should be approached much more cautiously. The sulfasalazine should again be discontinued for at least 2 weeks. The patient should then be started on one-eighth (⅛) tablet per day. The dose should be doubled every 7 days until a dose of 2 to 3 grams/day is reached. Minor recurrences of the sensitivity reaction (pruritus) may be treated with antihistamines with or without steroids. Close clinical follow up is imperative during the desensitization period.

Once desensitization has been achieved, the drug should be continued indefinitely to maintain it. The drug should be discontinued for severe hypersensitivity reactions during the desensitization process.

DRUG INTERACTIONS

Sulfasalazine, but not its metabolites, competitively inhibits the absorption of folic acid. Cholestyramine directly binds sulfasalazine in the gut lumen and markedly decreases the metabolism of the drug. A similar interaction has been reported between ferrous sulfate and sulfasalazine. Sulfasalazine decreases the bioavailability of digoxin. Sulfasalazine metabolism is diminished by the concurrent administration of broad-spectrum antibiotics.

NEW ANALOGUES

As previously stated, the active moiety of sulfasalazine is (5)-aminosalicylic acid, but most of its side effects are related to the sulfapyridine moiety. Analogues of sulfasalazine are now being investigated that do not contain the sulfapyridine moiety. These new analogues of sulfasalazine may prove to be of particular benefit in patients who are intolerant of or allergic to sulfasalazine.

Pentasa is a sustained-release tablet designed to release (5)-aminosalicylate in the small bowel and colon. It contains 250 milligrams of (5)-aminosalicylate in microgranules, coated with a semipermeable membrane of ethyl cellulose.

Sodium azo-disalicylate is a dimeric form of (5)-aminosalicylate consisting of two (5)-aminosalicylate molecules linked by a diazo bond. It is efficacious in the treatment of inflammatory bowel disease.

Poly-ASA is an oral formulation of (5)-aminosalicylate in a water-soluble polymer that links the moiety by an azo bond to an inert sulfanilamide ethylene polymer.

New forms of (5)-aminosalicylate can be delivered in enema form. (5)-aminosalicylate enemas are effective in distal ulcerative colitis. (4)-aminosalicylate enemas are also effective in distal ulcerative colitis. They have the advantage of being more stable and less expensive.

PEARLS AND PITFALLS

1. There is no place for sulfasalazine in the treatment of acute, severe flares of ulcerative colitis.
2. Megaloblastic anemia should alert the physician to the need to give supplemental folic acid, one milligram/day, to patients receiving sulfasalazine. Other drugs capable of inducing megaloblastic anemia include ethanol, methotrexate, and dilantin. Other conditions capable of causing a megaloblastic anemia include tropical sprue, terminal ileitis, pernicious anemia, and cirrhosis.
3. Sulfasalazine can be safely used in pregnant and nursing women.
4. Young men on sulfasalazine often experience significant decreases in sperm count and mobility. Sperm morphology is markedly abnormal. These changes may result in infertility. Sperm counts usually return to normal within 2 months of discontinuing the drug.
5. Desensitization should be attempted in patients who are intolerant of sulfasalazine or who have mild to moderate hypersensitivity or idiosyncratic reactions. Most patients can be successfully desensitized. Sulfasalazine analogues may be used in the patients who fail desensitization.
6. (5)-aminosalicylic acid or (4)-aminosalicylic acid enemas should be tried in patients with distal ulcerative colitis who have failed oral sulfasalazine and steroid enemas. These often obviate the need to go to oral steroids.
7. Sulfasalazine does not appear to be effective in Crohn's disease limited to the small bowel.

References

1. Azad Khan AK. Optimum dose of sulphasalazine for maintenance treatment in ulcerative colitis. Gut 1980; 21:232–240.

    A landmark clinical trial that established the optimum maintenance dose of sulfasalazine as 2 gms/day.

2. Bondesen S, Rasmussen SN, Rask-Madsen J. (5)-aminosalicylic acid in the treatment of inflammatory bowel disease. Ac Med Scand 1987; 221:227–242.

    A comprehensive review of the biochemistry and clinical use of (5)-aminosalicylate.

3. Collen MJ. Azulfidine-induced oligospermia. Am J Gastro 1980; 74:441–442.

    A case report and discussion.

4. Craven PA, Pfanstel J, Saito R. Actions of sulfasalazine and (5)-aminosalicylic acid as reactive oxygen scavengers in the suppression of bile acid-induced increases in colonic epithelial cell loss and proliferative activity. Gastroenterology 1987; 92:1998–2008.

    The study examines the mechanism of protective action of sulfasalazine in a rat model in which colonic epithelial cell loss and subsequent increases in epithelial proliferative

activity were induced by intracolonic instillation of sodium deoxycholate.
5. Das KM. Pharmacotherapy of inflammatory bowel disease I. Sulfasalazine. Postgrad Med 1983; 74:141–151.

   A comprehensive review of sulfasalazine use in inflammatory bowel disease.
6. Das KM, Chowdhury R, Fara JW. Small absorption of sulfasalazine and its hepatic metabolism in human beings, cats, and rats. Gastroenterology 1979; 77:280–284.

   The absorption and hepatic metabolism of sulfasalazine is discussed at length.
7. Donaldson RM. Management of medical problems in pregnancy—inflammatory bowel disease. NEJM 1985; 312:1616–1619.

   An excellent discussion of pregnancy in relationship to clinical, diagnostic, and therapeutic aspects of inflammatory bowel disease.
8. Friedman G. Sulfasalazine and new analogues. Am J Gastro 1986; 81:141–144.

   A discussion of new analogues and their side effects.
9. Haines JD. Hepatotoxicity after treatment with sulfasalazine. Postgrad Med 1986; 79:193–198.

   A case report and discussion.
10. Hoult JRS. Pharmacological and biochemical actions of sulphasalazine. Drugs 1986; 32(Suppl) 1:18–26.

    A review of the pharmacology and biochemistry of sulfasalazine.
11. Jacobson IM, Kelsey PB, Blyden GT. Sulfasalazine-induced agranulocytosis. Am J Gastro 1985; 80:118–121.

    A case report and discussion.
12. Korelitz B, et al. Desensitization to sulfasalazine after hypersensitivity reactions in patients with inflammatory bowel disease. J Clin Gastro 1984; 6:27–31.

    A report of 40 of 47 patients with hypersensitivity reactions successfully desensitized.
13. Margolin ML, et al. Clinical trials in ulcerative colitis II. Historical review. Am J Gastro 1988; 83:227–243.

    An exhaustive review of clinical trials in ulcerative colitis, with insightful comments by the authors on their significance.
14. Meyers S, et al. Olsalazine sodium in the treatment of ulcerative colitis among patients intolerant of sulfasalazine. Gastroenterology 1987; 93:1255–1262.

    A double-blind, randomized trial showing the benefit of Olsalazine over placebo in ulcerative colitis.
15. Miyachi Y, Yoshioka A, Imamura S. Effect of sulphasalazine and its metabolites on the generation of reactive oxygen species. Gut 1987; 28:190–195.

    The in vitro anti-oxidant effects of sulfasalazine and its metabolites is studied.
16. Moseley RH, Barwick KW. Sulfasalazine-induced pulmonary disease. Dig Dis Sci 1985; 30:901–904.

    A case report and discussion.
17. Pearl RK, Nelson RL. Serious complications of sulfasalazine. Dis Colon Rectum 1985; 29:201–202.

    A report of three serious complications of sulfasalazine.

18. Peppercorn MA. Sulfasalazine: Pharmacology, clinical use, toxicity, and related new drug development. Ann Int Med 1984; 101:377–386.

    An excellent review article on all aspects of sulfasalazine.

19. Peppercorn MA, Goldman P. Distribution studies of salicylazosulfapyridine and its metabolites. Gastroenterology 1973; 64:240–245.

    Distribution of sulfasalazine and its metabolites in humans and rats are discussed.

20. Peppercorn MA, Goldman P. The role of intestinal bacteria in the metabolism of salicylazosulfapyridine. J Pharm Exp Ther 1981; 181:555–562.

    The metabolism of sulfasalazine in conventional and germ-free rats is studied. Metabolism is directly related to the presence or absence of bacteria in the colon.

21. Ruderman WB, Farmer RG. Current management of inflammatory bowel disease. Rad Clin N Am 1987; 25:221–232.

    A concise but comprehensive review of medical therapy of inflammatory bowel disease.

22. Schroder H, Campbell DE. Absorption, metabolism, and excretion of salicylazosulfapyridine in man. Clin Pharm Ther 1972; 13:539–551.

    A study of the pharmacology of sulfasalazine in nine healthy patients on 4 gms/day for 10 days.

23. Shanahan F, Targan S. Sulfasalazine and salicylate-induced exacerbation of ulcerative colitis. NEJM 1987; 317:455.

    A letter attributing the rare acute hemorrhagic colitis side effect to the salicylate moiety.

24. Soldata PD, et al. A possible mechanism of action of sulfasalazine and 5-aminosalicylic acid in inflammatory bowel diseases: Interaction with oxygen-free radicals. Gastroenterology 1985; 89:1215–1216.

    The paper relates the in vivo anti-inflammatory action of sulfasalazine to its ability, through (5)-aminosalicylic acid, to scavenge oxygen-free radicals.

25. Summers RW, et al. National cooperative Crohn's disease study: Results of drug treatment 1979; 77:847–869.

    A double-blind, randomized trial that compared sulfasalazine (1 gm/15 mgs body weight) to placebo over 4 months in patients with various degrees of involvement of Crohn's disease.

26. Taffet SL, Das KM. Sulfasalazine: Adverse effects and desensitization. Dig Dis Sci 1983; 28:833–842.

    An excellent review article.

27. Taffet SL, Das KM. Desensitization in patients with inflammatory bowel disease to sulfasalazine. Am J Med 1982; 73:520–524.

    A presentation of one method of desensitization.

28. Watkinson G. Sulphasalazine: A review of 40 years' experience. Drugs 1986; 32(Suppl 1):1–11.

    An excellent review of clinical trials supporting the use of sulphasalazine in inflammatory bowel disease.

9
Antimetabolites
Michael M. Van Ness

The immunosuppressive drugs 6-mercaptopurine and azathioprine may benefit a selected group of patients with inflammatory bowel disease. Their use requires careful consideration by the physician of their risks, benefits, and limitations. Detailed instruction to the patient cannot be overemphasized. Signing of a doctor–patient "contract" is a useful tool to ensure complete understanding of the risks and benefits of these agents.

Brooke published the first anecedotal report of the benefit of azathioprine in six patients with Crohn's disease. Since then, seven controlled trials with azathioprine and one controlled trial with 6-mercaptopurine have been conducted and form the basis for use of these agents in inflammatory bowel disease.

PHARMACOLOGY

Both 6-mercaptopurine and azathioprine are antimetabolites that inhibit purine-ring biosynthesis, thereby decreasing DNA synthesis and impeding cellular division. Azathioprine is produced by conjugation of a free SH group to 6-mercaptopurine. It was developed in the hope of decreasing the toxicity of 6-mercaptopurine without decreasing its effectiveness. By weight, 6-mercaptopurine accounts for 54 percent of a dose of azathioprine. Both 6-mercaptopurine and azathioprine are metabolized by enzymatic oxidation by xanthine oxidase. Allopurinol, a powerful inhibitor of xanthine oxidase, greatly potentiates the cytotoxic action and toxic side effects of 6-mercaptopurine and azathioprine. Concurrent administration of allopurinal necessitates a 75 percent dose reduction of 6-mercaptopurine so as to avoid untoward side effects.

INDICATIONS

Based on the work of Present, Lennard-Jones, and Korelitz, indications for use of these drugs are strictly defined (Table 9–1). Patients who fail to achieve a remission on high-dose steroids (40–60 mgs/day), patients who fail to maintain a remission on sulfasalazine and require intermittent high-dose steroid use, patients who respond to steroids but who experience multiple early relapses, and patients who have active fistulous disease unresponsive to corticosteroids and metronidazole (Flagyl) are candidates for 6-mercaptopurine. Most authors favor use of 6-mercaptopurine instead of azathioprine, as 6-mercaptopurine is the active form of the pro-drug azathioprine and its effects are believed to be more predictable.

The largest clinical trial of 6-mercaptopurine in Crohn's disease was conducted by Present and his colleagues. They studied 83 patients with Crohn's disease active at the time

Table 9–1. Indications for use of 6-mercaptopurine in Crohn's disease

1. Active Crohn's disease unresponsive to maximal medical management, including sulfasalazine and corticosteroids.
2. Prolonged (>6 months) corticosteroid use or multiple, early relapses necessitating high-dose corticosteroid use.
3. Fistula unresponsive to maximal medical management, including metronidazole and corticosteroids.

of, or just prior to, entry into the study. These patients had had Crohn's disease for a mean of 4.3 years. Four groups were analyzed: patients with ileitis with fistulas, patients with ileitis without fistulas, patients with colitis or ileocolitis with fistulas, and patients with colitis or ileocolitis without fistulas. There was no arbitrary cessation of ongoing drug therapy at the time of entry into the study; in particular, corticosteroids were not arbitrarily stopped. Overall, between 67 percent and 79 percent of patients taking 6-mercaptopurine improved, compared to only 13 percent of patients taking placebo. Fistulas healed in 31 percent of patients taking 6-mercaptopurine, versus only 6 percent of patients taking placebo. In patients on 6-mercaptopurine, steroids were able to be discontinued in 55 percent and reduced in another 20 percent (total 75%), compared to steroid cessation or reduction in only 36 percent of patients receiving placebo. Clinical improvement after steroid cessation or reduction was maintained in 64 percent of patients receiving long-term therapy (up to 2 years in this study, up to 5 years in another). The mean time to response was 3.1 months (range 2 weeks to 9 months). There was a somewhat higher frequency of response (77%) in patients with ileocolonic disease compared to ileitis or colitis alone. The response to 6-mercaptopurine did not appear to be dose-related, with a mean dose of 70 milligrams/day in responders, compared to 89 milligrams/day in nonresponders.

Subsequent studies have added to our understanding of therapy of Crohn's disease with 6-mercaptopurine. Korelitz points out that patients who respond to the drug and subsequently stop the agent have a mean time to relapse of 12 months (0.5–42 months). Furthermore, in responders who stop the drug, relapse, and recommence therapy, the mean time until a second response is short (1.5 months compared to 3.1 months initially). The risk of malignancy from use of 6-mercaptopurine does not appear to be increased. Unlike renal transplant patients, who also receive combination immunosuppressive therapy, these patients receive relatively modest amounts of drug.

Fistulas have been shown to improve with treatment with 6-mercaptopurine. In a series reported by Korelitz and Present, improvement with fistula closure was seen in 39 percent and improvement in fistulas without complete closure in another 26 percent. Fistulas were more likely to heal in patients with no prior surgical history. The site of intes-

Table 9-2. Contraindications to use of 6-mercaptopurine in Crohn's disease

1. Pregnancy
2. Pancreatitis secondary to 6-mercaptopurine
3. Inability or unwillingness of the patient to cooperate with primary physician.

tinal involvement with Crohn's disease appeared unrelated to the likelihood of fistula healing. With continuous therapy, fistulas remained closed for up to 5 years.

CONTRAINDICATIONS

As outlined in Table 9-2, 6-mercaptopurine is contraindicated for use in the pregnant patient. Despite a dearth of knowledge about teratogenicity, therapeutic abortion is recommended by some authors if a patient taking 6-mercaptopurine becomes pregnant. On the other hand, uncomplicated pregnancies resulting in normal children are reported in women with malignant disease treated with chemotherapeutic agents.

6-mercaptopurine is contraindicated for use in the patient with a previous episode of 6-mercaptopurine-induced pancreatitis. Pancreatitis is a rare complication of 6-mercaptopurine use and is manifested by the development of abdominal pain, fever, nausea, and vomiting within the first month of therapy. In Haber's report of 13 cases, the incidence was 3.25 percent, the onset was within 8 to 32 days, and the amylase elevation averaged 6 times normal. With cessation of the drug, all signs and symptoms resolved rapidly (range 1–11 days) without complication. Of the seven patients rechallenged with the drug, all developed recurrent pancreatitis. All efforts to desensitize the patients to the agent by initiating therapy with very small doses were unsuccessful and led to recurrent pancreatitis. The authors conclude that once implicated as a cause of pancreatitis, 6-mercaptopurine should not be utilized again.

ADMINISTRATION

Prior to administration of 6-mercaptopurine, a clear understanding of the indications, dosing, side effects, and duration of therapy must be reached between the physician and the patient. This "contract" is best signed, with copies retained by both parties. An example of such a document is given in Figure 9-1.

6-mercaptopurine is best administered as a single daily oral dose, one milligram/kilogram of body weight. There is little benefit to increasing the dose beyond this level, as there is no known dose-response curve. On the other hand, the side effects of neutropenia and thrombosytopenia are clearly dose-related. Prior to the first dose, a complete blood cell count, platelet count, serum amylase determination,

DATE: _____

PATIENT'S NAME: _____

DIAGNOSIS: _____

MEDICATIONS: _____

I, _____
(patient's name)
have been informed by my doctor of the need to take the medication 6-mercaptopurine at a starting daily dose of _____ .
(number of the 50-milligram pills)

I understand that this drug can decrease the number of white blood cells in my blood.

I understand the need to have blood drawn weekly until my white blood cell count is stable.

I understand that this drug can cause pancreatitis and hepatitis.

I understand the need to inform my doctor as soon as possible of fever, abdominal pain, vomiting, or jaundice.

I understand that it may take as long as 3 to 6 months before I have any benefit from 6-mercaptopurine.

I understand that I may have no benefit whatsoever from this medication.

PATIENT'S SIGNATURE: _____

PHYICIAN'S SIGNATURE: _____

Fig. 9–1. Patient contract for treatment with 6-mercaptopurine.

and serum levels of serum alanine aminotransferase, aspartate aminotransferase, and alkaline phosphatase are required. Thereafter, weekly complete blood and platelet counts should be monitored to guide dose adjustments so as to keep the white blood cell counts above 4500 cells per cubic millimeter and platelet counts above 100,000 per cubic millimeter. Once stable, the frequency of blood studies can be decreased to a monthly basis. Abdominal pain, back pain, and elevated serum amylase, or fever alone, require abrupt cessation of 6-mercaptopurine therapy. If the diagnosis of pancreatitis is confirmed, 6-mercaptopurine should not be restarted. Rarely should 6-mercaptopurine be continued in the face of a known systemic infection.

PEARLS AND PITFALLS

1. Corticosteroid sparing is a known benefit of 6-mercaptopurine.
2. A trial of 6-mercaptopurine cannot be called a failure until the end of a trial period of at least 3 months.
3. There is little or no benefit to pushing the daily dose higher than 1.5 milligrams/kilogram body weight.
4. Pancreatitis from 6-mercaptopurine usually occurs within 30 days of initiation of therapy, usually is uncomplicated, and precludes future use of 6-mercaptopurine in that patient.
5. The signing of a "contract" by the patient minimizes the risk of misunderstandings in the use of this drug.

References

1. Bank L, Wright JP. 6-mercaptopurine-related pancreatitis in 2 patients with inflammatory bowel disease. Dig Dis Sci 1984; 29:357–359.

    Two cases of 6-MP-induced pancreatitis occurred within 21 days of initiation of therapy. Rechallenge led to recurrent pancreatitis within 3 hours of a single dose.

2. Blatt J, et al. Pregnancy outcome following cancer chemotherapy. Am J Med 1980; 69:828–832.

    A review of patients receiving cancer chemotherapy at the time of conception and organogenesis.

3. Brooke BN, Hoffman DC, and Swarbrick ET. Azathioprine for Crohn's disease. *Lancet* 1969; 2:612–614.

    These initial 6 cases are the basis for the subsequent trials of immunosuppressive agents for treatment of inflammatory bowel disease.

4. Haber CJ, et al. Nature and course of pancreatitis caused by 6-mercaptopurine in the treatment of inflammatory bowel disease. Gastroenterology 1986; 91:982–986.

    The authors report the clinical course of 13 cases of pancreatitis attributable to 6-MP in 400 (3.25%) patients with inflammatory bowel disease. The pancreatitis tends to occur early (within 30 days), is usually mild, and recurs with rechallenge.

5. Korelitz BI. Pharmacotherapy of inflammatory bowel disease. Postgrad Med J 1983; 74:165–172.

   A practical review of many of the salient points necessary to treat patients with anti-metabolites.

6. Korelitz BI, Present DH. Favorable effect of 6-mercaptopurine on fistulae of Crohn's disease. Dig Dis Sci 1985; 30:58–64.

   The authors present the data from the original NEJM report and add interesting long-term follow-up data supporting the claim that 6-MP is efficacious in the maintenance of fistulae closure for up to 5 years.

7. Lennard-Jones JE. Azathioprine and 6-mercaptopurine have a role in the treatment of Crohn's disease. Dig Dis Sci 1981; 26:364–367.

   The argument of a relatively enthusiastic proponent of 6-MP emphasizes the inadequacies of the NCCDS especially as to how they relate to azathioprine. He notes that all drug therapy ongoing at the time of initiation of the drug trial was stopped. This requirement may have unfairly biased the trial against azathioiprine and other immunosuppressive agents in general.

8. Present DH, et al. Treatment of Crohn's disease with 6-mercaptopurine. NEJM 1980; 302:981–987.

   The landmark article showing benefit of 6-MP. Reduction of steroid dosages, closure of fistulas, and clinical improvement in cases refractory to sulfasalazine and corticosteroids were demonstrated. The onset of response was often delayed as long as 3 months.

9. Singleton JW. Azathioprine has a very limited role in the treatment of Crohn's disease. Dig Dis Sci 1981; 26:368–371.

   The author reviews the NCCDS and concludes that azathioprine has no role as initial therapy for active Crohn's disease. Although he concedes it may be useful as an adjunct to prednisone in disease unresponsive to sulfasalazine and prednisone, he notes that the excess risk of cancer, as defined by Kinlen in patients given azathioprine for nontransplant, noncancer indications, is increased 1.6-fold.

10

Metronidazole

Thomas Dorsey

Metronidazole is an antimicrobial agent with antibacterial, antiprotozoal, and anti-inflammatory actions useful in the treatment of a variety of infectious diseases of the gastrointestinal tract and in specific forms of Crohn's disease.

The parent compound, azomysin, was discovered by Nakamura in 1955 and was shown to have antitrichomonal activity in 1956. In 1959, Cosar showed the azomysin derivative, metronidazole, to have both in vitro and in vivo antitrichomonal activity. Metronidazole was the first and remains the most widely used derivative. Its effectiveness against anaerobes was demonstrated in 1963 and it was subsequently shown highly effective in parasitic diseases of the gut, most notably against *Entamoeba histolytica* and *Giardia lamblia*. The first evidence of activity in inflammatory bowel disease was shown in 1975; since that time it has been actively studied.

PHARMACOLOGY

1-(B-hydroxyethyl)-2-methyl-5-nitroimidazole is a pale yellow, crystalline substance slightly soluble in water and alcohol. An oral dose is exceptionally well absorbed, yielding plasma levels similar to those achieved with an equal intravenous dose. It is also well absorbed rectally, although more variably and at a slower rate. Peak blood levels occur 1 to 2 hours after an oral dose. The drug circulates in the plasma less than 20 percent protein-bound. Serum half-life is 8 hours. It diffuses freely into total body water with levels in cerebrospinal fluid, saliva, bile, bone, and breast milk equivalent to serum levels. It appears rapidly on all mucosal surfaces, and bacteriocidal concentrations have been documented in pus from hepatic abscesses.

Nonhepatic metabolism in humans is negligible. The primary metabolic site is the liver via oxidation of side chains and glucuronide formation. Urinary excretion accounts for 60 to 80 percent of a given dose, with 80 percent as metabolites and 20 percent as unchanged drug. Stool excretion accounts for 6 to 15 percent. Metabolites may impart a reddish-brown discoloration to the urine but this has no clinical significance. Renal failure does not alter the distribution or metabolism of the drug and there is no need for dose reduction except in severe renal insufficiency. Hemodialysis removes 50 percent of a given dose. Patients with hepatic insufficiency as manifested by ascites, encephalopathy, low albumin levels, or a prolonged prothrombin time have decreased metabolism and require dose reduction.

MECHANISM OF ACTION, INDICATIONS, AND ADMINISTRATION

Anaerobic Bacteria and Protozoa

The drug is taken up by passive diffusion and rapidly metabolized, decreasing the intracellular concentration of unchanged drug and thus increasing the transmembrane concentration gradient leading to continuous uptake. Metabolism in bacteria is via reduction of the nitro group by nitroreductases, which play a major role in anaerobic energy metabolism. Metronidazole acts as an electron sink depriving the cells of reducing equivalent. In addition, the reduction of metronidazole yields free radicals, short-lived cytotoxic intermediates that interact with DNA and other intracellular macromolecules. These metabolites disrupt the helical structure of DNA and cause single- and double-stranded breaks.

Inflammatory Bowel Disease

The mode of action in inflammatory bowel disease is unknown. Possible mechanisms include its antimicrobial effect in eliminating bacterial overgrowth and reducing the load of bacterial antigens. In an animal model metronidazole has been shown to inhibit some parameters of cell-mediated immunity, specifically granuloma formation. Finally, metronidazole may have a direct tissue effect.

Ulcerative Colitis

There have been two prospective, randomized, double-blind controlled trials of metronidazole in ulcerative colitis. In 1977, Davies studied the effect of metronidazole suppositories in mild chronic proctitis. There was no evidence of benefit on clinical, endoscopic, or histologic parameters after 28 days of therapy. In the second study, a 5-day course of intravenous metronidazole failed to improve remission rate, need for urgent surgery, or late mortality in hospitalized patients with severe colitis requiring intravenous and topical steroids and total parenteral nutrition. Current evidence does not support the use of metronidazole in ulcerative colitis.

Crohn's Disease

Ursing and Kamme reported their experience with metronidazole in five patients with Crohn's disease in 1975. Four of the five improved clinically and biochemically within 4 weeks. Three of these were able to discontinue sulfasalazine and steroids. One patient had a more gradual response over 4 months.

Blichfeldt treated 22 patients with Crohn's disease requiring sulfasalazine and steroids with metronidazole for 2 months in a double-blind crossover trial compared with placebo. Small bowel Crohn's disease showed no response, but those with colitis showed a striking improvement in symptoms (diarrhea, abdominal pain, and sense of well-being) and biochemical markers (hematocrit and ESR).

Bernstein studied the effect of metronidazole in 21 patients with chronic, unremitting perianal Crohn's disease. Twenty improved on a dose of 20 milligrams/kilogram/day and 10 healed completely on chronic therapy. In a follow-up study, Brandt confirmed the beneficial effects and showed that (1) therapy could be discontinued in only 28 percent of patients without recurrence, (2) recurrences were fewer if the drug was tapered rather than stopped abruptly, (3) all recurrences responded to reinstitution of therapy at full dose, and (4) remissions were maintained for the duration of the study (36 months) on therapy.

Ursing compared metronidazole, 0.8 gram/day, to sulfasalazine, 3 grams/day, in a randomized, double-blind controlled trial and found no difference in efficacy. However, there was greater biochemical improvement in the metronidazole group. In addition, sulfasalazine nonresponders showed clinical response to metronidazole but metronidazole nonresponders showed no clinical or biochemical response to sulfasalazine. It was concluded that both are efficacious in Crohn's disease of the colon, with metronidazole demonstrating slightly more efficacy.

Current indications for metronidazole in Crohn's disease include (1) perianal disease (abscesses, ulcerations, and fistulae, including retrovaginal fistulae), (2) Crohn's colitis, (3) metastatic skin ulcerations of Crohn's, and (4) sulfasalazine intolerance or allergy. There may be a role in therapy of enterocutaneous fistulae and recalcitrant small bowel disease, but these indications have not been studied in clinical trials.

The drug should be continued until healing occurs, no additional benefits are seen, or side effects occur. The dose should be tapered in those who respond and if disease recurs the full dose should be reinstituted.

Bacterial Infections: Anaerobes

Metronidazole demonstrates activity against a wide variety of anaerobic organisms, including gram-negative rods (*Bacteroides* species such as *B. fragilis* and *Fusobacterium*), gram-positive rods (*Clostridia* species including *C. difficile* and *Eubacterium*), and gram-positive cocci (*peptococcus* and *peptostreptococcus*). *Bifidobacterium, Actinomyces, Arachini,* and *Propionibacterium* are resistant. *B. fragilis* is a common anaerobe causing life-threatening infections. It is often multiply resistant to other antibiotics. It may manifest a relative resistance to metronidazole that is mediated by a decreased nitroreductase activity. In practice, this resistance can be overcome by increasing the dose.

Metronidazole has been effective in meningitis, brain abscess, osteomyelitis, septic arthritis, and endocarditis caused by these organisms. It is also quite effective in pelvic and intra-abdominal abscesses, including diverticular abscesses.

A loading dose of 15 milligrams/kilogram is given over a period of 1 hour, followed by 7.5 milligrams/kilogram every 6 hours infused over 1 hour. When the patient is responding, therapy can be completed by oral administration of 7.5 milligrams/kilogram orally every 6 hours.

Clostridium Difficile–Associated Colitis

Teasley demonstrated in a prospective, randomized clinical trial that metronidazole has equivalent efficacy, relapse rates, and patient tolerance, compared to oral vancomycin therapy, in treatment of *C. difficile*–associated colitis. Metronidazole has the advantage of being much less expensive. Dosage is 500 milligrams orally twice a day for 10 days. It should be noted that in rare instances metronidazole has apparently caused *C. difficile*–associated colitis.

Surgical Prophylaxis

Metronidazole has also been used perioperatively in colon surgery, appendectomy, and hysterectomy to decrease the incidence of intra-abdominal and wound infections. It is as effective as other drugs in this setting.

Protozoal Infections

Amebiasis

Metronidazole is exceedingly active against *Entamoeba histolytica*. In culture, drug concentrations of 1 to 2 micrograms/milliliter kill 100 percent of organisms at 24 hours, and concentrations of 0.2 micrograms/milliliter kill 100 percent of organisms at 72 hours. There have been no reports of resistance, but asymptomatic cyst carriers are not adequately treated by metronidazole. The drug is active against dysenteric and hepatic forms of infection. Most hepatic abscesses respond dramatically with prompt reduction in size. Failure to respond after 48 hours may indicate the need for percutaneous or surgical drainage. In both dysentery and hepatic abscess, therapy must be followed by a lumbricidal agent (Iodoquinol) to ensure that no organisms persist. Adult dosage in dysentery and hepatic amebiasis is 750 milligrams orally 3 times a day for 10 days, followed by Iodoquinol, 650 milligrams orally 3 times a day for 20 days. In children, the correct dose is 35 to 50 milligrams/kilogram/day in three doses for 10 days, followed by Iodoquinol, 40 milligrams/kilogram/day (maximum 2 grams) in three divided doses for 20 days.

Balantidium coli

Balantidium coli is a parasite of hogs that can cause dysentery in humans and mimics *E. histolytica*. Metronidazole (500 milligrams orally 4 times a day for 10 days), followed by Iodoquinol (650 milligrams orally 3 times a day for 20 days) are effective. In children, the dose of metronidazole is 10 milligrams/kilogram 4 times a day for 10 days (maximum dose 2 grams/day), followed by Iodoquinol, 40 milligrams/kilogram/day (maximum 2 grams) in three divided doses for 20 days.

Entamoeba polecki

Entamoeba polecki is another porcine parasite, seen in immigrants from southeast Asia. It may be mistaken for *E. histolytica*. Therapy consists of metronidazole in doses used for *E. histolytica* followed by diloxanide furoate, 500 milligrams orally 3 times a day for 10 days in adults, and 20 milligrams/kilogram/day in three doses for 10 days in children.

Giardiasis

Metronidazole has not been approved by the FDA for the therapy of *Giardia lamblia*, but it is an effective and well-tolerated alternative to quinacrine. The recommended dose is 250 milligrams orally 3 times a day for 5 to 7 days in adults and 5 milligrams/kilogram 3 times a day for 7 days in children.

Blastocystis hominis

Blastocystis hominis is a protozoan that causes mild to moderate abdominal cramping and nonfebrile, nonbloody diarrhea that may be recurrent. Metronidazole, 750 milligrams orally 3 times a day for ten days in adults and 35 to 50 milligrams/kilogram/day in three divided doses for 10 days in children, results in 60 to 70 percent cure rates.

Dracunculiasis

Infestation by the guinia worm, *Dracuncula medinensis,* is seen worldwide in the tropics. Metronidazole, 250 milligrams orally 3 times a day for 7 days, is an effective alternative to thiabendazole or niridazole.

SIDE EFFECTS AND CONTRAINDICATIONS

Metronidazole is generally well tolerated and only rarely are side effects sufficiently severe to cause discontinuation. Most side effects are self-limited.

Contraindications to use include hypersensitivity to metronidazole or other imidazoles. Relative contraindications are pregnancy (first trimester), a history of a blood dyscrasia, or active neurologic disease (neuropathy or seizure disorder).

The most common side effects are gastrointestinal. A metallic taste occurs in 92 percent of patients. Glossitis, stomatitis, furry tongue, and dry mouth are not uncommon. Anorexia, nausea, vomiting, epigastric pain and discomfort, and cramps are also seen. Therapy can cause an exacerbation of candidiasis. As mentioned previously, it has rarely been implicated in causing *C. difficile* colitis.

Neurologic side effects, including headache, ataxia, vertigo, encephalopathy, and seizures, are not uncommon and warrant discontinuation of therapy. Peripheral neuropathy is common with prolonged use. It is commonly sensory with paresthesias involving lower extremities and is more prominent in the winter months. It is associated with higher doses and longer duration of therapy, with 50 percent of patients affected after 6 months of therapy. It is reversible if recognized early and the dose decreased or stopped. It can persist for a prolonged period after cessation of the drug.

Dermatologic side effects include urticaria, flushing, and pruritis.

Genitourinary complaints include vaginal dryness and burning, cystitis, urethritis, pelvic pressure, and discoloration of urine.

Hematologic manifestations include reversible neutropenia seen after long-term use. Complete blood counts are recommended during prolonged therapy. Phlebitis at the site of infusion has been reported.

Metronidazole causes an artifactural depression of SGOT levels.

Metronidazole and its metabolites are mutagenic in bacterial culture. It is oncogenic in mice and rats but not in hamsters. Its mechanism of action in bacteria and protozoa involves direct damage to cellular DNA. Despite these findings, no chromosomal abnormalities were demonstrated in humans receiving 20 milligrams/kilogram/day for prolonged periods. No teratogenicity has been demonstrated in human fetuses.

Several retrospective human studies have shown no increased incidence of malignancies in patients receiving metronidazole. The most recent study showed no increased cancer in a group of 771 women followed for 15 to 25 years after exposure.

Used in pregnancy, metronidazole crosses the placenta and rapidly enters the fetal circulation. Although no teratogenic effect has been noted in several small series of human pregnancies or in rodents, its use is relatively contraindicated in pregnancy because of the possibility of carcinogenic potential with a long latent period.

In nursing mothers, metronidazole achieves breast-milk concentrations similar to plasma levels. Although there are no known ill effects, the potential for carcingoenesis with a long latent period must be considered such that metronidazole's use in nursing mothers is relatively contraindicated.

Metronidazole is currently being investigated as a radiosensitizer to potentiate the effect of radiation on certain malignancies.

DRUG INTERACTIONS

Alcohol

Metronidazole can cause a disulfuramlike reaction, with cramps, headache, flushing, nausea, and vomiting. Alcohol should be strictly avoided until at least 24 hours after the last dose.

Sulfasalazine

Concern over metronidazole elimination of the bacterial population required for activation of sulfasalazine was dismissed by a study showing no change in blood sulfapyridine levels in 10 patients treated with both drugs over a 2-week period. Metronidazole does not decrease the bioavailability of sulfasalazine.

Warfarin

Metronidazole potentiates warfarin prolongation of prothrombin time. Prothrombin times should be monitored and doses adjusted accordingly when these two drugs are used together.

Cimetidine

Cimetidine decreases clearance of metronidazole. This drug interaction is of no significance in patients with intact liver and kidney function.

Anticonvulsants

Metronidazole decreases the clearance of Dilantin causing elevated serum Dilantin levels. Both Dilantin and phenobarbita increase metronidazole clearance.

PEARLS AND PITFALLS

1. Human metabolism of metronidazole is almost exclusively hepatic. Dose reduction is required only in severe renal insufficiency.
2. Metronidazole has shown no benefit in the therapy of ulcerative colitis.
3. Indications for use of metronidazole in Crohn's disease include perineal disease, Crohn's colitis, and sulfasalazine intolerance or allergy. The drug should be continued until healing occurs, benefit plateaus, or side effects occur. Dose reduction should be gradual in those patients who respond and full-dose therapy should be reinstituted for relapse.
4. Metronidazole is effective in a variety of bacterial and protozoal infections including *B. fragilis* infections, *C. difficile*–associated colitis, and as surgical prophylaxis. Amebiasis responds to metronidazole but a luminacidal agent (Iodoquinol) is necessary to ensure eradication.
5. Side effects are uncommon and well tolerated. A metallic taste is common and harmless. Neurological side effects are serious and warrant discontinuation of drug.
6. Laboratory abnormalities include a reversible neutropenia after long-term use and artifactual depression of SGOT levels.
7. Drug interactions of significance include a disulfiramlike reaction with alcohol use. Metronidazole potentiates the effects of warfarin and Dilantin. Concomitant use with sulfasalazine does not diminish bioavailability of sulfasalazine.
8. Although there is no evidence of carcinogenicity or teratogenicity in humans, the use of metronidazole in pregnant and nursing mothers is relatively contraindicated.

References

1. Beard CM, et al. Cancer after exposure to metronidazole. Mayo Clin Proc 1988; 63:147–153.

    A follow-up study of 771 women exposed to metronidazole from 1960–1969 showing no increased risk of cancer.

2. Bernstein LH, et al. Healing of perineal Crohn's disease with metronidazole. Gastroenterology 1980; 79:357–365.

    A study demonstrating the effectiveness of metronidazole in patients with chronic, unremitting perineal Crohn's disease.

3. Blichfeldt P, et al. Metronidazole in Crohn's disease. Scand J Gastro 1978; 13:123–127.

    A beneficial effect of metronidazole was noted on the clinical and biochemical markers in patients with Crohn's colitis.

4. Brandt LJ, et al. Metronidazole therapy for perineal Crohn's disease. Gastroenterology 1982; 83:383–387.

    A follow-up study further defining the activity of metronidazole in perineal disease.

5. Chapman RW, Selby WS, Jewell DP. Controlled trial of intravenous metronidazole as an adjunct to corticosteroids in severe ulcerative colitis. Gut 1986; 27:1210–1212.

    No benefit of intravenous metronidazole was seen after 5 days of therapy.

6. Davies PS, et al. Metronidazole in the treatment of chronic proctitis. Gut 1977; 18:680–681.

    No benefit with metronidazole suppositories after 28 days of therapy.

7. Goldman P. Metronidazole. NEJM 1980; 303:1212–1218.

    A comprehensive review of the indications and adverse effects of metronidazole.

8. Grove DI, Mahmoud AAF, Warren KS. Suppression of cell-mediated immunity by metronidazole. Int Arch Allerg Immunol 1977; 54:422–427.

    Metronidazole inhibits granuloma formation in mice.

9. Rissing JP, Newman C, Moore WL. Artifactual depression of serum glutamic oxaloacetic transaminase by metronidazole. Antimicrob Ag Chemo 1978; 14:636–638.

    Falsely low SGOT values in patients on metronidazole were noted.

10. Rosenblatt JE, Edson RS. Metronidazole. Mayo Clin Proc 1987; 62:1013–1017.

    A concise review of metronidazole as an antibacterial agent.

11. Saginur R, Hawley DR, Bartlett JG. Colitis associated with metronidazole therapy. J Infect Dis 1980; 141:772–774.

    A case report of *C. difficile* colitis in a patient receiving metronidazole.

12. Scully BE. Metronidazole. Med Clin N Am 1988; 72:613–621.

    A comprehensive review emphasizing that surgical drainage of intra-abdominal abscesses is the key to successful treatment, that metronidazole's role in Crohn's disease has not stood up in controlled trials, and that the true mecha-

nism of action of metronidazole is unknown but presumed to be binding of toxic metronidazole intermediates to bacterial intracellular DNA.
13. Tanowitz HB, Weiss LM, Wittner M. Diagnosis and treatment of protozoan diarrhea. Am J Gastro 1988; 83:339–350.

    A clinical review of amebiasis and giardiasis with specific recommendations on therapy.
14. Teasley DG, et al. Prospective randomized trial of metronidazole versus vancomycin for *Clostridium difficile*–associated diarrhea and colitis. *Lancet* 1983; 2:1043–1046.

    Metronidazole is as effective as vancomycin in the treatment of pseudomembranous enterocolitis.
15. Ursing B, Kamme C. Metronidazole for Crohn's disease. *Lancet* 1975; 1:775–777.

    The first report of efficacy of metronidazole in inflammatory bowel disease.
16. Ursing B, et al. A comparative study of metronidazole and sulfasalazine for active Crohn's disease. Gastroenterology 1982; 83:550–562.

    A follow-up study to the initial case report demonstrating benefit in a larger cohort.
17. Urtasun RC, Rabin HR, Partington J. Human pharmacokinetics and toxicity of high-dose metronidazole administered orally and intravenously. Surgery 1983; 93:145–148.

    The first of five articles covering pharmacokinetics, toxicity, and mode of action in normals and patients with renal insufficiency.

11

5-ASA and 4-ASA

Edward Fox

5-ASA

Sulfasalazine (SAS) is the drug most commonly used to treat mild to moderate ulcerative colitis. 5-aminosalicylic acid or 5-ASA is the active ingredient of sulfasalazine. The other component of sulfasalazine, sulfapyridine, is a carrier molecule linked to 5-ASA by an azo bond, has no activity against ulcerative colitis, and is released in the colon by the lysis of the azo bond by colonic bacteria. By virtue of the presence of 5-ASA, sulfasalazine is an effective drug for both inducing and maintaining remissions in cases of mild to moderate ulcerative colitis. Over the years its use in a large number of patients has been limited by the frequency (up to 25% of cases) of side effects. These side effects were mostly due to the sulfapyridine which, in contrast to the 5-ASA, was systemically well absorbed. Because 5-ASA given orally is completely absorbed in the proximal small bowel, thus preventing it from working topically on the colonic inflammation, recent efforts to sidestep the problem of sulfapyridine toxicity have led researchers to look for other ways of delivering 5-ASA unaltered to the colon. Recently several new carriers have been demonstrated as effective in delivering intact ASA. Similarly, because 5-ASA is felt to work topically, several studies have looked at the utility of 5-ASA given as a retention enema.

PHARMACOLOGY

5-ASA is a salicylate analogue that can be readily bound to other moieties, including itself. In looking for another carrier, four drugs have demonstrated effectiveness in clinical trials (Table 11–1). Pentasa is 250 milligrams of 5-ASA microgranules within a semipermeable ethylcellulose membrane. Asacol is 400 milligrams of 5-ASA coated with an acrylic resin that dissolves in a pH greater than 7. This formulation allows the 5-ASA to transit intact until it reaches the terminal ileum and colon. Salofalk is 250 milligrams of 5-ASA coated first with an ethylcellulose membrane followed with an acrylic resin that breaks down in a pH greater than 5.6. Finally, Dipentum takes another approach by linking two 5-ASA molecules with an azo bond. Like sulfasalazine, this azo bond remains intact until it is destroyed by anaerobic and aerobic colonic bacteria, thus freeing two molecules of 5-ASA. All of the above compounds are effective in delivering most of the acetylsalicylic acid (>75%) to the colon where it is poorly absorbed and excreted in the feces. The fraction of 5-ASA that is absorbed (approximately 10%) is rapidly acetylated by the liver and excreted in the urine. A fraction of the 5-ASA is also acetylated by the colonic mucosa and excreted in that form in the feces.

Table 11–1. Formulations of 5-ASA

Drug	Type	Dose (daily)	How supplied
Pentasa	ECM	1.5 gms	250-mg tablets
Asacol	ARC	2.0 gms	400-mg tablets
Salofalk	ECM + ARC	1.5 gms	250-mg tablets
Dipentum	Azodisalicylate	2.0 gms	1000-mg tablets

ECM = Ethylcellulose membrane
ARC = Acrylic resin coating

Retention enemas have also been studied as a method of safely delivering the 5-ASA to the colon. The 5-ASA is suspended in 60 to 100 milliliters of a neutral base solution and instilled in the rectum, usually overnight. Radiotracer-labeled 5-ASA studies have shown that 100-milliliter enemas distribute consistently from the rectum to the splenic flexure, correlating well with the demonstrated benefit in proctosigmoiditis. Spread to the other areas of the colon can be variably enhanced by increasing the volume of the enema, and by increased mucosal inflammation. Most of the 5-ASA is excreted unchanged in the feces.

MECHANISM OF ACTION

The mechanism of action of 5-ASA has not yet been elucidated. Not surprisingly, any purported mechanism can only be inferential since to date the pathophysiology of ulcerative colitis is unknown. What seems clear is that 5-ASA acts topically. This action is supported by the observations that (1) the drug is effective in proportion to the amount delivered intact to the colon, (2) there is no relation between the blood levels and efficacy, and (3) direct colonic installation with almost no systemic absorption is highly effective. Numerous mechanisms have been proposed, ranging from inhibition of cyclooxygenase and inhibition of neutrophil and monocyte chemotaxis, to inhibition of oxidation of short-chain fatty acids, none of which has been fully supported. More recent studies have implicated leukotrienes B4 and C4 in the mucosal inflammation of ulcerative colitis; the synthesis of both are inhibited by 5-ASA.

INDICATIONS

Oral 5-ASA is indicated for the treatment of mild to moderate ulcerative colitis, both to induce and maintain remission. As outlined in Table 11–2 to date not all forms of oral 5-ASA have been studied in acute attacks, to induce remission, and in maintaining remission of ulcerative colitis. However, given that all preparations seem to deliver approximately equal amounts of 5-ASA to the colon, it will likely only be a matter of time before all compounds are shown to be similarly effective.

Table 11–2. Indications for 5-ASA

Drug	Ulcerative acute	Colitis chronic	Crohn's colitis
Pentasa	NS	NS	Yes
Asacol	NS	Yes	NS
Salofalk	Yes	NS	Yes
Dipentum	Yes	NS	NS

NS = Not studied
Yes = Demonstrated efficacy in clinical trials

In treatment of Crohn's disease involving the colon, both Pentasa and Salofalk have been effective for mild to moderate flares of the disease. No 5-ASA compound is indicated for or has been effective in maintaining remissions of Crohn's disease.

5-ASA enemas are indicated in the treatment of mild to moderate left-sided proctocolitis. Controlled studies have shown 5-ASA to be superior to placebo and to SAS enemas, effecting remission in 60 to 70 percent of acute flares. Recurrence rates are similar to those of sulfasalazine. In that some studies have shown less effective delivery of oral 5-ASA to the distal colon, enemas can be used in conjunction with oral 5-ASA. They can also be used in conjunction with systemic steroids in more refractory cases of ulcerative proctocolitis.

DOSAGE

For oral 5-ASA, standard dosing regimens have not yet been developed. Clinical trials have used doses ranging from 1.5 grams/day to 3 grams/day. It appears that 2 grams/day is likely to be the standard oral dose, combining the greatest efficacy with the lowest side effects and lowest cost. 5-ASA enemas are generally 4 grams of ASA in 100 milliliters of buffered solution given as an overnight retention enema. It appears that tapering the doses when stopping the drug alleviates acute flares occasionally associated with abrupt cessation of therapy.

SIDE EFFECTS

In marked contrast to sulfasalazine, oral 5-ASA compounds have been remarkably free of side effects. In fact, oral 5-ASA compounds have been studied in patients unable to tolerate sulfasalazine, and approximately 90 percent of sulfasalazine-intolerant patients were able to use 5-ASA without problems. Infrequently reported complaints have included headache, nausea, and indigestion. Two patients on Asacol reportedly had acute flares of the disease shortly after starting the drug, one requiring colectomy, the other subsiding after stopping the drug. To date none of the dermatologic, hematologic, or biochemical abnormalities reported with sulfasalazine have been reported with 5-ASA. It must be kept in mind, though, that only Asacol has been given for as long as 6 months; thus the long-term sequelae of chronic 5-ASA use are unknown. The experience to date, however, does not suggest these types of problems.

To date there have been no side effects attributed to the 5-ASA enemas, other than the local anal trauma associated with repeated insertion of the enema tube. This problem can be minimized by proper instruction and anal care. 5-ASA enemas in the dosages recommended appear exceedingly safe and trouble-free. In one study, the placebo group reported more side effects than did the treatment group.

No known drug interactions have been recognized and reported to date.

PEARLS AND PITFALLS

1. 5-ASA in the oral or enema form is not indicated for severe flares of ulcerative colitis, for chronic suppressive therapy of Crohn's disease, or for small bowel Crohn's disease.
2. Because of its safety profile, one should strongly consider oral 5-ASA in lieu of sulfasalazine in those patients intolerant of sulfasalazine.
3. With the availability of the oral 5-ASA compounds, in a patient you suspect is not tolerating sulfasalazine well, do not rechallenge the patient with sulfasalazine but switch instead to 5-ASA.
4. 5-ASA enemas have been shown to be effective when retained for as little as 30 minutes, so if your patient is having difficulty with overnight retention but appears to be responding, try decreasing the enema-retention time.
5. 5-ASA does not appear to affect male fertility.

4-ASA

Another salicylate analogue useful in topical treatment of inflammatory bowel disease is 4-aminosalicylic acid, para-aminosalicylic acid, or 4-ASA. For years it has been used orally as an antituberculous drug and through that experience it has demonstrated a good safety profile. 4-ASA has the advantage over 5-ASA in that it is relatively cheap, available, and considerably more stable. Recently there has been interest in 4-ASA enemas in the treatment of distal proctocolitis.

Clinical studies with 4-ASA have so far been limited to topical treatment of distal proctocolitis. Trials have compared 4-ASA to placebo and 5-ASA. These studies indicate that 4-ASA is active and superior to placebo. Further, direct comparison shows that the response rate of patients with distal (<60 cms of inflamed mucosa) proctosigmoiditis to 4-ASA and 5-ASA are identical. As with 5-ASA, the mechanism of action of 4-ASA is not understood. Side effects have been absent in the 2 gram/day recommended dosage. Comments made above regarding Pearls and Pitfalls for 5-ASA enemas above apply equally to 4-ASA enemas.

In summary, 4-ASA retention enemas 2 grams in 60 milliliters of water, are indicated for the same clinical settings where one would order 5-ASA enemas. Though they are equally efficacious, 4-ASA offers the advantage of being less expensive, chemically more stable, and more readily available. Despite the fact that much effort has recently been directed toward 5-ASA, in the long run 4-ASA's advantages should become more readily apparent and allow it to become the drug of choice for topical treatment of left-sided proctosigmoiditis.

References

5-ASA

1. Barber GB, et al. Refractory distal ulcerative colitis responsive to 5-aminosalicylate enemas. Am J Gastro 80:612–614.

    In a group of six patients failing therapy with topical corticosteroids and sulfasalazine therapy, five of the six responded to topical 5-ASA, most likely because of higher concentrations of 5-aminosalicylate at the mucosal level.

2. Biddle WL, et al. 5-aminosalicylic acid enemas: Effective agent in maintaining remission in left-sided ulcerative colitis. Gastroenterology 1988; 94:1075–1079.

    This randomized, double-blind, placebo-controlled trial demonstrates the efficacy of 5-ASA enemas in the maintenance of remission for 1 year in 75% of patients receiving drug, versus an 85% relapse rate within 16 weeks for patients receiving placebo.

3. Bondesen S. Topical 5-aminosalicylic acid (5-ASA) versus prednisolone (Pred) in ulcerative proctosigmoiditis (abstr). Gastroenterology 1984; 90:1350.

    A 1-gm 5-ASA (Pentasa) enema was at least as effective as topical corticosteroid enemas for inducing remission in 114 patients with left-sided disease. Treatment duration of at least 14 days was often required to induce remission.

4. Campieri M, et al. Treatment of ulcerative colitis with high-dose 5-ASA enemas. *Lancet* 1981; ii:270–271.

    A randomized, blinded trial of 5-ASA versus hydrocortisone enemas in volunteer patients, which showed 5-ASA to be superior, giving a 93% clinical remission rate, compared to a 57% remission rate for the hydrocortisone group. There were no side effects reported, and all disease was distal to the splenic flexure.

5. Campieri M, et al. A controlled trial on the efficacy and compliance of 5-ASA enemas versus 5-ASA suppositories in distal ulcerative sigmoiditis (abstr). Gastroenterology 1984; 90:1364.

    The authors studied two treatment-delivery systems in patients with ulcerative sigmoiditis and found that suppositories and enemas were both well tolerated but that suppositories were somewhat more easily tolerated.

6. Campieri M, et al. Efficacy of 5-aminosalicylic acid enemas

versus hydrocortisone enemas in ulcerative colitis. Dig Dis Sci 1987; 32:67S–70S.

This study showed clinical response rates almost identical to the 1981 Lancet article. Further, they demonstrated with radiolabeled 5-ASA that the 100-ml enemas consistently reach the splenic flexure. Larger volumes (200 mls) inconsistently passed beyond the splenic flexure.

7. Dew MJ, et al. Maintenance of remission in ulcerative colitis with oral preparation of 5-aminosalicylic acid. BMJ 1982; 285:1012.

A study of 72 patients demonstrating that oral 5-ASA, 1.2 gms/day, and sulfasalazine, 2 gms/day, were equivalent in that nine of the 5-ASA patients and six of the sulfasalazine patients relapsed during the 16 weeks of the study.

8. Dew MJ, et al. Maintenance of remission in ulcerative colitis: 5-aminosalicylic acid in high doses by mouth. BMJ 1983; 287:23–24.

In this trial the patients received in a double-blind fashion either 5-ASA or sulfasalazine to maintain remission in ulcerative colitis (including extensive disease and left-sided disease). The 32 patients receiving 5-ASA took a mean daily dose of 2.7 gms/day, compared to a mean daily dose of 2.3 gms of sulfasalazine. Seven of the 32 patients taking 5-ASA (22%) and five of the 25 patients taking sulfasalazine (20%) relapsed. Four of the patients developed such severe headache on sulfasalazine that they were withdrawn from the study.

9. Garretto M, Riddell RH, Winans CS. Treatment of chronic ulcerative colitis with poly-ASA: A new nonabsorbable carrier for release of 5-aminosalicylate in the colon (abstr). Gastroenterology 1983; 84:1162.

An initial report documenting that eight patients intolerant to sulfasalazine can tolerate and respond to a new drug, poly-ASA, or 5-ASA diazotized to a nonabsorbable sulfanilamidoethylene polymer.

10. Habal FM, Greenberg GR. Treatment of ulcerative colitis with oral 5-aminosalicylic acid including patients with adverse reactions to sulfasalazine. Am J Gastro 1988; 83:15–19.

This study from Toronto looks at both acute treatment of ulcerative colitis flares and maintenance therapy with oral 5-ASA. Fifty-one of the 85 patients previously had adverse reactions to sulfasalazine. Sixty-four percent achieved remission and 78% of those eligible for the maintenance arm were in remission 1 year later. Only six had adverse reactions: one with pericarditis and bronchospasm, one with fever, one with a marked increase in stool volume, and three with noncardiac retrosternal chest pain.

11. Hanauer SB, Schultz PA, Kirsner JB. Treatment of refractory proctitis with 5-ASA enemas (abstr). Gastroenterology 1982; 88:1412.

A study of 22 patients with proctosigmoiditis either unresponsive to or intolerant of sulfasalazine showed that 13 of the 22 (56%) responded to 5-ASA enemas. The authors note that disease proximal to the sigmoid colon was a predictor of nonresponsiveness.

12. Janssens J, et al. 5-aminosalicylic acid (5-ASA) enemas are effective in patients with resistant ulcerative rectosigmoiditis (abstr). Gastroenterology 1978; 84:1198.

   The addition of 5-ASA enemas to the treatment regimen of 20 patients with refractory rectosigmoiditis resulted in improvement in 75 percent of the cohort.

13. Klotz V, Maier KE. Pharmacology and pharmacokinetics of 5-aminosalicylic acid. Dig Dis Sci 1987; 32:46S–50S.

   After liberation of 5-ASA in the terminal ileum or colon, it is only partly absorbed. A major part of it is presystemically eliminated by N-acetylation during its first passage through the intestinal mucosa and liver. Mean steady-state plasma levels of unchanged 5-ASA are low as it is eliminated at the renal level more quickly than N-acetyl-5-ASA.

14. Levinson RA. Disodium azodisalicylate. Am J Gastro 1985; 80:203–205.

   A comprehensive review of the disodium azodisalicylate form of 5-ASA finds that the drug, while holding promise for those patients intolerant of sulfasalazine, may not have efficacy beyond that of sulfasalazine.

15. Martin F. Oral 5-aminosalicylic acid preparations in treatment of inflammatory bowel disease. Dig Dis Sci 1987; 32:57S–63S.

   The author notes that in the treatment of acute flares of Crohn's disease, the 5-ASA preparations Pentasa and Salofalk appear more effective than placebo. Likewise, in the treatment of acute ulcerative colitis and maintenance of remission, 5-ASA preparations appear as efficacious as sulfasalazine, without significant side effects.

16. McPhee MS, et al. Proctocolitis unresponsive to conventional therapy Dig Dis Sci 1987; 32:76S–81S.

   Forty-one of 47 patients unresponsive to oral sulfasalazine, steroid enemas, or oral steroid medication achieved a good response to therapy with daily 5-ASA enemas, one 4-gm 5-ASA enema at bedtime.

17. Peskar BM, et al. Possible mode of action of 5-aminosalicylic acid. Dig Dis Sci 1987; 32:51S–56S.

   The authors' results demonstrate that like the parent compound, sulfasalazine, 5-ASA in a dose-dependent manner inhibits release of LTB4 (leukotriene B4) and sulfidopeptide-LT, 5-lipoxygenase products, from normal human mucosa.

18. Riley SA, et al. A comparison of delayed-release 5-aminosalicylic acid and sulfasalazine as maintenance treatment of ulcerative colitis (abstr). Gastroenterology 1987; 92:1596.

   Delayed-release 5-ASA was as effective as sulfasalazine in maintaining remission in 100 patients with ulcerative colitis, and had fewer side effects.

19. Sutherland LR, et al. 5-aminosalicylic acid enema in the treatment of distal ulcerative colitis, proctosigmoiditis, and proctitis. Gastroenterology 1987; 92:1894–1898.

   A randomized, double-blind, placebo-controlled study of 153 patients with left-sided ulcerative colitis. The 5-ASA patients had a clinical improvement rate of 63% from 4-gm nighttime enemas. These data are important in that drop-

outs were included in the final calculation of the intent-to-treat success rate.
20. Williams CN, Haber G, Aquino JA. Double-blind, placebo-controlled evaluation of 5-ASA suppositories in active distal proctitis and measurement of extent of spread using 99m Tc-labeled 5-ASA suppositories. Dig Dis Sci 1987; 32:71S–75S.

    This study reiterates the utility of 5-ASA, 500-mg suppositories 3 times a day, in active proctitis. The suppositories deliver the 5-ASA to the rectum alone.

4-ASA

1. Campieri M, et al. A double-blind clinical trial to compare the effects of 4-aminosalicylic acid to 5-aminosalicylic acid in topical treatment of ulcerative colitis. Digestion 1984; 29: 204–208.

    This randomized trial of topical 4-ASA versus 5-ASA demonstrated clearly that the two drugs were equal in the treatment of left-sided ulcerative colitis. The response rates were virtually identical when judged by clinical, sigmoidoscopic, and histologic criteria. These authors turned to 4-ASA in searching for a less expensive, more stable alternative to 5-ASA.

2. Gandolfo J, et al. 4-aminosalicylic acid retention enemas in treatment of distal colitis. Dig Dis Sci 1987; 32:700–704.

    A study demonstrating the benefits of 2-gm/day enema treatment for distal colitis. Interestingly, higher doses of 4 gms/day were no better than placebo in the treatment of distal colitis.

3. Ginsberg AL, Steinberg WM, Nochomovitz LE. Evaluation of 4-aminosalicylic acid enemas in patients with left-sided ulcerative colitis (abstr). Gastroenterology 1984; 90:1089.

    The report of the initial open-label study attesting to the efficacy of 4-ASA in the treatment of mildly active colitis. Although only five of the 12 patients responded to the drug, the stringent study requirements included the necessity of cessation of all other medications for 3 weeks prior to initiation of 4-ASA, with the likelihood of bias against the drug. Subsequent studies have confirmed this negative bias and have confirmed the utility of 4-ASA enemas in the treatment of left-sided ulcerative colitis.

4. Ginsberg AL, et al. A placebo-controlled trial of 4-aminosalicylic acid enemas in left-sided ulcerative colitis (abstr). Gastroenterology 1986; 92:1406.

    The initial report demonstrating efficacy of 4-ASA in a blinded trial. Ten of the 12 patients in the treatment group improved in all clinical, sigmoidoscopic, and histologic parameters, with 2 gms of 4-ASA in a volume of 60 mls as a nightly retention enema. Of the 11 placebo-treated patients, eight were subsequently treated with 4-ASA and showed improvement.

5. Ginsberg AL, et al. Treatment of left-sided ulcerative colitis with 4-aminosalicylic acid enemas: A double-blind, placebo-controlled trial. Ann Int Med 1988; 108:195–199.

    In this trial, the efficacy of 4-ASA is evident. Though not

compared directly to 5-ASA, the response rate cited for 4-ASA is similar to other reported rates for topical 4-ASA and 5-ASA.

6. Selby WS, Bennett MK, Jewell DP. Topical treatment of distal ulcerative colitis with 4-aminosalicylic acid enemas. Digestion 1984; 29:231–234.

These authors looked at 4-ASA in both 1- and 2-gm enema doses. Because of the small numbers of patients and the short duration of treatment, the study could not reach statistical significance, though the trend was toward improvement in the treatment group. Subsequent to this early study, the accepted dose for 4-ASA enemas has been 2 gms.

Central Vein Feedings

1. Patients are unable to tolerate enteral intake for greater than 7 days
2. In moderately to severely elevated metabolic rate
3. In moderate to severe malnutrition not correctable with enteral feedings
4. In cardiac, renal, or hepatic failure or other conditions necessitating fluid restrictions
5. When there is limited access to peripheral veins

Curtailing the imbalance of metabolic homeostasis and loss of lean body mass are the major objectives of adjunctive TPN in various GI disorders. Specific clinical settings in which TPN should be a part of routine care are: (1) massive (> 70%) small bowel resection, (2) impaired intestinal motility or absorption, as in scleroderma, SLE, sprue, and ischemia, (3) radiation enteritis, (4) severe, intractable diarrhea, vomiting in chemotherapy patients, or severe pancreatitis, (5) severely catabolic patients (> 50% body surface-area burns, multiple trauma, extensive surgery, and sepsis), and (6) severe inflammatory bowel disease.

Clinical settings where TPN would be helpful are: (1) major surgery, (2) moderate stress (30–50% body surface area burns, trauma, moderately severe pancreatitis, neurologic trauma, and other similar stresses), (3) enterocutaneous fistulae, (4) hyperemesis gravidarum, (5) moderate malnutrition in patients who require medical and surgical intervention, and (6) inflammatory adhesions with small bowel obstruction.

NUTRITION AND DIET THERAPY IN INFLAMMATORY BOWEL DISEASE

Malnutrition is a common complication of Crohn's disease and ulcerative colitis. The etiology is multifactorial and includes inadequate intake, excess intestinal losses, malabsorption, and increased requirements. The medical therapy of inflammatory bowel disease has long included bowel rest, either for therapeutic intent or because the severity of disease precludes oral intake. The efficacy of parenteral and enteral nutrition as primary therapy is unproven, but there are clear indications for employing nutritional therapy, which include supportive care, growth failure, and as an adjunct to surgical intervention.

Nutritional support is a valuable tool for Crohn's patients with inflammatory strictures or for those with diffuse disease that is not surgically correctable, including those patients who are otherwise unable to sustain themselves due to anorexia, nausea, vomiting, or postprandial pain. There is no evidence that nutritional therapy obviates the ultimate need for surgery some time in a patient's course, but some patients sustain a prolonged remission on medical therapy alone, thus postponing surgical intervention. Supportive therapy has been most useful in patients with short-bowel syndrome, whether from Crohn's disease or other causes. These patients are able to be maintained long term

12

Total Parenteral Nutrition

Joel Sabangan, Steven Swartz, and Michael M. Van Ness

Intravenous hyperalimentation was first utilized by Sir Christopher Wren in 1656. Using goose quill connected to a pig's bladder, he was able to introduce ale, opium, and wine into dogs' veins. The 1800s refined this method to treat diarrhea and shock. By the early 1900s, intravenous use of glucose was recognized for surgical patients. It was in the early 1950s that central venous infusion via the subclavian vein was started by the French surgeon Aubaniac as a means of administering blood rapidly to battle casualties in the French-Indochina war. In 1965, Dudrik and his colleagues applied this concept to total parenteral nutrition (TPN) to deliver essential nutrients and calories for nutritional support.

Enteral alimentation is the preferred method of nutritional support in clinically functioning gastrointestinal tracts. The advantages of enteral alimentation include physiologic maintenance of intestinal structure and function by the trophic effects of intraluminal nutrients, augmented insulin response to enterally administered carbohydrates, and delivery of more nutritionally complete feeding solutions than is possible by parenteral formulas. There are relative and absolute contraindications, however, in the use of enteral alimentation. As an alternative, total parenteral nutrition may be used.

INDICATIONS

Total parenteral nutrition (TPN) provides varying amounts of carbohydrates, protein, fat, vitamins, and minerals intravenously to individuals who are unable to assimilate nutrients via the GI tract because of gut dysfunction. TPN may be delivered via central or peripheral vein, and the decision to provide central versus peripheral TPN is related to several factors: (1) duration of the treatment plan, (2) the energy requirements of the patient, (3) the overall goal of treatment (i.e., to minimize weight loss, maintain weight, or gain weight), and (4) the availability of adequate routes of administration. Indications of each mode are the following:

Peripheral Vein Feedings

1. When enteral intake is interrupted, but expected to resume within 5 to 7 days
2. As supplementation to enteral feedings or transitional phase until enteral feedings meet needs
3. In mild to moderate malnutrition, necessitating intervention in order to prevent further protein depletion
4. In normal or mildly elevated metabolic rate
5. When there is no organ failure
6. When you are unable to access a central vein

on parenteral and enteral nutrition, allowing them mobility and survival previously not available.

Nutritional therapy is useful as an adjuvant to surgical intervention. Due to malnutrition, many inflammatory bowel disease patients require preoperative and postoperative nutritional support. The routine use of parenteral nutrition has not decreased the need for surgery, but a decrease in postoperative complications has been documented in malnourished ulcerative colitis patients receiving preoperative parenteral nutrition. Parenteral nutrition has historically been used with good success in the treatment of non-Crohn's enterocutaneous fistulae, but this efficacy has not carried over to Crohn's fistulae except when combined with surgical excision. Wound healing and general recovery are enhanced by the maintenance of good nutritional status.

The least controversial use of nutritional support is in the reversal of growth arrest in children with inflammatory bowel disease. Twenty to 40 percent of children with inflammatory bowel disease suffer from growth retardation or delayed puberty. It is well documented that this growth retardation can be reversed if they are provided with adequate caloric, protein, mineral, and vitamin intake. The supplementation does not provide long-term remission of disease, but the caloric boost provides for weight gain and linear growth while it is maintained. These improvements have been noted despite concurrent medical therapy, including steroids, and have been unrelated to the activity of the disease.

Several recent reports have documented remission of uncomplicated Crohn's disease using elemental diets as the primary therapy. They have compared favorably to steroids in a controlled trial. The patients were treated with Vivonex orally to provide 40 to 60 kilocalories/kilogram/day and 8 to 12 grams/day of protein. After 4 weeks, food was slowly reintroduced into the diet. The decreased morbidity of diet therapy as compared to steroid therapy with the same results make this therapy an attractive alternative, but it needs to be confirmed by other investigators before it is more widely applied.

The mechanisms by which nutritional therapy is of benefit in these patients include correction of inadequate intake of nutrients, reversal of loss of enteral protein, and enhanced absorption of all nutrients after restitution of adequate oral intake. Even utilizing enteral nutrition, protein losses in the stool are shown to stabilize or decrease during therapy. Elemental feedings cause little stimulation of digestive hormones as compared to whole proteins. Other benefits of enteral and parenteral diets are postulated but less well documented. These include decreased mucosal exposure to antigens, decreased mechanical irritation, altered bowel flora, and alterations of microbial metabolism.

The administration of nutritional supplements has by no means been standardized. Generally, enteral nutrition is preferable to parenteral because of fewer complications. Several commercial elemental diets are available and as yet none has been definitively shown to be more efficacious than the others. Elemental feedings are absorbed high in the intestinal tract and thus are often suitable even in patients with tight strictures secondary to Crohn's disease. Most patients can be maintained on elemental diets either orally or by nasogastric tube. Potential complications limiting their use include unpalatability, bloating, dumping syndrome, and abdominal pain. These problems can sometimes be avoided by advancing from one-third-strength to full-strength feedings over 3 days to allow the gut to adapt to the hyperosmolar fluid. Enteral supplementation can be utilized in the hospital and at home and can be administered during sleeping hours through a nasogastric tube to allow for more normal daytime activity.

Parenteral nutrition has not been shown to have any therapeutic benefit over enteral nutrition in the treatment of patients with inflammatory bowel disease. It is extremely useful, however, in patients unable to tolerate enteral nutrition or who must be maintained NPO. Some patients with short-bowel syndrome can be maintained on parenteral nutrition until they recover enough gut function to tolerate enteral feedings.

The drawbacks of parenteral nutrition are that it must be administered through a central venous catheter, with all the attendant complications of placing and maintaining the catheter. Despite the increased difficulty, home parenteral nutrition has been successful utilizing subcutaneously tunneled indwelling catheters in patients requiring long-term therapy. To be successful, these programs require the support of a coordinated nutrition team that works to supply, maintain, and monitor these patients. This multidisciplinary or team approach requires members to serve a distinct role in the management of the TPN patient. The members of the team should include a physician, a registered nurse, a dietician, and a pharmacist dedicated to optimize nutritional support of patients during hospitalization and rehabilitation. This team can best ensure a smooth transition from hospital to home care, if necessary. One major advantage of this concerted effort is the significant reduction of complications of catheter sepsis, thrombosis, and metabolic derangements. Adhering strictly to protocols with firm guidelines also lessens risk and rate of complications.

ADMINISTRATION

TPN solutions generally contain calories (concentrated dextrose), a nitrogen source, electrolytes, vitamins, minerals, and an essential fatty acid source.

1. *Calories*—The calorie requirement should be met mainly as glucose and protein supplemented by fat. Traditionally, using formulas such as the Harris-Benedict equation, the basal metabolic rate (BMR) is calculated with the total calorie requirement being a multiple of the BMR, depending on the clinical condition of the patient. The baseline caloric requirements in the adult range from

40 to 45 kilocalories/kilogram/day. In hypermetabolic states, energy requirements are increased. For example, in febrile states, there is a 12-percent increase with each degree above 37°, a 20- to 30-percent increase with major surgery, a 40- to 50-percent increase with severe sepsis, and a 100 percent or greater increase with major burns. Alternate caloric sources not frequently used are fructose, sorbitol, and xylitol.

2. *Proteins*—The recommended daily adult requirement with normal liver and kidney function is 1 to 1.5 grams/kilogram/day. Crystalline amino acid solutions are given to provide 42.5 grams of protein (e.g., aminosin, 8.5% in 500 cc.) and 25 grams of protein (aminosin, 5% in 500 cc.) via the central route and peripheral route, respectively. These solutions provide essential and nonessential amino acids. Branched chain amino acids are usually in higher concentration than the rest of the essential amino acids, as some studies suggest benefit in the treatment of patients with hepatic encephalopathy. In contrast, the aromatic amino acids phenylalanine and tryptophan are in lower concentration, as they are thought to aggravate hepatic coma.

3. *Dextrose*—Dextrose is the major source of calories and by far the least expensive. Usually a 50-percent solution is employed in central venous hyperalimentation while a 10-percent solution is appropriate for peripheral use. A concomitant infusion of fat emulsion or slowing the rate of infusion can decrease peripheral vein irritation. Patients with diabetes mellitus or resistance to insulin require a lower dextrose concentration. In contrast, a higher concentration (70%) can be used in patients whose total volume intake must be restricted. Each gram of dextrose has 3.4 kilocalories.

4. *Electrolytes*—The electrolyte ranges in Table 12–1 are recommended in each bottle of solution on a daily basis unless contraindicated:

5. *Vitamins*—Parenterally administered vitamin doses should meet the American Medical Association guidelines for vitamin therapy except for Vitamin K. Because of its allergic and cardiac effects (palpitations and blood pressure changes), Vitamin K is frequently left out of the solution unless specifically ordered. Vitamin supplements are given as needed in single doses of separate vitamins. Biotin and Vitamin B_{12} may need to be specifically ordered.

6. *Trace elements*—Trace elements include zinc, copper, manganese, and chromium and are usually added to solutions by the pharmacy. Individual minerals can be added in suspected deficiencies.

7. *Lipid emulsions*—The two major indications for fat emulsions are the treatment and prevention of essential fatty acid deficiency and the provision of calories. Fat emulsions are increasingly used to deliver concentrated calories. Solutions are composed of fat (soybean and safflower), an emulsified (1.2% egg yolk) phospholipid, and glycerol (2.5%). All three compounds provide calories.

Table 12–1. Electrolyte ranges

Calcium	10–15 mEq/day (5 mEq/l)
Magnesium	8–24 mEq/day (8 mEq/l)
Potassium[1]	90–240 mEq/day (20–50 mEq/l)
Sodium	60–150 mEq/day (20–50 mEq/l)
Acetate[1]	80–120 mEq/day (30–50 mEq/l)
Chloride[1]	60–150 mEq/day (20–50 mEq/l)
Phosphorous[2]	30–50 mM/day (10–15 mM/l)

[1]Amino acid solution 5% (Aminosyn 5%–500 ml) provides 43 mEq acetate and 2.7 mEq potassium.
Amino acid solution 8.5% (Aminosyn 8.5%–500 ml) provides 45 mEq acetate, 17.5 mEq chloride and 2.7 mEq potassium.
Amino acid solution 10% (Aminosyn 10%–500 ml) provides 74 mEq acetate and 2.7 mEq potassium.
Essential amino acid solution 5.2% (Aminosyn RF 5.2%–300 ml) provides 31.5 mEq acetate and 1.5 mEq potassium.
[2]When ordered as potassium phosphate, each prescribed millimole of phosphorous will contribute 1.47 mEq of potassium. Likewise 1 mM of sodium phosphate will contribute 1.3 mEq of sodium.
Reprinted from *The University of Michigan Hospitals Parenteral and Enteral Nutrition Manual,* 1980, The Regents of the University of Michigan, p. 24.

Available preparations provide a caloric density of 1.1–2 kilocalories/cubic centimeter and obviate the need for excessive intravenous volume in patients.

8. *Other additives*—Heparin in a concentration of 1 unit/cubic centimeter of parenteral nutrition solution should be given to prevent fibrin-sheath formation on the catheter (which can lead to venous thrombosis). Regular insulin can be added to the solution to prevent glucosuria and hyperglycemia.

How to Order TPN Solutions

Most patients' protein and calorie requirements are met with standard solutions containing 25 percent dextrose, 4 percent crystalline amino acids, electrolytes, minerals, trace elements, and vitamins. The total caloric value is approximately 1000 kilocalorie/liter or 1 kilocalorie/cubic centimeter. The nonprotein calorie per gram of nitrogen ratio is 127:1. A sample of TPN formulation is shown in Table 12–2.

Most hospitals and institutions have their own standard orders and administration forms. TPN solution should be given in sequential order as long as the patient is on parenteral nutrition. Orders to increase or decrease any ingredient should be filled 24 hours in advance of the change in order to minimize the economic burden of TPN therapy.

Generally therapy is instituted slowly by administering 1 liter for the first 24 hours. The rate of delivery can be subsequently increased by a liter per day until the volume that satisfies the patient's protein and caloric needs is achieved.

Ch 12. Total Parenteral Nutrition   149

Table 12–2. Mixed amino acid formulation

Amino acids (4.25%)	42.5 g	**Approximate volume**	
Dextrose (25%)	250 g	1050 ml	
Calcium	4.5 mEq	**Approximate osmolarity**	
Magnesium	5 mEq	1825 mOsm	
Potassium	40 mEq	**Total caloric value**	
Sodium	35 mEq	1020 kcal	
Acetate	74.5 mEq	(approx. 1 kcal/ml)	
Chloride	52.5 mEq	**Nitrogen content**	
Phosphorus	12 mM	6.7 g	
Heparin sodium	1000 units	**Nonprotein calorie/g nitrogen**	
Multivitamins with biotin, B_{12} and folic acid	10 ml	127:1	
Trace elements	5 ml		

Reprinted from *The University of Michigan Hospitals Parenteral and Enteral Nutrition Manual*, 1980, The Regents of the University of Michigan.

Alterations of TPN solutions for specific diseases require knowledge of their pathophysiology and tailoring solutions to nutrient requirements and tolerances. For example, in patients with pancreatitis, hypertriglyceridemia is contradicted and lipid infusion should be omitted. The severe malabsorption or diarrhea seen in inflammatory bowel disease often results in electrolyte and mineral losses, especially potassium, magnesium, zinc, and bicarbonate. Repletion of these essential elements requires electrolyte supplementation. As another example, calcium, lipid, and fat soluble vitamins are often deficient in patients with inflammatory disease and thus require parenteral supplementation to normalize calcium, essential fatty-acid, and fat-soluble-vitamin levels. Other potential modifications of standard TPN solutions are shown in Table 12–3.

Catheter maintenance requires meticulous aseptic techniques and dry, sterile, and air-occlusive dressings that are applied to the catheter insertion site and changed every 48 hours. Administration sets and tubings are changed every 24 hours to prevent contamination and infection.

Monitoring

Before parenteral nutrition is begun, several parameters are assessed:*

Baseline Laboratory Evaluation:
  SMA-20: Serum electrolytes and pH
Serum Ca++, inorganic phosphorus
Blood urea nitrogen (BUN)

---

*Reprinted from SH Krey and RL Murray, eds, *Dynamics of Nutrition Support: Assessment, Implementation, Evaluation* (New York: Appleton-Century-Crofts, 1986), p. 387.

Table 12-3. Potential modulation of standard TPN (4.25% AA/25% dextrose) with standard electrolytes, multivitamins, and trace minerals in various diseases[a]

	Dextrose	Amino acids	Fat	Electrolyte	Vitamins	Trace minerals
Pancreatitis	NM	↑ (5%)	Daily if glucose intolerance Omit if ↑ TG	↑ NaCl if NG losses are excessive	↑ B-vit, folate if ETOH ↑ A,D,E,K if steatorrhea	NM
Renal failure	↑ (35%) if fluid restriction	↓ (2.1% mixed EAA and non-EAA) or (EAA only 1.35–2.7%) ↑ (5%) if dialysis	Daily if glucose intolerance Omit if ↑ TG	↓ Na+ ↓ other electrolytes per labs and renal function	Provide ↑ B-vits if dialysis	Omit
Cardiac disease	↑ (35%) if fluid restriction	NM	Omit if ↑ TG	↓ Na ↑ K+, Mg++, Ca++ if diuretic therapy ↑ PO4=	NM	Se supplementation ↑ Zinc if diuresis
Pulmonary disease	↑ (35%) if fluid restriction Carb should provide no > 50% calories	NM	Daily → Fat should provide 50% kcal	↓ Na+ if fluid balance is + ↑ PO4=	NM	NM

Liver disease	↑ (35%) if fluid restriction	↑ (5%) If encephalopathy ↓ (2.1%) or ↓ (4%–↑ BCAA/ ↓ AAA)	Daily if glucose intolerance √ TG level	↓ Na$^+$ ↑ K$^+$, Mg^{++}, Ca^{++} if lactulose therapy ↑ bicarb if lactulose therapy	↑ A, D, E, K if steatorrhea ↑ B$_1$ ↑ folate	Omit Cu and Mn if cholestasis
Stress	In ebb/complicated stress ↓ (15–20%)	↑ (5–7%) or provide ↑ BCAA Solution ↑ (5%)	Daily if glucose intolerance Omit if ↑ TG	↑ Mg, K$^+$, PO$_4^=$	NM	↑ Zn
Gastrointestinal disease	NM	↑ (5%)	NM	↑ NaCl if ↑ NG losses ↑ bicarb, K$^+$, Mg^{++} if lower GI losses are excessive	↑ Biotin, Vit K ↑ Vitamin C	↑ Zn with high fistula/ileostomy output/diarrhea

↑ ( ), increase concentration to; ↓ ( ), decrease concentration to; NM, no modulation necessary; ↑, increase; ↓, decrease; TG, triglyceride; EAA, essential amino acids; NEAA, nonessential amino acids.
[a]Standard electrolytes, multivitamins, and trace minerals: Na, 45 mEq/L; Cl, 4.5 mEq/L; Ca, 4.5 mEq/L; PO$_4$, 35 mEq/L; K, 20 mEq/L; Mg, 5 mEq/L; Acetate, 29.5 mEq/L; MVI-12, 1 amp; Trace minerals, 1 amp providing the 4 following minerals: Zinc, 3 mg; Copper, 1 mg; Manganese, 0.4 mg; Chromium, 0.001 mg.
Reprinted from SH Krey and RL Murray, eds., *Dynamics of Nutrition Support: Assessment, Implementation, Evaluation.* (New York: Appleton-Century-Crofts, 1986), p. 430.

Serum creatinine
Liver function tests
Total protein/albumin
Serum glucose
CO_2
PT, PTT
Serum magnesium
Complete blood count (CBC) with differential
Serum iron, total iron-binding capacity
Serum triglycerides (if fat emulsion is used)
Urine analysis
Serum and urine osmolarity
Additional tests for central vein infusions: serum levels of B_{12}, folate, trace elements (Mn, Cu, Zn)

These parameters allow assessment of the appropriateness and adequacy of nutrient regimes.

The ultimate goal of monitoring during parenteral nutrition is the avoidance of complications. Once TPN has begun, the following ongoing monitoring procedures are indicated:*

Every 4 to 6 hours: vital signs; urine glucose and ketones
Daily: serum electrolytes, BUN, CO_2, serum glucose, pH, fluid intake and output, weight
Twice per week: SMA-20, CBC with differential (when the patient is stable, these may be ordered weekly)
Weekly: serum magnesium, serum and urine osmolarity, urine analysis, serum triglycerides (until fat emulsion is discontinued), other serum vitamin and mineral levels as needed

The length of therapy is variable and mainly dependent on the clinical situation. As an adjunct to medical care, it should be continued until the patient is able to take adequate nutrition orally. One or 2 weeks of therapy preoperatively replaces nutrients and enables body stores to be replenished. Growth failure in children requires 6 weeks or more of therapy, depending on disease activity and treatment goals. Elemental diet therapy for Crohn's disease has been used for 4 weeks with the gradual introduction of oral intake after that.

Growth failure in children has been treated with 60 to 80 kilocalories/kilogram/day and 2 to 3 grams/kilogram/day of protein. Adults in all groups are usually given 40 to 60 kilocalories/kilogram/day of calories and 1 to 2 grams/kilogram/day of protein. These should be accompanied by vitamins and minerals to meet the daily requirements. Therapy can be monitored by weight gain, growth, standard nutritional indicators (albumin, transferring, absolute lymphocyte count), anthropometric measurements, or clinical response.

---

*Reprinted from SH Krey and RL Murray, eds, *Dynamics of Nutrition Support: Assessment, Implementation, Evaluation* (New York: Appleton-Century-Crofts, 1986), p. 387.

COMPLICATIONS

Catheter-Related Complications

Mechanical

1. Pneumothorax—The most prevalent complication of subclavian venipuncture, occurring in up to 5 percent of attempted catheterizations
2. Subclavian artery puncture—The second most frequent complication
3. Carotid artery puncture—The most common complication of percutaneous internal jugular catheterization; a resulting hematoma may lead to tracheal compression and respiratory compromise
4. Air embolism
5. Brachial plexus injury

Septic

The catheter may become contaminated due to improper care (improper handling of solutions) or seeding from a distant site of infection.

Metabolic Complications

1. Hyperglycemia—Usually self correcting; treat only if 4+ glucosuria or significant osmotic diuresis is present. Ten units of regular insulin/liter may be added. If untreated, hyperosmolar hyperglycemic nonketotic coma may develop.
2. Hypoglycemia—Due to sudden decrease or cessation of solution infusion secondary to iatrogenic or mechanical problems. Substitution of 10-percent dextrose as a temporizing measure can be lifesaving.
3. Hyperkalemia—Secondary to underutilization of administered potassium in the inadequately anabolic patient
4. Hypokalemia—Requirement increases as patient begins to synthesize protein and becomes anabolic.
5. Hypercalcemia, hypermagnesemia, or hyperphosphatemia—These are due to underutilization.
6. Hypocalcemia—Secondary to decreased total serum albumin; asymptomatic because of normal ionized calcium level
7. Hypomagnesemia—Increased requirement during increased anabolism and protein synthesis
8. Hypophosphatemia—Needed for synthesis of intracellular high-energy phosphate compounds, metabolic structure, and bone formation, thus increased requirement in anabolic state
9. Hyperlipidemia—Secondary to rapid infusion of lipid emulsion
10. Essential fatty acid deficiency—Increased needs during anabolic states that cannot be met by limited stores of linoleic acid
11. Mineral deficiency—Well documented; should be repleted on a daily basis

Organ-Related Complications

1. Lungs—Increased oxygen consumption and carbon dioxide production in hypermetabolic patients is associated with high glucose loads of TPN.
2. Liver—Fatty liver, cholestasis, and nonspecific triaditis.

References

1. American Society for Parenteral and Enteral Nutrition Board of Directors. Guidelines for use of total parenteral nutrition in the hospitalized adult patient. J Parent Ent Nut 1986; 10:441–445.
   Guidelines for the role of TPN in different clinical settings.
2. Askanazi J, et al. Respiratory changes induced by the large glucose loads of total parenteral nutrition. JAMA 1980; 243:1444–1447.
   A study of the adverse effects of high glucose loads of TPN on O_2 consumption and CO_2 production.
3. Baker AL, Rosenberg IH. Hepatic complications of total parenteral nutrition: Need for prospective investigation. Am J Med 1987; 82:489–497.
   A summary of the current understanding of the pathogenesis and management of liver injury during short-term TPN.
4. Dean RE. *Total Parenteral Nutrition: Standard Techniques.* Chicago: Pluribus Press, 1983.
   A review of standard techniques in TPN.
5. Eastwood MA. Nutrition overview. *Current Opinion in Gastroenterology* 1988; 4:287–288.
   A brief overview.
6. Elson CO, et al. An evaluation of total parenteral nutrition in the management of inflammatory bowel disease. Dig Dis Sci 1980; 25:42–48.
   Assessing the role of TPN as an adjunct in the therapy of inflammatory bowel disease.
7. Hoover HC, et al. Nutritional benefits of immediate postoperative jejunal feeding of an elemental diet. Am J Surg 1980; 139:153–159.
   The beneficial effects of postoperative jejunal feeding gauged by nitrogen balance and weight assessment.
8. Keohane PP, et al. Effect of catheter tunneling and a nutrition nurse on catheter sepsis during parenteral nutrition. *Lancet* 1983; 2:1388–1390.
   The importance of the role of nursing care and catheter tunneling in the reduction of TPN catheter sepsis.
9. Krey SH, Murray RL, eds., *Dynamics of Nutritional Support: Assessment, Implementation, Evaluation.* New York: Appleton-Century-Crofts, 1986.
   A comprehensive review of nutritional support.
10. Mizock BA. Critical care nutrition. Affiliated hospitals at Canton combined medical grand rounds 1988; 11:41–52.
    A comprehensive overview of critical care nutrition.
11. Muggia-Sullam M, et al. Postoperative enteral versus par-

enteral nutritional support in gastrointestinal surgery. Am J Surg 1985; 149:106–112.

This study does not lend support to the commonly held belief that enteral nutrition is superior to TPN.

12. Nehme AE. Nutritional support of the hospitalized patient: The team concept. JAMA 1980; 243:1906–1908.

    A comparison of two groups of patients undergoing TPN. The first group was managed by a nutrition support team; the second, by a variety of physicians. The complication rate was significantly higher in the second group.

13. Reilly JJ, Gerhardt AL. Modern surgical nutrition. Curr Prob Surg. October, 1985.

    A look at nutrition for the surgical patient.

14. Shanbhogue LKR, et al. Parenteral nutrition in the surgical patient. Br J Surg 1987; 74:172–180.

    A discussion of all aspects of parenteral nutrition in the surgical patient.

15. University of Michigan hospitals parenteral and enteral nutrition manual, 1980, The Regents of the University of Michigan, Ann Arbor, Michigan.

    A straightforward review of parenteral and enteral nutrition.

16. Winters C. Parenteral nutrition. In SJ Chobanian, MM Van Ness (eds.), *Manual of Clinical Problems in Gastroenterology*. Boston: Little, Brown, 1988.

    A quick review of parenteral nutrition.

III
Acute Infectious Gastrointestinal Disease Drugs

The gastrointestinal tract is exposed to the environment at both ends and hence is subject to a great number of infectious agents and their toxins. It is no surprise, therefore, that the average individual suffers an infection of the gastrointestinal tract from 1 to 6 times a year, depending on location, living conditions, and age. When one considers the world as a whole, the problem is enormous. Cuckler calculated in 1975 that there were more cases of parasitic infections in the world than there were people. Despite medical progress, the problem is increasing. Only *Schistosoma japonicum* and *Trichinella spiralis* infections have decreased in numbers over the last 40 years. The recent AIDS epidemic has only exacerbated this problem further.

Acute infectious diarrhea is the second most common clinical illness in our society, and few maladies cause an otherwise healthy individual to seek medical attention faster than this affliction. Infectious diarrhea is defined as the abrupt onset of three or more watery or unformed stools per day caused by an infectious agent. Dysentery is defined as the passage of diarrhea stools with blood, leukocytes, and mucus. Dysentery usually implies bacterial invasion of the intestinal wall or destruction of the mucosal surface from a toxin.

When confronted by acute infectious diarrhea, the patient's history is important. A good differential diagnosis can be made by the presence or absence of associated cases, the timing of onset, relation to particular meals, and the presence of fever, vomiting, or dysentery. Questions of particular importance that should be asked of all patients are the possibility of recent travel, recent antibiotic use, rectal intercourse, or exposure to day care or institutionalized populations. Affirmative answers to these questions significantly alter the differential diagnosis and thus the clinical approach.

The patient with mild diarrhea generally needs little more than a clinical assessment, symptomatic relief, and reassurance. In moderate or more severe diarrhea, some laboratory testing is indicated. The most valuable is a fecal leukocyte test, which if positive, confirms the presence of diffuse inflammation of the colonic mucosa. A negative test does not rule out the presence of a bacterial pathogen. Shigella, for instance, often has no fecal leukocytes during the early, small bowel phase.

A stool culture need not be submitted in every case of diarrhea. Rather, only those patients with moderate or severe diarrhea, fever, dysentery, fecal leukocyte–positive stools, or symptoms for more than a week, need to be cultured. This approach significantly reduces cost and allows the laboratory to give more attention to those cultures that are clinically important.

Sigmoidoscopy can be useful in selected patients; for most cases, however, it is only able to confirm or deny the presence of inflammation—the same information obtainable from the less expensive and less invasive fecal leukocyte test. It can be helpful in suspected pseudomembranous colitis, amoebic colitis (selective biopsy and culturing of ulcers), villous adenoma, or where inflammatory bowel disease is possible (culture-negative diarrhea with prolonged symptoms).

The most important initial decision facing the clinician is whether to hospitalize the patient. The presence of significant dehydration, intractable vomiting, serious underlying medical problems, severe toxicity, or extremes of age are all indications for hospitalization. Most patients with infectious diarrhea heal themselves without antibiosis if adequate attention is paid to fluid and electrolyte management. Oral rehydration is best accomplished with a glucose and electrolyte solution, and is reasonable and time-tested. It relies on the principle of solvent drag, the passive absorption of water and sodium following active transport of glucose. A recipe for a homemade solution is in the section on cholera. Good commercial solutions are Pedialyte, Gatorade, and Exceed.

Antibiotics are useful for most of the more severe cases of infectious diarrhea. Organisms that respond to antibiotics include enterotoxigenic and enteropathogenic *E. coli*, *Shigella*, and *Campylobacter*. Antibiotics given late in the course of *Campylobacter* are of dubious value. Only compromised or toxic patients with *Salmonella* should be treated; this issue is well discussed in the Shigella/Salmonella section. The antibiotic treatment of enteric infections will probably change over the next several years because of increasing resistance patterns and the development of newer drugs, such as the quinolones. For this reason, a separate section specifically addresses the use of the newest quinolone, ciprofloxacin, which was recently approved for use in bacterial diarrhea.

Viral and fungal diseases have become important clinical entities because of the more frequent use of immunosuppressive drugs and the AIDS epidemic. Both of those classes of pathogens primarily cause esophageal disease. Infections of the esophagus are readily localized to that organ because the usual symptoms, dysphagia and odynophagia, are fortunately relatively specific. Detection of the actual pathogen is a more difficult task. It requires isolation of the particular virus or fungus, or demonstration of the appropriate morphologic change. Fiberoptic endoscopy is the best study to provide this information since it affords the opportunity to observe the morphology as well as to obtain specimens for culture, histology, and microscopy.

The treatment of protozoal and parasitic infections is well covered in the chapters to follow. The parasitic infections are not commonly encountered in the United States, but in the homosexual, institutionalized individual, world traveler, and military population, these are important causes of disease. In these cases, the clinical suspicion of the physician and the technical ability of the laboratory are the cornerstones of diagnosis. It must be remembered that barium studies, antacids, antidiarrheal drugs, and even antimicrobials can hinder the laboratory diagnosis of protozoal and parasitic infections. The clinician must rely on perseverance and serology or biopsy in such cases to reach a diagnosis.

Many chapters in this part are necessarily more disease-oriented than in the other parts of the book. In the management of infectious gastrointestinal illness, the identification of the actual pathogen is the critical step in the treatment regimen. The ability to expeditiously arrive at the correct diagnosis is thus the first step in drug therapy for these diseases. Nevertheless, every attempt has been made to help the reader with the newest aspects and the basic pharmacology of drug therapy for these infections.

Michael S. Gurney

References

1. Cook GC. The clinical significance of gastrointestinal helminths—A review. Trans R Soc Trop Med Hyg 1986; 80:675.
   A comprehensive review of the significant clinical gastrointestinal helminthic infections in humans.
2. Cuckler AC. Estimated incidence of worldwide parasitic infections. J Parasitol 1976; 61:55.
   Cuckler estimates and tabulates the numbers of various parasitic infections worldwide.
3. DuPont, HL, et al. Current problems in antimicrobial therapy for bacterial enteric infections. Am J Med 1987; 82(Supp 4A):324.
   DuPont discusses some of the current problems in antibiotic therapy of GI acute bacterial infections.
3. DuPont HL. Acute nonparasitic diarrhea. In JE Berk (ed.), *Bockus Gastroenterology* vol 3 (4th ed). Philadelphia: Saunders, 1985.
   An excellent discussion of the diagnosis and therapy of infectious diarrhea by one of the leaders in the field.
4. Lolekha S. Consequences of treatment of gastrointestinal infections. Scan J Infec Dis 1986; Supp 49:154.
   A good discussion of the negative aspects of antibiotic treatment of diarrhea.
5. Mehta MN, Subramanian S. Comparison of rice water, rice electrolyte solution, and glucose electrolyte solution in the management of infantile diarrhea. *Lancet* 1986; 1:843.
   Akternative, and often more convenient, oral rehydration solutions are compared.
6. Monroe LS. Gastrointestinal Parasites. In JE Berk (ed.), *Bockus Gastroenterology* vol 7 (4th ed). Philadelphia: Saunders, 1985.
   An outstanding discussion of gastrointestinal parasitic infections and their therapy.
7. Pichler HET. Clinical efficacy of ciprofloxacin compared with placebo in bacterial diarrhea. Am J Med 1987; 28(Supp 4A):324.
   The efficacy of the new quinolone, ciprofloxacin, is proven in a placebo-controlled trial.
8. Surawicz CM, et al. Spectrum of rectal-biopsy abnormalities in homosexual men with intestinal symptoms. Gastroenterology 1986; 91:652.
   A useful study of the utility of rectal biopsy in the homosexual population.

Bacterial Infections

John Malone and Michael S. Gurney

Salmonella

Salmonella are gram-negative bacilli of the *Enterobacteriacae* tribe that can cause four separate clinical entities: gastroenteritis, bacteremia, typhoid fever (enteric fever), and a chronic carrier state. Gastroenteritis, the most common, is characterized by several days of diarrhea with polymorphonuclear leuckocytes present on fecal smear and positive stool cultures. The *Salmonella enteritidis* group is the usual pathogen in gastroenteritis. This group, the largest, contains 1400 biotypes such as *typhimurium, caterititis,* and *heidelberg*. Antibiotics may prolong illness and result in persistent positive stool cultures. Bacteremia related to *S. cholerasuis* presents with fever and chills without gastrointestinal symptoms and accounts for 8 to 15 percent of all *Salmonella* infections. Localized infections are common, causing infected aortic aneurysms or osteomyelitis. Typhoid fever (usually due to *S. typhi* or *paratyphi*) is a systemic illness characterized by high intermittant fevers and prostration. Antecedent diarrhea is infrequent. Constipation and hepatosplenomegaly may be important clinical clues. Untreated, mortality is 15 to 20 percent. Approximately 400 cases per year occur in the United States, with hundreds of thousands in underdeveloped countries. The fourth clinical entity is an asymptomatic chronic carrier state, defined when stools are positive for *S. typhi* paratyphi for 1 year. This is due to colonization of the liver and biliary tract.

TRANSMISSION

In the U.S., contaminated poultry and meat processing are major sources. Chickens and turkeys acquire *Salmonella* early in life. Eggs are infected before the shell calcifies; therefore, heating in the shell for 3 minutes may not kill organisms. Water contaminated with fecal waste is common in the underdeveloped world and a risk in flood situations. Since humans are the only reservoir of *Salmonella* typhi, chronic carriers pose a public health risk, especially in food workers with poor handwashing habits after defecation.

An innoculum of 10^5 organisms results in a 30-percent infection rate, in contrast to *Shigella,* where only 100 organisms are necessary. *Salmonella* are destroyed by a pH of 2.0 and unaffected by a pH greater than 5. Individuals with partial gastrectomies are at increased risk due to absent acid and rapid gastric emptying time. Normal bacterial flora are also partially protective since they compete for metabolic growth requirements. A slow bowel transit time (as occurs with antimotility agents) may also increase infection potential by allowing for increased mucosal barrier penetration.

Besides those with low gastric acid production, typhoid fever–susceptible individuals include those with sickle cell disease (decreased phagocytic opsonizing capacity), leukemia lymphoma (impaired cellular prevention mechanisms), and schistosomiasis (adherence of *Salmonella* to fluke tegument). Bartonellosis- and malaria-infected individuals are also prone.

TREATMENT—TRADITIONAL

Typhoid fever has traditionally been treated with Chloramphenicol, which is primarily used in underdeveloped countries due to its effectiveness and minimal expense; resistance has occurred in Southeast Asia, the Middle East, and Mexico (1972 large epidemic). Currently 30 percent of South American strains are resistant. Besides resistance, concern over the possibility of severe hematologic toxicity has minimized United States usage. Drug levels are recommended. Ampicillin, amoxicillin, and trimethoprim/sulfa have been investigated and are effective alternatives. Single-dose dexamethasone in high doses (3 mg/kg/body weight) intravenously has definitely been shown to improve survival in severe typhoid fever manifested by delirium, obtundation, stupors, coma, or shock).

Typhoid fever—all therapies require 12 to 14 days of treatment.

Chloramphenicol

Adults and Children: 50 to 100 milligrams/kilogram of body weight every 6 hours
Infants less than 2 weeks old: 25 milligrams/kilogram of body weight every 6 hours
Higher doses are used in the first 48 hours, then decreased to 50 milligrams/kilogram of body weight every 6 hours.

Ampicillin

Adults: 6 to 8 grams/day intravenously every 6 hours (No oral usage due to increase failure. Defervescence slower than chloramphenicol; relapse may be higher.)
Children: 200 milligrams/kilogram of body weight/day every 6 hours.

Amoxicillin

Adults: 4 to 6 grams/day
Children: 100 milligrams/kilogram of body weight/day every 6 hours
Satisfactory oral substitute

Trimethoprim (TMP) and Sulfamethoxazole (SXT)

Adults: 160 milligrams TMP and 800 milligrams SXT (one double-strength tablet) twice a day for 14 days
Children: 185 milligrams/mole TMP and 925 milligrams/mole SXT each 24 hours

Choramphenicol plasmid–mediated resistance also codes for SXT, therefore TMP may be the only active component. If a patient shows no response in 72 hours, antibiotics should be changed. Ineffective drugs (even if in-vitro sensitive) include Aminoglycosides and tetracycline; first-generation cephalosporins are questionable.

TREATMENT—NEW DEVELOPMENTS

Ciprofloxacin and third-generation cephalosporins show in-vitro bacteriacidal activity 12 times greater than ampicillin and 500 times greater than chloramphenicol while obtaining intracellular penetration.

Cefoperazone: 100 milligrams/kilogram of body weight/day every 12 hours for 12 to 14 days (Effectiveness was shown in children with severe shock. Randomized clinical trial in Haiti resulted in 22 individuals becoming afebrile in 4 days, compared with 6 days in chloromphenical-treated patients.)

Ceftriaxone: Dose-finding studies have shown good results with 1.5 grams twice a day or 3 to 4 grams every day.

Ciprofloxacin: 500 milligrams every 12 hours for 14 days was effective in 36 out of 38 patients.

PEARLS AND PITFALLS

1. *Salmonella* gastroenteritis is usually due to *Salmonella* enteridites group (1400 biotypes). Antibiotics are contraindicated, in most settings, and adequate hydration recommended.
2. New alternatives for enteric (typhoid) fever include cefoperazone, ceftriaxone, and ciprofloxacin. These drugs have proved exceedingly effective in clinical trials. Steroids in high doses improve survival in severe cases. Enteric isolation is necessary. Bone marrow and liver biopsy have a higher yield than blood culture.
3. Chronic carriers of *Salmonella* typhi or paratyphi are defined when stool cultures are positive for 1 year. Cholelithiasis is a possible underlying cause, and cholecystectomy may be indicated. Ciprofloxacin, 750 milligrams twice a day for 30 days, may be an alternative.
4. Differential diagnostic points
   a. Pulse or temperature deficit may occur with typhoid fever
   b. Other diseases reported include Brucellosis, tularemia, rheumatic fever, infectious mononucleosis, leptospirosis, tuberculosis, Hodgkins lymphoma, and Rickattsial infections (Rocky Mountain spotted fever)
5. Clinical clues to enteral infection
   a. Salmonellosis: Group outbreak following a certain meal; incubation approximately 24 hours
   b. Staphylococcal: Exotoxic induction—severe vomiting and diarrhea within 20 to 60 minutes of ingestion
   c. *Shigella*: Toxicity greater than *Salmonella*, fever higher, stools bloody, increased number of fecal leukocytes compared to other bacterial infections
   d. *Vibrio parahemolyticus*: Shellfish-associated, with mild watery diarrhea

e. *Bacillas cereas*: Watery diarrhea after contaminated food (rice)
  f. Calicivirus: Involves teenage children in clusters; fever lasts 1.5 to 3 days
  g. Rotavirus: Involves children 4 to 5 years old
  h. Enterotoxigenic *E. coli*: Occurs in travelers to underdeveloped countries; 3-day illness with cramps and diarrhea (nonbloody), low-grade fever, and nausea
  i. *Giardia*: Onset 10 days after exposure to water from mountain streams; malodorous stools
  j. *Campylobacter*: Bloody diarrhea lasting 3 days; puppy in household with diarrhea

Shigellosis

Shigellosis is due to a gram-negative, nonmotile rod of the tribe *Eschericheae*, genus *Shigella*, and is the common cause of bacillary dysentery. The term *dysentery* describes frequent stools containing blood and mucous. Transmission is through fecal and oral routes involving contaminated food, water, hands, and flies. Outbreaks associated with poor sanitation have occurred in day care centers, Indian reservations, institutionalized mentally retarded individuals, military campaigns, and travelers to underdeveloped countries. Infection may occur with inoculums as small as 100 viable cells, as compared with *Salmonella typhi*, requiring 10^5 for infection, or Enterotoxigenic *E. coli* and *Vibrio cholerae* with 10^7 organisms needed for infection.

Four species of *Shigella* exist: *S. dysenteria, S. flexneri, S. boydii,* and *S. sonnei*. *Shigella*, along with *Salmonella*, are differentiated from other common nonpathogenic gram-negative rods such as *E. coli* by the inability to ferment lactose and produce acid. Because dye indicators are not changed by a lowered pH on the MacConkey bacterial screening agar, colonies appear clear and colorless. More selective media such as salmonella/shigella agar containing a high bile salt content that inhibits the growth of most other coliforms can also be utilized. Currently *S. sonnei* is isolated 60 percent of the time and *S. flexneri* in 36 percent of cases. *S. dysenteriae* was the most common species in the early 1900s. Changing patterns probably reflect building immunity.

Pathogenesis involves the ability of a small inoculum to resist gastric acidity and multiply in the small bowel causing upper abdominal distress and watery stools. Individuals with low gastric acid production (vagotomy and pyloroplasty, H2-blockers, antacids) or on steroid suppression are more susceptible. Bacteria pass to the colon where mucosal cell invasion results in acute onset of dysentery. Incubation ranges from 1 to 3 days for *S. dysenteriae*, to 3 to 7 days for *S. sonnei* and *S. flexneria*. Shiga toxin produced by *S. dysenteriae* is cytotoxic in tissue culture and also causes transudation of fluid in tissue cells through adenylate cyclase activation. Prostaglandin stimulation may also contribute to secretory activity.

Disease may be self-limited over a 7- to 10-day period. However, attention to fluid and electrolytes (especially in children) is stressed since dehydration is a major cause of mortality. Antibiotic treatment definitely shortens the length and severity of disease. In contrast to *salmonella* infections, development of a chronic carrier state is very infrequent and not related to treatment. Therefore, antibiotic treatment of all shigellosis is generally recommended.

TREATMENT

With respect to drug therapy, antibacterial plasmid-mediated resistance to sulfas, tetracycline, ampicillin, and trimethoprim-sulfamethoxazole has developed through the decades. Individuals with foreign-travel exposure have a high rate of resistant *Shigella,* including multidrug resistance. In the United States, resistance patterns on 252 *Shigella* isolates randomly collected by the Centers for Disease Control in 1985 and 1986 were as follows: tetracycline, 43 percent resistant; ampicillin, 32 percent; TMP-SXT, 7 percent; chloramphenicol, 5 percent; and gentamycin, 4 percent. A rapid rise in the resistance to naldixic acid has been reported from an American Indian reservation.

Treatment recommendations are as follows:

Ampicillin

Adults: 1 gram orally every 6 hours for 5 days
Children: 50 to 100 milligrams/kilogram of body weight orally, divided, every 6 hours for 5 days
A large amount of resistance is present.

Trimethoprim (TMP) and Sulfamethoxazole (SXT)

Adults: 160 milligrams TMP and 800 milligrams SXT (one double-strength tablet) orally twice a day for 5 days
Children: 10 milligrams/kilogram of body weight TMP and 50 milligrams/kilogram SXT per day orally twice a day for 5 days
Best choice if medication allergy is not a problem.

Tetracycline

2.5 grams orally in a single dose, or 500 milligrams orally every 6 hours for 5 days
Not for use in children less than 10 years old due to dental staining; *Shigella* resistance is high

Fluoroquinolones

Ciprofloxacin: 500 milligrams orally twice a day for 5 days
Norfloxacin: 400 milligrams orally twice a day for 5 days
Use in adults only, due to possible cartilage damage in developing children. Consider these drugs when resistance to Trimethoprim-Sulfamethoxazole is likely. The chief disadvantage is expense.

Oral Cephalosporins

Not effective

PEARLS AND PITFALLS

1. Resistance to ampicillin is common, and resistance to Trimethoprim/Sulfamethoxazole is increasing, especially in foreign countries (Mexico and Thailand particularly).
2. Bloody diarrhea of sudden onset containing fecal leukocytes may also characterize other pathogens such as *Campylobacter* (most common), *Enteropathogenic E. coli*, *Salmonella, Yersinia,* and *Entameba histolitica*. Inflammatory bowel disease (ulcerative colitis or regional enteritis) is also a possibility.
3. For the laboratory, fresh stools (preferably less than 4 hours old) should be submitted. Alert the laboratory with a differential diagnosis of pathogens written on the laboratory slip to ensure appropriate evaluation—not just "diarrhea" or "stool culture."
4. Opiate derivatives such as diphenoxylate (Lomotil) and loperamide hydrochloride (Imodium) lead to increased tissue destruction and are contraindicated. Pectin compounds (Kaopectate) offer no additional benefit.
5. A bivalent vaccine may be released soon. Candidates include institutionalized mentally retarded individuals, military populations, and American Indians on reservations with poor sanitation. Individuals planning to live in underdeveloped countries where compromised sanitation conditions exist (Peace Corps workers and missionaries) should also be included.
6. Transmission is by the fecal-oral route. Humans are the only reservoir. High transmission rates occur in families, especially among young siblings. For hospitalized individuals, appropriate precautions would include thorough handwashing. Centers for Disease Control Guidelines of Enteric Precautions are indicated.
7. The rare chronic carrier is difficult to treat. Antibiotics are seldom effective. Lactulose may be of assistance. Ciprofloxacin, 750 milligrams twice a day for 30 days, has been found to be effective in *Salmonella* typhi carriers.

Vibrio Cholera

Vibrio cholera has been epidemic in India since the beginning of recorded history, and has been responsible for seven pandemics since 1817. Although it is an important cause of morbidity and mortality in Asia and Africa, it is uncommon in the United States and is limited to the Gulf Coast area. Nevertheless, it has great potential for epidemics, and the last pandemic in 1961 did extend to the United States.

Cholera produces a classic secretory diarrhea by production of a toxin that binds irreversibly to the small intestinal mucosa and stimulates cyclic AMP production. The increased intracellular cyclic AMP leads to secretion of water and electrolytes into the gut. The volume of fluid produced can be most impressive; well-hydrated patients with severe cholera have been known to produce an amount of diarrheal fluid equal to their own weight. Inability to replace the gut fluid losses in severe cases leads to the traditional outcome of cholera before rehydration therapy: dehydration, shock, and death (70 to 80 percent of cases). Cholera is virtually the only infectious diarrhea able to cause circulatory collapse in adults.

In reality, most cases of cholera are subclinical or indistinguishable from other infectious diarrheas. Seven to 25 percent (depending on biotype) require medical attention and 2 to 11 percent require hospitalization. The usual case of cholera begins abruptly and the first few stools contain fecal material. However, the stools rapidly become clear and liquid, with flecks of mucus (rice-water stools). Vomiting may occur initially but usually ceases as the infection progresses. If the patient is not rehydrated, the consequences of dehydration rapidly ensue. Dehydration is the most devastating consequence of cholera, but metabolic acidosis and hypokalemia may occur due to loss of bicarbonate and potassium in the stool.

Diagnosis is made by the clinical setting, by dark-field microscopy revealing the characteristic motility pattern, by stool culture, and by serology, which becomes positive four days after the onset of symptoms.

Rapid rehydration with fluid and electrolytes is the critical element in cholera treatment. Patients who are severely dehydrated or unable to take fluids orally need rapid intravenous fluid replacement. Most other patients can be successfully treated with oral rehydration solutions. The rate of intravenous replacement for severely dehydrated adults is 2 liters over the first 30 minutes. If improvement is noted, the rate can be slowed to 110 milliliters/kilogram of body weight over the next 4 hours. Children in shock need 30 milligrams/kilogram in the first hour and an additional 40 milliliters/kilogram in the next 2 hours. Ringer's lactate with 10 milliequivalents/liter of added potassium is the proper intravenous solution. In both children and adults, oral rehydration solution can then be ingested if the patient is stable.

The formula for oral rehydration solution recommended by the World Health Organization is sodium, 90 millimoles/liter; potassium, 20 millimoles/liter; chloride, 80 millimoles/liter; bicarbonate, 30 millimoles/liter; and glucose, 111 millimoles/liter. A number of clinical trials have shown that this solution is safe and clinically useful in the treatment of all types of diarrhea in all groups of patients. For mild dehydration, the solution should be given at the rate of 50 milligrams/kilogram of body weight within the first 4 hours. For moderate dehydration, 100 milliliters/kilogram should be given in the same time period. Vomiting rarely prevents successful use of oral rehydration solution. Occasionally the diarrhea is so severe that both intravenous and oral routes must be utilized.

Antibiotics are not a substitute for rehydration therapy, but reduce the volume and duration of diarrhea and shorten the period of *Vibrio* excretion. Tetracycline, 500 milligrams every 6 hours for 3 days, is the drug of choice. Chloramphenicol and erythromycin are acceptable alternatives.

Furazolidone (5–7 mg/kg), a nonabsorbable antibiotic, may be preferable in children and pregnant women but requires a longer course of treatment. Antibiotic resistance has not been a problem except in outbreaks in Bangladesh and Kenya.

Atropine and steroids are unnecessary and may be harmful. Kaolin and antispasmodics are of no clinical value. Chlorpromazine and nicotinic acid inhibit intestinal secretion and may be of small benefit.

In recent years, several non-cholera *vibrios* have become clinically important. *Vibrio parahemolyticus* has been identified as a food-borne cause of gastroenteritis. It is usually caused by mishandling of seafood after cooking. Clinical manifestations include diarrhea (98%), nausea (71%), vomiting (52%), headache (42%), and low-grade fever (27%). The incubation period is from 4 to 96 hours, and the illness usually subsides within 3 days. Therapy is primarily supportive, with replacement of fluid and electrolyte losses. There are no good data on antibiotic efficacy but tetracycline would be a reasonable choice if antimicrobials are needed.

Vibrio vulnificus has recently been identified as a cause of wound infections and primary septicemia, particularly in patients with chronic illnesses. Chronic liver disease patients seem to be the group at greatest risk. *Vibrio vulnificus* infections are most remarkable for their virulence: A recent study showed a 55-percent mortality rate for septicemia, and a 24-percent mortality rate for wound infections. Almost all septicemia cases occurred after ingestion of raw oysters. The wound infections occurred after exposure of preexisting wounds to seawater. Tetracycline is the most effective agent but early treatment is mandatory. Since this organism is so devastating, prevention by avoidance of raw seafood and protection of wounds from warm seawater (particularly estuaries) is the prudent course to follow.

PEARLS AND PITFALLS

1. Patients with low gastric acid output, either from medications (H2-blockers), surgery, or gastric atrophy, are much more vulnerable to cholera infection. If a patient is on chronic acid suppression and is traveling to an endemic area, it would be prudent to temporarily stop the medication or change to a medication such as Carafate.
2. Cholera is virtually the only infectious diarrhea that can cause shock in a healthy adult.
3. Hypotension from cholera should *not* be treated with vasopressors or cardiac stimulants. The proper therapy is fluid, fluid, fluid.
4. Existing vaccines are only 60 percent effective in preventing cholera. Since the efficacy of vaccines is low, the side effects significant, and the usual traveler is at low risk, routine cholera immunization for travel to an endemic area is not recommended.
5. If oral rehydration solution is not available, a homemade recipe for temporary oral rehydration solution is 1 teaspoon of salt, 1 teaspoon of bicarbonate, and 4 teaspoons

of table sugar dissolved in 1 liter of water. Commercial electrolyte and sugar solutions such as Pedialyte, Gatorade, and Exceed are also good substitutes.

Campylobacter

Campylobacter's name is derived from the Greek terms for curved (campylo) and rod (bacter), and it describes these motile, nonspore-forming, comma-shaped gram-negative rods, which are some of the most common bacterial pathogens in humans. When first isolated in 1909, they were called *vibrio fetus* because of their appearance, but a separate genus was recently created when DNA studies identified their unique characteristics. The most common species causing enteritis in humans are *C. fetus ss. fetus* and *C. jejuni*. There has been a great deal of recent interest in *C. pylori*, which may be involved in the pathogenesis of inflammatory and ulcerative diseases of the stomach and duodenum. This chapter focuses on the treatment of the organisms causing enteritis; the section on acid peptic disorders discusses treatment of *C. pylori*.

Campylobacter comprises a worldwide zoonosis with reservoirs in cattle, sheep, swine, foul, dogs, cats, and rodents. Human infection frequently occurs after slaughter-house contamination of undercooked meats, particularly poultry products. Consumption of raw (unpasteurized) milk and untreated water (as by backpackers and campers); and contamination of municipal water systems have resulted in outbreaks. Raw clams, cake icing, and salads have been reported to cause infection. Contact with household pets, especially young dogs and cats with diarrhea, has been implicated. Some cases of traveler's diarrhea are also caused by *Campylobacter jejuni*.

CAMPYLOBACTER JEJUNI

Campylobacter jejuni is isolated more often from diarrhea stool specimens than are *salmonella* or *shigella*. Intestinal infection results in enteritis, with fever, malaise, crampy abdominal pain, and diarrhea ranging from loose stools to voluminous movements of water and gross blood. Disease is self-limited in a majority of patients; however, 10 to 20 percent have symptoms longer than 1 week. The relapse rate is 5 to 10 percent. Severe infections may occur, with large amounts of blood in the stool, tenesmus, high fevers, and toxic megacolon. In *C. jejuni,* bacteremia occurs in less than 1 percent, usually in infants and the elderly. Complications such as meningitis, endocarditis, pancreatitis, and cholecystitis are extremely rare. A reactive arthritis can occur in individuals who are HLA-B27 positive.

CAMPYLOBACTER FETUS

In contrast, *Campylobacter fetus* is frequently associated with bacteremia. Intermittent diarrhea and nonspecific abdominal pain occurs in 35 percent of patients. However, more systemic signs of relapsing fevers, chills, myalgias, and night sweats are more typical. A predilection for seeding of vascular sites results in mycotic aneurysms of the abdominal aorta, thrombophlebitis, and endocarditis. Other localized infections from bacteremia include septic arthritis, lung abscess, cholecystitis, and meningoencephalitis. Most patients recover with necessary antibiotic therapy. Self-limiting bacteremias have also been observed.

Diagnosis usually involves culture of the organism. *Campylobacters* require reduced oxygen tension and special media with additional antibiotics to inhibit other enteric flora and prevent overgrowth of the slow-growing *Campylobacters*. Specimen labels should alert the laboratory to the possibility of *Campylobacter*. While all can develop at the usual incubator temperature of 37°C, *C. jejuni* (the most common isolate) grows best at 42°C. Due to their slow growth characteristic, blood cultures of *Campylobacter fetus* are often not positive until days 5 to 14. Serological tests have a low specificity and sensitivity.

THERAPY

Many *Campylobacter* intestinal infections are self-limited, with resolution of bloody diarrhea, cramps, and fevers by the time cultures return. Several studies have not shown any benefit of antibiotics over placebo; however, patient numbers were small and treatment started late. Individuals needing treatment are those with high fever and bloody diarrhea, and those with worsening or unimproved symptoms at the time of bacterial culture confirmation. Erythromycin eliminates *Campylobacter* in 72 hours and has few serious side effects. A chronic carrier state does not occur. In children, early treatment may diminish spread in households, day care settings, or nursery schools.

Treatment

Enteritis:

1. Erythromycin: Adults, 250 milligrams 4 times a day orally for 5 to 7 days
   Children, 40 milligrams/kilogram/every 24 hours for 5 to 7 days
   Treatment of choice due to efficacy and few side effects. Resistance from 1 to 8 percent in Southeast Asia and Sweden.
2. Ciprofloxacin: Adults, 500 milligrams twice a day orally for 5 days
   Exceedingly effective but expensive. Broad spectrum against bacterial enteric pathogens. Use in adults only.
3. Tetracycline: Adults, 250 to 500 milligrams 4 times a day orally for 5 days
   Children greater than 10 years old, 50 milligrams/kilogram/24 hours for 5 days
   Plasmid-mediated resistance 15 percent in Canada.

4. Furazolidone: 5 milligrams/kilogram per 24 hours
   Useful in children due to oral preparation.

Septicemia: Gentamicin—4 week-course to be considered; endovascular infections common.
Meningitis: Chloramphenicol has the most experience.

PEARLS AND PITFALLS

1. Erythromycin is the treatment of choice for *Campylobacter* enteritis but must be given early for greatest efficacy.
2. Symptoms of abdominal cramps and bloody diarrhea may represent *shigella* or *salmonella*; however, *Campylobacter* is more common. Ciprofloxacin is effective with all these pathogens.
3. Stool cultures need to be labeled for *Campylobacter* since special medium and lowered oxygen are required for growth.
4. Historical aspects indicating possible *Campylobacter* enteritis would include exposure to young dogs or cats with diarrhea, unpasturized milk consumption, poorly cooked meats, and fresh surface water consumption.
5. Ineffective medications in *Campylobacter* enteritis include:
   a. Trimethoprin/sulfamethoxazole
   b. Vancomycin
   c. Metronidazole
   d. Unprotected beta lactam rings (Ampicillin, penicillin, cephalosporins, ticarcillin)

Addition of an clavulinic acid to amoxicillin and ticarcillin furnishes in-vitro sensitivity.

Clostridia Difficile

Pseudomembranous colitis from *Clostridia difficile* is a distinct clinical entity characterized by inflammatory plaques and pseudomembranes in the large intestine, associated with diarrhea. It was first described in 1893 and was occasionally reported over the next 70 years as a rare complication of surgery, uremia, malignancy, and other conditions. The incidence of pseudomembranous colitis rose dramatically in the 1970s due to increased sensitivity to it by physicians and to the advent of clindamycin and lincomycin as antimicrobials. In the late 1970s, the association with *Clostridia difficile* was shown conclusively by Bartlett and others.

Pseudomembranous colitis should be suspected in any patient who develops diarrhea within 10 weeks of antibiotic therapy. Specific findings include nonbloody, water diarrhea (90–95%), bloody diarrhea (5–10%), fever (80%), leukocytosis (80%), fecal leukocytes (50%), and rebound tenderness (10–20%). The diagnosis is based on the clinical setting, the endoscopic appearance (85–90% have pseudomembranes on flexible sigmoidoscopy; 10% have pseudomembranes only in the right colon), a positive toxin assay (90% have toxin; false-positive rate, 5%), or a positive culture. The culture is more difficult to perform, requires more time, and is less sensitive and less specific.

TREATMENT

The natural course of pseudomembranous colitis is usually self-limited if the offending antibiotic is discontinued. However, one-third of patients require hospitalization or extension of their hospital stay for this complication. The first step in therapy is to stop the antibiotic. If an infection exists that requires further treatment, change to a different antimicrobial. For mild cases of colitis, a resin that binds the toxin such as colestipol (5 gms tid), or cholestyramine (4 gms tid) can be used. Colestipol is more palatable and binds 4 times more toxin per gram in vitro, but the two have not been compared clinically. Moderate to severe colitis does not improve with a binding resin, and antibiotics should be used.

The standard of antibiotic therapy is oral vancomycin, 125 milligrams every 6 hours for 1 to 2 weeks. The clinical response is usually within 2 to 3 days. Disadvantages include bad taste, expense (up to $500 for a 10-day course), and a relapse rate of approximately 20 percent. Vancomycin is only minimally absorbed when given orally; therefore, systemic toxicity is not usually a problem. However, with prolonged therapy in patients with renal failure, elevated serum levels have occurred and toxicity reported. Such patients should have drug levels monitored.

Alternative antibiotics are metronidazole or bacitracin. Each drug has been shown to be as effective as vancomycin and have the same relapse rate. The cost of either drug is one-tenth of vancomycin's for a 10-day course. Bacitracin is given orally, 25,000 units every 6 hours for 7 to 10 days. Metronidazole is given orally, 250 milligrams every 6 hours for 7 to 10 days. If the patient has an ileus, or is too ill to take oral medications, metronidazole is the drug of choice and should be given intravenously, 500 milligrams every 6 hours. There is good evidence that parenteral metronidazole is secreted into the bowel and achieves intraluminal concentrations adequate to inhibit *C. difficile*. Although it is a very effective therapeutic agent, metronidazole has been reported to cause pseudomembranous colitis itself. Occasionally patients are unresponsive to therapy and progress to toxic megacolon or perforation. The only recourse in such patients is surgery.

A significant problem is recurrence of the infection. This may be due to persistence of *C. difficile* spores in the colon or by reinfection from the environment. Recurrence usually responds to another course of treatment but multiple relapses can occur. In such cases, Tedesco has shown that the following schedule is effective: vancomycin, 125 milligrams every 6 hours for 1 week; then 125 milligrams every 12 hours for 1 week; then 125 milligrams daily for 1 week; then 125 milligrams every other day for 1 week; then, finally, 125 milligrams every third day for 2 weeks. This regimen was designed to deal with the possibility of *C. difficile* spores in the colon. None of Tedesco's 22 patients had another relapse after this course. Another recent regimen to deal with relapses used combined vancomycin, 125 milligrams 4 times a day, and rifampin, 600 milligrams twice a day for 1 week. Clinical outcome was good in the seven patients treated, but stool cultures in all seven became positive again 1 month after therapy.

PEARLS AND PITFALLS

1. Never give antimotility agents to patients with documented or suspected pseudomembranous colitis. Such drugs are associated with the development of toxic megacolon.
2. Do not give steroids (if possible) to patients with pseudomembranous colitis. Steroids are associated with a high perforation rate in animal models.
3. If patients do not respond to a resin-binding agent, do not simply add an antibiotic. The resin must be discontinued since it binds the antibiotic in the gut lumen.
4. Higher doses of vancomycin (up to 500 mg every 6 hours) are no more effective than recommended ones, cost more, and may be associated with a higher relapse rate.
5. Pseudomembranes observed by sigmoidoscopy are not specific for *C. difficile* infection. They can also be seen in shigellosis, amebiasis, ischemic colitis, and in *Yersinia* infections. Conversely, a sigmoidoscopy negative for pseudomembranes does not mean the absence of infection. The pseudomembranes may be right-sided only in 10 percent of cases, or they may be microscopic.
6. Normal patients can have both a positive *C. difficile* toxin (1–5%) or culture (up to 20%).

References

SALMONELLA

1. Bryan JP, Rocha H. Problems in salmonellosis: Rationale for clinical trials with newer Beta-Lactam agents and quinolones. Rev Inf Dis 1986; 8:189.

    The use of third-generation cephalosporins and quinolones in the treatment of bacteremia enteric fever, osteomyelitis, and the chronic carrier state is discussed in depth.

2. Gilman RH, Terminel M. Comparison of trimethoprim-sulfamethoxazole and amoxicillin in therapy of chloramphenicol-resistant and chloramphenicol-sensitive typhoid fever. J Inf Dis 1975; 132:630.

    Trimethoprim-sulfamethoxazole is effective therapy for chloramphenicol-resistant and probably of ampicillin-amoxicillin–resistant typhoid fever.

3. Goldstein EW, Chumpitaz JC. Plasmid-mediated resistance to multiple antibiotics in *Salmonella* typhi. J Inf Dis 1986; 153:261.

Two hundred forty-one strains of *Salmonella* typhi from Lima, Peru, underwent in vitro testing. Thirty percent were resistant to chloramphenicol, ampicillin, sulfonamides, and trimethoprim. Isolated strains were exceedingly sensitive to cefoperazone, ceftriaxone, and quinolone compounds.

4. Hornick RB. Salmonella infections. In RD Feigin, JD Cherry (eds), *Textbook of Pediatric Infectious Diseases* (2nd ed.). Philadelphia: Saunders, 1987.

   An in-depth discussion of all forms of *Salmonella* infections.

5. Keusch GT. Antimicrobial therapy for enteric infections and typhoid fever: State of the art. Rev Inf Dis 1988; 10(Suppl. 1):S199.

   Resistance patterns are discussed along with treatment utilizing quinolone compounds.

6. Pope JW, Gerde H. Typhoid fever: Successful therapy with cefoperazone. J Inf Dis 1986; 153:272.

   A randomized trial involving 25 Haitian children with severe typhoid fever found cefoperazone as effective as chloramphenicol.

SHIGELLA

1. Dupont HL. Shigella species (bacillary dysentary). In GL Mandell, RG Douglas, JE Bennet (eds), *Principles and Practice of Infectious Disease* (2nd ed.). New York: Wiley, 1985.

   An in-depth but concise synopsis with 63 references.

2. Gots RE, Formal SB, Giannella BA. Indomethacin inhibition of *Salmonella typhimurium, Shigella flexneri* and cholera-mediated rabbit ileal secretion. J Infect Dis 1974; 130:280.

   Prostaglandins are involved in enteropathogenic-stimulated secretory states, possibly through adenyl cyclase activation.

3. Hornick RB. *Shigella* infections. In RD Feign and JD Cherry (eds), *Textbook of Pediatric Infectious Diseases* (2nd ed.) Philadelphia: Saunders, 1987.

   Excellent in-depth synopsis of *Shigella*, also pertinent to adults; 25 references.

4. Nelson J, et al. Trimethoprim-Sulfamethoxazole therapy for *Shigellosis*. JAMA 1976; 235:1239.

   Twenty-eight infants and children hospitalized for severe *Shigellosis* responded in 1.6 days. Diarrhea abated in 3 days. Ampicillin resistance occurred in 4 patients but responded later to Trimethoprim-Sulfamethoxazole.

5. Schaffer N, Tauxe RV. Rapid emergence of nalidixic acid–resistant *Shigella* on the Navajo reservation. Twenty-seventh interscience conference on antimicrobial agents and chemotherapy (abs 290). Atlanta, Ga.: Centers for Disease Control, 1987.

   Trimethoprim-Sulfamethoxazole–resistant *Shigella* emerged when nalidixic acid was introduced. Within 8 months, 23% of *Shigella* strains became nalidixic acid–resistant, along with resistance to ampicillin and streptomycin. Isolates remained sensitive to Norfloxacin and Ciprofloxacin.

6. Tauxe RV, et al. Antimicrobial resistance in *Shigella*. Twenty-seventh interscience conference on antimicrobial agents and chemotherapy (abs 289). Atlanta, Ga.: Centers for Disease Control, 1987.

   This abstract describes types of *Shigella* species and resistance patterns of 252 isolates sent to the Centers for Disease Control in 1985 and 1986.

CHOLERA

1. Blake PA. *Vibrios* on the half-shell: What the walrus and the carpenter didn't know. Ann Intern Med 1983; 99:558.

   A short but pertinent warning about the dangers of raw seafood ingestion. This is even more important today.

2. Bonner JR, et al. Spectrum of *Vibrio* infections in a Gulf Coast community. Ann Intern Med 1983; 99:464.

   An excellent article on the various manifestations of *Vibrio* infection.

3. Holmberg SD. *Vibrios* and *Aeromonas*. Infect Dis Clin N Am 1988; 2:655.

   An excellent review of the various species of *vibrio* and their illnesses. Holmberg also discusses the non-vibrio *Vibrionaceae* such as *Aeromonas hydrophilia* and *Pleisiomonas shigelloides*.

4. Johnston JM, et al. Cholera on a Gulf Coast oil rig. NEJM 1983; 309:523.

   A description of the various manifestations of a cholera "epidemic" on an oil rig.

5. Klontz KC, et al. Syndromes of *vibrio vulnificus* infections. Ann Intern Med 1988; 109:318.

   A compilation of 62 cases of *V. vulnificus* infections from Florida is reported. The virulence of the organism is stressed.

6. Morris JG Jr. *Vibrio vulnificus:* A new monster of the deep? Ann Intern Med 1988; 109:261.

   An editorial in the same issue as Klontz's article. Morris stresses the need for prevention.

7. Morris JG Jr. Vibrio and Aeromones. In SL Gorbach (ed.), *Infectious Diarrhea*. Boston: Blackwell Scientific Publications, 1986.

   A well-written review by one of the leading authorities in the field.

CAMPYLOBACTER

1. Blaser MT, Laforce FM. Reservoirs for human campylobacteriosis. J Infect Dis 1980; 141:655.

   Sixty-six percent of household contacts with diarrhea had stool cultures positive for *Campylobacter*. Domestic animals, especially puppies with diarrhea, were frequently infected with *Campylobacter*.

2. Blaser MT, Reller LB. *Campylobacter* enteritis. NEJM 1981; 305:1444.

   A complete review of *Campylobacter jejuni*, including historical background, epidemiology, pathogenesis, clinical features, and treatment.

3. Drake AA, Gilchrist MJ. Diarrhea due to *Campylobacter fetus* subspecies *jejuni*: A clinical review of 63 cases. Mayo Clin Proc 1981; 56:414–423.

   Clinical features included a prodrome of malaise, followed by abdominal cramps, diarrhea, anorexia, fever, nausea, and vomiting. Bloody diarrhea occurred in 53 cases.

4. Francoli P, Herzstein J. *Campylobacter fetus* subspecies *fetus* bacteremia. Arch Internal Med 1985; 145:289.

   Lower-extremity phlebitis and cellulitis occurred in four of eight patients. Relapse and osteomyelitis progression were seen on erythromycin therapy and clinical failures occurred with ceftriaxone, cefazolin, and tobramycin. Gentamicin or chloramphenicol for several weeks should be considered.

5. Gaudreau CL, Lariviere LA. Effects of clavulinic acid on susceptibility of *Campylobacter jejuni* and *Campylobacter coli* to eight Beta-lactam antibiotics. Antimicrob Ag Chemo 1987; 31:940.

   Thirty-two strains of *Campylobacter jejuni* and *Campylobacter coli* became sensitive in vitro to amoxacillin and ticarcillin with the addition of clavulinic acid.

6. Klein BS, Vergeront JM. *Campylobacter* infection associated with raw milk: An outbreak of gastroenteritis due to *Campylobacter jejuni* and thermotolerant *Campylobacter fetus* subspecies *fetus*. JAMA 1986; 225:361.

   Unpasturized milk and heat-tolerant strains were identified in source outbreaks.

CLOSTRIDIA DIFFICILE

1. Buggy BP, Fekety R, Siliva J Jr. Therapy of relapsing *Clostridium difficile*–associated diarrhea and colitis with the combination of vancomycin and rifampin. J Clin Gastro 1987; 9:155.

   Buggy used a combined 7-day course of vancomycin, 125 mgs qid, and rifampin, 600 mgs bid, for seven patients with relapsing pseudomembranous colitis. There was good clinical improvement and no relapses, but all stool cultures returned positive for *C. difficile* 1 month after therapy.

2. Bartlett JG. Treatment of *Clostridium difficile* colitis. Gastroenterology 1985; 89:1192.

   An excellent, concise discussion of treatment issues.

3. Burke GW, Wilson ME, Mehrez IO. Absence of diarrhea in toxic megacolon complicating *Clostridium difficile* pseudomembranous colitis. Am J Gastro 1988; 83:304.

   This case report makes an important point: Occasionally pseudomembranous colitis presents as an ileus or megacolon without antecedent diarrhea.

4. Chang TW, Onderdonk AB, Bartlett JG. Anion-exchange resins in antibiotic-associated colitis. Lancet 1978; 2:258.

   The in vitro binding of the toxin to the resins is studied.

5. Finegold SM, Dowell VR. *Clostridium difficile*–associated colitis: A monograph. San Diego: Marion Laboratories, 1977.

   An excellent monograph summarizing epidemiology, pathogenesis, diagnosis, and treatment.

6. Kleinfeld DI, Sharpe RJ, Donta ST. Parenteral therapy for antibiotic-associated pseudomembranous colitis. J Infect Dis 1988; 157:389.

    Kleinfeld reports success using intravenous metronidazole in one patient and reviews the pertinent literature.

7. Teasley DE, et al. Prospective randomized trial of metronidazole versus vancomycin for *Clostridium difficile*–associated diarrhea and colitis. *Lancet* 1983; 2:1043.

    Metronidazole had equivalent efficacy and relapse rates in this randomized trial of 101 patients, but the cost of metronidazole is dramatically lower.

8. Tedesco FJ, Gordon D, Fortson WC. Approach to patients with multiple relapses of antibiotic-associated pseudomembranous colitis. Am J Gastro 1985; 80:867.

    The best study of treatment for relapse. A tapering 21-day course of vancomycin followed by 21 days of pulse vancomycin cured 22 patients with prior multiple relapses.

9. Wolke AM. Pseudomembranous colitis. In SJ Chobanian, MM Van Ness (eds.), *Manual of Clinical Problems in Gastroenterology*. Boston: Little, Brown, 1988.

10. Young GP, et al. Antibiotic-associated colitis due to *Clostridium difficile*: Double-blind comparison of vancomycin with bacitracin. Gastroenterology 1985; 89:1038.

    Bacitracin was equal to vancomycin in clinical response, but was not as effective in clearing the stool culture or the toxin. The relapse rate was similar.

14

Fungal Infections

Marsha G. Pierdinock

Candida albicans is a commensal organism of man and is commonly found in the gastrointestinal tract. Gorbach cultured the organism in 50 percent of oropharyngeal and 90 percent of fecal samples from healthy adults. When host defenses are altered, the organism can invade tissues, resulting in infection. Predisposing factors include use of antibiotics, steroids, chemotherapy, and radiation; diabetes; acquired immunodeficiency syndrome (AIDS); and malnutrition. The oral pharynx and esophagus are the most common gastrointestinal sites of *Candida* infection. Several antifungal agents are available for the treatment of oral or esophageal Candidiasis. Nystatin and clotrimazole are commonly used as first-line agents. If these topical agents fail, oral systemic treatment with ketoconazole is initiated. Amphotericin B is available in intravenous form for those unable to swallow, those unresponsive to ketoconazole, or those with evidence of disseminated or deep infection.

Nystatin and Clotrimazole

Nystatin is a polyene antibiotic derived from cultures of *Streptomyces noursei*. It acts by binding to sterols in the cell membrane of the fungus, resulting in altered cell membrane permeability and leakage of intracellular components.

Clotrimazole is an imidazole derivative that disturbs fungal cell membrane integrity by interfering with the biosynthesis of ergosterol, the primary sterol in fungal membranes.

PHARMACOKINETICS

Nystatin is poorly absorbed from the gastrointestinal tract and almost entirely excreted unchanged in the feces. Detectable blood levels are obtained only after massive doses. After administration of a 10-milligram clotrimazole troche, approximately 30 minutes are required for dissolution of the tablet. Concentrations of clotrimazole sufficient to inhibit *Candida* persist in the saliva for approximately 3 hours, apparently due to the binding of the drug to the oral mucosa.

INDICATIONS

Both nystatin and clotrimazole are commonly used in the treatment of oral and esophageal candidiasis. A randomized, double-blind study by Lawson demonstrated equal effectiveness of clotrimazole troches and nystatin vaginal tablets against oral candidiasis. A clinical improvement rate of 97 percent and clinical cure rate of 83 percent were reported.

SIDE EFFECTS AND CONTRAINDICATIONS

Adverse reactions to nystatin are rare, even with prolonged administration. High doses may produce diarrhea, nausea, and vomiting. Hypersensitivity reactions are extremely rare.

Minimal elevations of hepatic transaminases have been reported with the use of clotrimazole troches. Nausea and vomiting occur in approximately one in 20 patients.

DOSAGE AND ADMINISTRATION

Nystatin is available in oral suspension and tablet forms. The suspension has a bitter taste and is not as well tolerated as the tablet form. Recommended dosage for the oral suspension is 500,000 units (5 mls) of nystatin 5 times daily for 14 days. The suspension should be swished in the mouth for at least 30 seconds before swallowing. Each nystatin pastille contains 200,000 units of nystatin, with a recommended dosage of one pastille dissolved in the mouth 5 times daily for 14 days. A 10-milligram nystatin vaginal tablet may also be used as a troche 5 times daily for 14 days. Both tablets have the advantage of prolonged contact of nystatin with the oral mucosa. The recommended dose of clotrimazole is 1 10-milligram troche dissolved in the mouth 5 times daily for 14 days.

Ketoconazole

Ketoconazole is a synthetic imidazole that has broad-spectrum antifungal activity. It alters cell membrane permeability by interfering with the formation of membrane sterols.

PHARMACOKINETICS

Ketoconazole is readily absorbed through the gastrointestinal tract, with peak plasma levels of 3 to 4 milligrams/milliliter obtained within 1 to 2 hours after ingestion of a 200-milligram tablet. Gastric acidity, required for absorption, transforms the basic ketoconazole into the hydrochloric salt that is then absorbed. Plasma elimination is biphasic, with initial serum half-life of 1.5 to 2 hours and beta-phase half-life about 8 hours after a 200-milligram dose. Ketoconazole is approximately 99 percent bound to plasma proteins, with poor penetration of the blood–brain barrier. Extensive metabolism occurs in the liver, with the inactive metabolites excreted in the bile. About 13 percent is excreted by the kidneys, of which 2 to 4 percent is active drug.

INDICATIONS

Ketoconazole is indicated for patients with oral or esophageal candidiasis who fail to respond to nystatin or clotrimazole. It may also be used as first-line therapy of esophageal candidiasis in patients who demonstrate no evidence of dissemination or deep-organ involvement.

SIDE EFFECTS AND CONTRAINDICATIONS

The most common adverse effects are anorexia, nausea, and vomiting, which occur in approximately 3 percent of patients. Abdominal pain and pruritis occur in 1 to 2 percent. Other minor side effects such as headache, dizziness, somnolence, photophobia, and diarrhea occur in less than 1 percent of patients. Rare cases of anaphylaxis have been reported after the first dose. Ketoconazole can suppress plasma testosterone levels and cause gynecomastia and impotency in men. Lewis reports a mean incidence of mild asymptomatic hepatic enzyme abnormalities of approximately 12 percent. Symptomatic liver dysfunction occurs in 0.01 percent of patients. Rare cases of fatal hepatic necrosis have been reported. Mean duration of therapy in patients who developed symptomatic hepatotoxicity was 7 weeks, with a range of 1.5 to 24 weeks.

High doses of ketoconazole may depress plasma cortisol levels, although no cases of clinical adrenal insufficiency have been reported. Animal studies have demonstrated ketoconazole to be teratogenic in rats and its use is contraindicated during pregnancy.

DOSAGE AND ADMINISTRATION

The usual adult dose for treatment of *Candida esophagitis* is 200 to 400 milligrams once daily for 2 weeks. Taking the drug with food decreases the incidence of anorexia, nausea, and vomiting. Since gastric acidity is required for absorption, the drug should not be taken with antacids or histamine antagonists. In patients with achlorhydria, the tablets should be dissolved in 4 milliliters of 0.2 N HCl, drunk through a straw to protect the teeth, and followed by a glass of water. Concomitant use of nifampin or isoniazid may decrease serum ketoconazole concentration. Use of ketoconazole may alter the metabolism of phenytoin and drug levels should be monitored. The anticoagulant effect of coumadin may be enhanced and prothrombin time levels should be carefully followed. Serum levels of cyclosporin may increase with concomitant use of ketoconazole. Drug dosage in patients with renal or hepatic impairment need not be altered; however, those with underlying hepatic injury from receiving other potential hepatotoxic drugs should have close monitoring. In all patients, hepatic enzymes should be measured prior to therapy and at frequent intervals during treatment. Minor asymptomatic elevation of serum transaminases or alkaline phosphatase are common and usually are transient despite continued drug use. These patients should be followed closely. If enzyme levels continue to rise or patients become symptomatic, ketoconazole should be stopped.

Amphotericin B

Amphotericin B is an antifungal antibiotic derived from a strain of the acitnomycete *Streptomyces nodosus*. It binds to sterols in the fungal cell membrane altering membrane permeability and allowing leakage of cell contents.

PHARMACOKINETICS

Detailed information concerning the pharmacokinetics of amphotericin B is not known. The plasma half-life is approximately 24 hours. Amphotericin B appears to bind to plasma proteins and tissues, with subsequent slow release. There is poor penetration of the blood–brain barrier. After multiple doses, approximately 2 to 5 percent of the drug can be detected in the urine. Up to 7 weeks after therapy has been discontinued, amphotericin B can still be detected in the urine. The primary pathway for excretion of amphotericin B is not known.

INDICATIONS

Amphotericin B is indicated in those patients with Candidiasis who are unresponsive to nystatin, clotrimazole, or ketoconazole, unable to swallow, or demonstrate evidence of dissemination or deep infection.

SIDE EFFECTS AND CONTRAINDICATIONS

Adverse reactions to amphotericin B are common. Fever and chills are almost universal. Headache and anorexia occur in approximately 45 percent and vomiting in 20 percent of patients. Other common adverse reactions include myalgias, pain and phlebitis at the injection site, malaise, and abdominal pain. Serious nephrotoxicity is common and associated with hypokalemia, renal tubular acidosis, azotemia, nephrocalcinosis, and hyposthenuria. Normochromic, normocytic anemia is also commonly seen. A partial list of less common adverse reactions are thrombocytopenia, agranulocytosis, tinnitus, hearing loss, arrhythmias including ventricular fibrillation and cardiac arrest, hypotension, visual changes, and seizures.

DOSAGE AND ADMINISTRATION

It is estimated that an amphotericin B dosage of 0.3 to 0.5 milligrams/kilogram of body weight daily for 7 to 10 days is effective for the treatment of esophagitis. An initial test dose of 1 milligram amphotericin B in 20 milligrams 5% D/W should be given intravenously over 20 minutes, with monitoring of temperature and blood pressure every 30 minutes for 4 hours. If the test dose is tolerated, an initial dose of 0.25 milligrams/kilogram of body weight intravenously should be administered over 4 to 6 hours. The dose may be advanced to 0.5 milligrams/kilogram of body weight by the fifth day.

PEARLS AND PITFALLS

1. The addition of 5 to 50 milligrams of heparin to the infusion of amphotericin B helps diminish local phlebitis. Fever and chills can be reduced by giving 25 milligrams of hydrocortisone intravenously. Meperidine may also be effective in controlling amphotericin B–induced chills.
2. Advanced esophageal Candidiasis can affect nerve ends, and occasionally patients notice a reduction of pain as the disease progresses.
3. If a patient presents with Candidiasis, a search must be undertaken for predisposing diseases or drugs.
4. The absence of oral thrush does not rule out esophageal Candidiasis. Anywhere from 20 to 80 percent of patients with *Candida* esophagitis also have oral thrush.

References

1. Bodey GP. Topical and systemic antifungal agents. Med Clin N Am 1988; 72:637.
   Practical applications for use of the antifungal agents.
2. Borgers M. Mechanism of action of antifungal drugs, with special reference to the imidazole derivatives. Rev Infect Dis 1980; 2:520.
   A comprehensive review of the mechanisms of action of ketoconazole, clotrimazole, miconazole, and flacytosine.
3. Chretien JH, Garagusi VF. Current management of fungal enteritis. Med Clin N Am 1982; 66:675.
   A review of fungal infections of the GI tract.
4. Drutz DJ. Newer antifungal agents and their use, including an update on amphotericin B and flucytosine. Curr Clin Topics in Infect Dis 1982; 3:97.
   An excellent review of amphotericin B.
5. Fazio RA, Wickremesinghe PC, Arsura EL. Ketoconazole treatment of *Candida* esophagitis: A prospective study of 12 cases. Am J Gastro 1983; 78:261.
   A study of 12 patients treated with 200 mg ketoconazole daily for 14 days for candida esophagus. All had complete symptomatic relief within 8 days. One patient discontinued drug at 1 week due to nausea and vomiting. Re-endoscopy 3 weeks later showed uniform disappearance of Candidial lesions.
6. Gorbach SL, Nahas L, Lerner PI. Studies of intestinal microflora I. Gastroenterology 1967; 53:845.
   The first article reviewing intestinal microflora.
7. Gorbach SL, et al. Studies of intestinal microflora II. Gastroenterology 1967; 53:856.
   The second article reviewing intestinal microflora.
8. Huang YC, et al. Pharmacokinetics and dose proportionality of ketoconazole in normal volunteers. Antimicrob Ag Chemo 1986; 30:206.

A comprehensive review of pharmacokinetics and bioavailability of ketoconazole.

9. Lake-Bakaar G, Scheuer PJ, Sherlock S. Hepatic reactions associated with ketoconazole in the United Kingdom. BMJ 1987; 294:419.

An analysis of 72 cases of possible hepatotoxicity associated with ketoconazole reported to the Committee on Safety of Medicines.

10. Lawson RD, Bodey GP. Comparison of clotrimazole troche and nystatin vaginal tablet in the treatment of oropharyngeal candidiasis. Curr Therapy Res 1980; 27:774.

A randomized double-blind study demonstrating equal effectiveness of clotrimazole troches and nystatin vaginal tablets in the treatment of oropharyngeal candidiasis.

11. Lewis JH, et al. Hepatic injury associated with ketoconazole therapy. Gastroenterology 1984; 86:503.

An analysis of 33 cases of ketoconazole-induced hepatitis.

12. Mathieson R, Dutta SK. *Candida* esophagitis. Dig Dis Sci 1983; 28:365.

An excellent clinically oriented review article of *candida* esophagitis.

13. Abramowicz M (ed). Ketoconazole (Nizoral), a new antifungal agent. Medical Letter 1981; 23:85.

A general review of ketoconazole.

15

Viral Infections

Marsha G. Pierdinock

Viral infections of the gastrointestinal system are being recognized with increasing frequency. Anorectal herpes simplex virus infection is the most common cause of nongonococcal proctitis in the male homosexual. In a recent prospective study of 20 homosexual men with AIDS and diarrhea, cytomegalovirus was found to be the most frequently identified intestinal pathogen. Antiviral drugs such as acyclovir and the investigational drug ganciclovir have made significant impacts on the treatment of these diseases.

Acyclovir

MECHANISM OF ACTION

Acyclovir, an acyclic purine nucleoside analogue, is highly effective against herpes simplex virus replication while having little effect on normal cells. Once taken up by infected cells, acyclovir is phosphorylated to a monophosphate form by herpes virus–specific thrymidine kinase. Normal cellular enzymes then cause transformation to the triphosphate form. Acyclovir triphosphate inhibits herpes virus DNA polymerase and viral DNA replication.

PHARMACOKINETICS

Acyclovir is almost entirely excreted unchanged through the kidneys by glomerular filtration and tubular secretion. The half-life and total body clearance of acyclovir is dependent on renal function. In the adult patient with normal renal function (Clcr >80 ml/min) the half-life of acyclovir is 2.5 ± 0.6 hours, while in the anuric patient it may increase to 19.5 hours.

The bioavailability of oral acyclovir is approximately 20 percent. Steady-state plasma levels are reached after 1 day of therapy. Acyclovir achieves a concentration in the cerebrospinal fluid of approximately 50 percent of plasma levels. It achieves good penetration into most tissues and body fluids, including vaginal secretions and herpetic vesicular fluid.

INDICATIONS

Acyclovir has been shown to be effective in decreasing the duration and severity of mucocutaneous herpes infections. The efficacy of acyclovir in the treatment of herpes simplex virus proctitis has only recently been studied. Rompalo and her colleagues conducted a prospective, randomized, double-blind study of 29 patients with their first episode of rectal herpes simplex virus infection. Oral acyclovir was shown to decrease the duration of rectal lesions. Duration of local symptoms associated with proctitis tended to be lower in the acyclovir recipients; however, these differences were not statistically significant.

SIDE EFFECTS

Acyclovir is generally well tolerated, with a wide margin of safety. When used orally, most side effects are related to the gastrointestinal system, with nausea and vomiting occurring in some patients (2–3%). Headache may occur in rare patients (<1%). Diarrhea, fatigue, dizziness, skin rash, arthralgia, and adenopathy are also rare side effects.

The potential risk for nephrotoxicity appears to be related to higher serum levels achieved following intravenous administration. Acyclovir may precipitate within the renal tubules and cause a rise in blood urea nitrogen (BVN) and serum creatinine with a decrease in creatinine clearance. In most cases the impairment in renal function is reversible following dosage adjustment or discontinuation of acyclovir. The renal toxicity is largely avoidable if attention is given to adequate patient hydration and dose adjustment based on creatinine clearance. Preexisting renal disease, use of other nephrotoxic drugs, dehydration, and intravenous bolus administration are risk factors for the development of renal toxicity.

Encephalopathic changes such as lethargy, tremors, confusion, hallucinations, agitation, seizure, coma, and obtundation have been reported in rare patients receiving intravenous acyclovir (1%). The drug should be used with caution in patients with underlying neurologic abnormalities or those simultaneously receiving intrathecal methotrexate or interferon.

Concurrent use of acyclovir with probenecid has been shown to increase the half-life and reduce the urinary excretion and renal clearance of acyclovir.

ADMINISTRATION

Rompalo used 2 grams of oral acyclovir (400 mgs 5 times daily) for 10 days in the treatment of herpes simplex proctitis. Lower-dose regimens of 1 gram/day may be effective, but further studies are needed. Intravenous therapy may be indicated, depending on the severity of disease and the ability of the patient to tolerate oral medication.

Ganciclovir

MECHANISM OF ACTION

Ganciclovir (9-(1,3-Dihydroxy-2-Propoxymethyl) guanine), an acyclic nucleoside analogue, is structurally similar to acyclovir, differing only by the addition of a hydroxymethyl group. It is a prodrug and must first be converted to a triphosphate form which then acts by inhibiting viral DNA polymerase. The marked increase in activity of ganciclovir against cytomegalovirus compared to acyclovir appears in part due to the more efficient conversion to the monophosphate form in cytomegalovirus-infected cells.

PHARMAKOKINETICS

Ganciclovir is almost entirely excreted unchanged by the kidneys. Its plasma half-life is 3.3 hours and oral bioavailability is 3.6 percent.

INDICATIONS

At the time of this writing, ganciclovir is available only for investigational use. It appears promising in the treatment of cytomegalovirus gastrointestinal disease. Uncontrolled studies demonstrate that induction treatment and maintenance therapy with ganciclovir are effective in reducing dysphagia, diarrhea, abdominal pain, nausea, and vomiting.

SIDE EFFECTS

The most common side effect is neutropenia, which occurs in 25 percent to 68 percent of patients receiving induction or maintenance therapy. This neutropenia almost always resolves within days after therapy is discontinued. Subsequent dosage reduction and titration of ganciclovir dose to absolute neutrophil count usually allows patients to continue ganciclovir therapy. Dose-related thrombocytopenic and eosinophilia are also seen. Other adverse reactions include nausea, vomiting, skin rash, anorexia, inhibition of spermatogenesis, disorientation, and psychosis.

ADMINISTRATION

Induction ganciclovir treatment consists of the administration of 2.5 milligrams/kilogram of body weight intravenously every 12 hours for a 10- to 14-day period. Each infusion is given over 1 hour. Maintenance therapy is usually given as a single intravenous dose of ganciclovir, 5 to 7.5 milligrams/kilogram of body weight 5 to 7 days per week. Oral maintenance ganciclovir regimens are being investigated. Dosage reductions are required for patients with underlying renal impairment.

References

1. Baker DA, Milch PO. Acyclovir for genital herpes simplex virus infections. J Reprod Med 1986; 31(suppl 5):433–438.
   Excellent overall review of acyclovir.
2. Bridgen D, Whiteman P. The clinical pharmacology of acyclovir and its prodrugs. Scand J Infect Dis 1985; 47(suppl):33–39.
   Thorough review of clinical pharmacology of acyclovir.

3. Chacova A, et al. 9-(1,3-dihydroxy-2-propoxymethyl) guanine (ganciclovir) in the treatment of cytomegalovirus gastrointestinal disease with the acquired immunodeficiency syndrome. Ann Intern Med 1987; 107:133–137.

    Prospective therapeutic trial using ganciclovir in the treatment of 41 AIDS patients with cytomegalovirus gastrointestinal infection.

4. Jacobson M, Mills J. Serious cytomegalovirus disease in the acquired immunodeficiency syndrome (AIDS). Ann Intern Med 1988; 108:585–594.

    Excellent review of the clinical findings, diagnosis, and treatment of cytomegalovirus infections.

5. Laeum OD. Toxicology of acyclovir. Scand J Infect Dis 1985; 47(suppl):40–43.

    In-depth review of available toxicological data of acyclovir.

6. Masur H, et al. Effect of 9-(1,3-dihydroxy-2-propoxymethyl) guanine on serious cytomegalovirus disease in eight immunosuppressed homosexual men. Ann Intern Med 1986; 104:41–44.

    Uncontrolled clinical trial using ganciclovir in the treatment of 8 immunocompromised patients with cytomegalovirus infections.

7. Miranda P, Blum R. Pharmacokinetics of acyclovir after intravenous and oral administration. J Antimicrob Chemo 1983; 12(suppl B): 29–37.

    Comprehensive review of pharmacokinetics of acyclovir.

8. Reines E, Gross P. Antiviral agents. Med Clin N Am 1988; 72:691–715.

    Practical review of antiviral agents focusing on clinical use.

Protozoal Infections

Marsha G. Pierdinock

Giardiasis

Giardia lamblia is the most commonly diagnosed pathogenic intestinal parasite in the United States and the most frequent cause of water-borne epidemic diarrheal disease. The spectrum of infection ranges from asymptomatic cyst carrier, to mild, self-limited diarrhea, and on to chronic diarrhea associated with weight loss, steatorrhea, abdominal bloating, and flatulence. Three drugs are available in the United States for the treatment of *G. lamblia*. Quinacrine remains the drug of choice with reported cure rates of 90 to 95 percent. Metronidazole, though not approved by the FDA for the treatment of giardiasis, is frequently prescribed, with reported cure rates of 85 to 90 percent. Furafolidone is available in suspension form and may be useful in the treatment of young children. Cure rates range from 75 to 90 percent.

QUINACRINE (ATABRINE)

Quinacrine hydrochloride is an acridine dye originally used as an antimalarial agent during World War II. Its mechanism of action is unclear, but it is believed to affect protein synthesis by intercalation into DNA.

Pharmacokinetics

Quinacrine is water soluble and readily absorbed from the gastrointestinal tract. Peak serum levels are achieved 8 hours after oral administration. The drug binds extensively to plasma proteins and metabolically active tissues, achieving high concentrations in the liver, spleen, epidermis, and lung. Quinacrine crosses the placenta, with fetal drug levels approaching maternal levels. It is excreted very slowly through the kidneys. The drug may be detected in the urine for at least 2 months after therapy has been discontinued.

Indications

Treatment should be instituted for symptomatic infected individuals. There is some controversy as to whether asymptomatic cyst passers should receive treatment. Although clinically well, the potential exists for transmission of their infection to others, especially when the cyst passer is a food handler, a homosexual, or a child. Cyst passers may also develop intermittent chronic symptoms. For these reasons, most authors recommend treating *all* infected individuals as long as there are no contraindications to the use of available drugs.

Side Effects and Contraindications

Quinacrine is available in tablet form and has a bitter taste. Common side effects include nausea and vomiting (especially in young children), headache, dizziness, and insomnia. Quinacrine causes yellow discoloration of the urine and can cause yellow discoloration of the skin, which becomes fluorescent when exposed to ultraviolet light. This skin discoloration occurs in approximately 4 percent of patients treated for giardiasis. It appears 1 to 2 weeks after beginning therapy and persists for 2 to 8 weeks. More serious side effects are infrequent. A transient toxic psychosis has been reported in 1 to 2 percent of patients receiving quinacrine for giardiasis, and its use is contraindicated in those with a history of psychosis. Quinacrine rarely causes severe exfoliative dermatitis and is contraindicated for use in patients with psoriasis. It should not be given together with primaquine, since it displaces primaquine from tissue-binding sites, thereby increasing plasma primaquine levels and its toxicity. Since quinacrine concentrates in the liver, it should be given with caution to a patient with underlying hepatic disease. It should not be given to a pregnant patient because of the ability of quinacrine to cross the placenta. Mild hemolysis may be seen in patients with glucose-6-phosphate dehydrogenase deficiency.

Dosage and Administration

The recommended dose for adults and children older than 8 years of age is 100 milligrams twice a day for 5 days. For younger children, the dose is 2 milligrams/kilogram of body weight for 5 days (maximum, 300 mg/day).

METRONIDAZOLE (FLAGYL)

Recommended dosage of metronidazole for giardiasis in adults is 250 milligrams twice a day for 5 days, and in children 5 milligrams/kilogram of body weight twice a day for 5 days. (Metronidazole is reviewed more extensively in Chapter 17, Amebiasis.)

FURAZOLIDONE (FUROXONE)

Furazolidone is a nitrofuran derivative that interferes with various parasitic enzyme systems. It is active against *Giardia lamblia* as well as *Salmonella*, *Shigella*, and *Vibrio cholerae*. It is the only anti-Giardial drug formulated as an oral suspension, making it particularly useful in young children. Side effects are common and include nausea, vomiting, hypersensitivity reactions, and headache. Mild hemolysis may occur in the G-6-PD deficient patient. When combined with alcohol, furazolidone may cause a disulfiramlike reaction. It is a monoamine-oxidase inhibitor so caution should be used when given with other MAO inhibitors, tyramine-containing foods, and sympathomimetic amines. Metabolic degradation products of furazolidone may turn the urine brown. Animal studies have demonstrated increased incidence of lung tumors in mice and mammary neoplasia in rats. The recommended dosage for adults is 100 milligrams 4 times a day for 7 to 10 days, and for children, 1.25 milligrams/kilogram of body weight 4 times a day for 7 to 10 days.

SUMMARY

There is no ideal drug available for the treatment of giardiasis. Quinacrine is the drug of choice, but side effects are common and it is poorly tolerated in the pediatric population. Metronidazole is not approved in the United States for the treatment of giardiasis. It is generally better tolerated than quinacrine; however, there is concern for potential mutagenicity. Furazolidone is well tolerated, especially in the pediatric population. However, it is less effective than quinacrine or metronidazole and has potential carcinogenicity. None of the three drugs discussed is safe for use during pregnancy. Their use in the pregnant patient should be reserved for the situation in which symptoms from infection are severe and benefit outweighs potential risk.

PEARLS AND PITFALLS

1. Giardiasis is rarely associated with fever and bloody diarrhea, helping to distinguish it from bacterial dysentery and amebiasis.
2. Disaccharidase deficiency is commonly caused by *Giardia* and may persist for several weeks after treatment. Consider lactose intolerance in patients who continue to have excessive flatus, bloating, and foul stools after treatment for giardiasis.
3. In a patient who has taken quinacrine for giardiasis, yellow discoloration of the skin may be confused with hyperbilirubinemia. A Wood's lamp examination of the skin demonstrates a brilliant yellow-green fluorescence when discoloration is due to quinacrine.

Cryptosporidiosis

Cryptosporidium is a protozoan that originally was a well-recognized cause of enteritis only in domestic animals. In 1976, the first reported infection in humans occurred in an immunocompromised patient. Since the advent of AIDS, *Cryptosporidium* has become a well-recognized cause of enteritis. It is estimated that approximately 4 percent of patients with AIDS have cryptosporidium enteritis. In the immunocompromised patient, cryptosporidiosis is characterized by prolonged, severe, watery diarrhea, abdominal cramping, weight loss, anorexia, nausea, and myalgias. Conversely, in the immunocompetent patient, cryptosporidiosis presents as an acute, self-limited enteritis manifested by nausea, vomiting, abdominal cramping, anorexia, and watery, frothy bowel movements. Symptoms resolve within 10 to 14 days without therapy.

Unfortunately, there is no known effective therapy for the immunocompromised patient with cryptosporidiosis. Promising anecdotal reports using spiramycin have been published. Currently underway is a multicenter, controlled clinical trial using spiramycin for the treatment of cryptosporidiosis in patients with AIDS. Spiramycin is not available in the United States except from the Food and Drug Administration, phone number (301) 443–4310.

References

GIARDIASIS

1. Abramowicz M (ed.). Drugs for Parasitic Infections. *Medical Letter* 1988; 759:15.

    Recommended drugs and dosages for most parasitic infections.

2. Bassily S, et al. The treatment of *Giardia lamblia* infection with mepacrine, metronidazole, and furazolidone. J Trop Med Hyd 1970; 73:15.

    A comparative study of drug therapy for giardiasis in 80 Egyptian adults. Quinacrine cured 100%, metronidazole 95%, and furazolidone 80%.

3. Craft JC, Murphy T, Nelson JD. Furazolidone and quinacrine. Am J Dis Child 1981; 135:164.

    A comparative study of therapy for giardiasis in children.

4. Gorski ED. Management of giardiasis. Am Fam Phys 1985; 32:157.

    A practical, clinically oriented review of *G. lamblia* infection.

5. Holtan NR. Giardiasis. Postgrad Med J 1988; 83:54.

    An excellent review of Giardiasis focusing on diagnosis, treatment, and prevention.

6. James JJ, et al. Quinacrine-induced toxic psychosis in a child. Pediatr Infect Dis J 1987; 6:427.

    A case report of quinacrine-induced toxic psychosis in a child treated for giardiasis.

7. Lerman SJ, Walker RA. Treatment of giardiasis. Clin Pediatr 1982; 21:409.

    A review of the administration, efficacy, and toxicity of quinacrine, metronidazole, and furazolidone.

8. Murphy TV, Nelson JD. Five- versus ten days' therapy with furazolidone for giardiasis. Am J Dis Child 1983; 137:267.

    A prospective, randomized trial of 22 children with giardiasis demonstrating that 5-day therapy for most children is inadequate.

9. Smith JW. Giardiasis. Ann Rev Med 1980; 31:373.

    A review of giardiasis, with a focus on diagnosis and treatment.

10. Tanenbaum L, Tuffanelli DL. Antimalarial agents, chloroquine, hydroxychloroquine, and quinacrine. Arch Dermatol 1980; 116:587.

The pharmacokinetics, mechanism of action, and toxicity of quinacrine are reviewed.
11. Wolfe MS. Giardiasis. JAMA 1975; 233:1362.
A clinically oriented review of giardiasis.

CRYPTOSPORIDIOSIS

1. Meisel JL, et al. Overwhelming watery diarrhea associated with a *Cryptosporidium* in an immunosuppressed patient. Gastroenterology 1976; 70:1156.
    The first reported case of cryptosporidiosis in humans.
2. Portnoy D, et al. Treatment of intestinal cryptospiridiosis with spiramycin. Ann Intern Med 1984; 101:202.
    A study of 10 patients treated with spiramycin. After 1 week of therapy, five patients had resolution of diarrhea and four patients had symptomatic improvement. One patient required 30 days of treatment for resolution of diarrhea.
3. Quinn TC. Clinical approach to intestinal infections in homosexual men. Med Clin N Am 1986; 70:611.
    A practical, clinically oriented review.
4. Soave R. Cryptosporidiosis and isosporiasis in patients with AIDS. Infec Dis Clin N Am 1988; 2:485.
    An excellent clinically oriented review.

Amebiasis

Marsha G. Pierdinock

Approximately 10 percent of the world's population is infected with *Entamoeba histolytica*. In the United States the prevalence is about 5 percent. At greatest risk are those in areas of poor sanitation, in institutions, and in the homosexual population. The spectrum of infection ranges from asymptomatic cyst passers, through mild or moderate intestinal amebiases and amebic dysentery, to disseminated amebiases with liver or other tissue abscesses. The choice of medication depends on the stage of infection. Drug selection is further dependent on availability: Several amebicidal drugs are either unavailable in the United States or obtainable only from the Centers for Disease Control. Fortunately, metronidazole and iodoquinol, which are the drugs of first choice for all types of amebic infections, are well tolerated and relatively easy to obtain.

Metronidazole (Flagyl)

Metronidazole is a synthetic 5-nitronimidazole compound that is amebicidal at both the intestinal mucosa and extraintestinal sites. The mechanism of action of metronidazole is not fully understood. It is believed that metronidazole enters the pathogenic protozoa where it undergoes reduction and activation. Short-lived toxic intermediate products are thought to bind to and damage DNA. These are quickly metabolized to inactive end products.

PHARMACOKINETICS

Metronidazole achieves excellent and rapid absorption after oral administration, achieving peak plasma concentrations in 1 to 2 hours. Absorption is delayed when taken with food, but total bioavailability is unchanged. The serum half-life is approximately 7 hours and serum levels are proportionate to the dose administered. Metronidazole is lipid-soluble and has a large volume of distribution, achieving excellent tissue penetration, including good levels in the cerebrospinal fluid.

Metronidazole is metabolized in the liver. The kidneys excrete approximately 77 percent of the dose given as both intact metronidazole and its metabolites. Fourteen percent is eliminated from the feces and the remainder presumed to be degraded in the body.

INDICATIONS

Metronidazole is the drug of choice for mild to moderate intestinal amebiases, severe amebic dysentery, and amebic abscesses. Therapy with metronidazole should always be followed by the luminally active drug iodoquinol to eradi-

Table 17–1. Treatment of choice in infections of *Entamoeba hystolytica*

Severity of infection	Drug of choice	Adult dose
Asymptomatic cyst passer	Iodoquinol	650 mg po tid × 20 days
Mild to severe intestinal disease or hepatic abscess	Metronidazole followed by iodoquinol	750 mg po tid × 10 days 650 mg po tid × 20 days

Adapted from Abramowicz, M (ed.) Drugs for parasitic infections. *Medical Letter*, 1988; 759:15.

cate trophozoites and cysts within the intestinal lumen, thereby preventing relapse. The treatment regimens are summarized in Table 17–1. These regimens should cure 95 percent or more of cases.

SIDE EFFECTS AND CONTRAINDICATIONS

The most common side effects of metronidazole are related to the gastrointestinal tract. Nausea, vomiting, and a metallic taste occur in 5 to 10 percent of patients. Other, less common reactions include burning of the tongue, rash, vaginal and urethral burning, reversible neutropenia, and dark urine. Central nervous system toxicity is rare but more serious. Peripheral neuropathy (characterized primarily by numbness or paresthesias), seizure, encephalopathy, and cerebellar dysfunction have been reported. These effects are rare unless high doses or prolonged therapy is used. If abnormal neurologic symptoms are observed, the medication should be discontinued immediately. Isolated cases of metronidazole-induced pancreatitis and gynecomastia have been published.

Metronidazole is structurally similar to antabuse and may cause a disulfiramlike reaction when alcohol is imbibed. Additionally, metronidazole may potentiate the effect of warfarin by inhibiting its metabolism. When warfarin is given concomitantly, the dose should be reduced and the prothrombin time followed closely.

Metronidazole has been shown to be mutagenic in some bacteria and lung cancer has occurred in mice with long-term use. The risk of cancer in patients receiving standard short courses of metronidazole is negligible. However, further studies are needed to fully evaluate the potential teratogenicity of metronidazole in humans when used on a long-term basis. Metronidazole has been used without adverse outcome in pregnancy but routine use in gestational patients is discouraged, especially in the first trimester, because of the concern for teratogenicity. In patients with chronic liver disease, especially in the presence of concurrent impaired renal function, plasma clearance of metronidazole is decreased. Dosage reduction may be required and it is advisable to monitor serum drug levels.

DOSAGE AND ADMINISTRATION

The dosages for the various phases of amebic infections are summarized in Table 17–1. For patients unable to take metronidazole orally, a parenteral preparation is available. It should be given as a loading dose of 15 milligrams/kilogram infused over 1 hour, followed by 7.5 milligrams/kilogram every 6 hours. Alternative regimens include emetine, 1 milligram/kilogram/day, or dehydroemetine, 1 to 1.5 milligram/kilogram/day intramuscularly for 5 days. The emetines have frequent adverse side effects, the most serious of which are mycardial depression and rhythm disturbances. They should always be considered second-line drugs and used with great caution.

Patients should be advised not to take alcohol while taking metronidazole. If a patient is taking warfarin, the dose should be reduced and the prothrombin time closely monitored. Dosage adjustment is not usually required in patients with renal impairment, but if significant concomitant liver disease exists, dose reduction is advisable.

Iodoquinol

Iodoquinol (diidohydroxyquin) is a halogenated oxyquinole that is amebicidal against both trophozoites and cysts. The mechanism of action is unknown. It is poorly absorbed from the gastrointestinal tract and therefore is not effective in extraintestinal amebiases. Side effects are uncommon and include diarrhea, abdominal pain, and rash. Iodoquinol contains 64 percent organically bound iodine and can interfere with thyroid function testing or cause iodine dermatitis. It is contraindicated in patients with iodine intolerance or hepatic disease.

A related drug, iodochlorhydroxyquin, is readily absorbed and can lead to a syndrome of subacute myelo-optic neuropathy. This compound is no longer available in the United States. In doses recommended for the treatment of intestinal amebiasis, iodoquinol has not been shown to cause optic atrophy, although it has been reported with long-term use in large doses.

An alternative to iodoquinol is diloxanide furanoate, which is only available from the Centers for Disease Control. It is effective in eliminating intraluminal amebae in over 90 percent of patients. The dose regimen is 500 milligrams 3 times daily for 10 days. It is well tolerated, with the primary complaint being an increase in flatulence.

PEARLS AND PITFALLS

1. Serologic testing for amebiasis may remain positive up to 20 years after initial infection. This should be considered when interpreting a positive test.
2. Bismuth, barium, gallbladder dye, kaolin, nonabsorbable antacids, and antibiotics may interfere with stool examination for amebiases.

3. Ulcerative colitis and amebiases may appear identical on barium enema or proctosigmoidoscopy. Amebic serologic testing and stool examination are critical to distinguish between the two conditions, as corticosteroids exacerbate amebic colitis.
4. Due to the disulfiramlike reaction when metronidazole is combined with alcohol, patients should avoid *all* products with alcohol. These include many cough syrups, mouthwashes, liquid medications, paint solvents, and foods prepared with alcohol or liqueurs.
5. For further information regarding drug therapy, contact the Parasitic Disease Division of the Centers for Disease Control, Atlanta, GA 30333; (404) 329–3670.

References

1. Abramowicz M (ed.). Drugs for parasitic infections. *Medical Letter* 1988; 759:150.
   The recommended drugs and dosages for most parasitic infections.
2. Fagan TC, Hohnson DG, Gross DS. Metronidazole-induced gynecomastia. JAMA 1985; 254:3217.
   A case report of Metronidazole-induced gynecomastia 4 weeks after induction of metronidazole. Rechallenge led to breast tenderness within 3 weeks.
3. Finegold SM. Metronidazole. Ann Int Med 1980; 93:585.
   A general review of metronidazole use.
4. Finegold SM, Mathisen GE. Metronidazole in the treatment of anaerobic bacterial infections. Curr Clin Top Inf Dis 1985; 6:156.
   An excellent review of the pharmacokinetics, spectrum of activity, and clinical use of metronidazole.
5. Plotnick BH, et al. Metronidazole-induced pancreatis. Ann Int Med 1985; 196:891.
   A case report of metronidazole-induced pancreatitis 4 days after institution of metronidazole. Rechallenge led to recurrent pancreatitis.
6. Scully BE. Metronidazole. Med Clin N Am 1988; 72:613.
   Practical applications for the use of metronidazole.
7. Wolfe MS. Treatment of intestinal protozoan infections. Med Clin N Am 1988; 66:707.
   A practical, clinically oriented review of intestinal protozoan infections.

18

Intestinal Nematodes

David G. Litaker

Infection with gastrointestinal nematodes represents a major public health concern both in developed and developing nations throughout the world. It has been estimated that between one and two billion people are infected with *Ascaris lumbricoides,* hookworm, *Trichuris trichiura,* and *Strongyloides stercoralis.* It is fortunate, therefore, that most anthelminthics available today have a broad range of action and can be used as single agents in the patient with multiple parasite infections (Table 18–1). The focus of this chapter is the treatment of intestinal nematodes commonly encountered in the United States, the common elements of their life cycles, and the mechanisms of action of the drugs employed to eradicate these infections.

Ascaris lumbricoides

Infection with roundworm in humans follows the ingestion of an embryonated egg, usually found in fecally contaminated food or soil. Eggs hatch in the intestine and mature into larvae, which penetrate the intestinal wall and migrate to the capillary beds of the lung. Further migration from the pulmonary parenchyma, up the trachea, and back into the gastrointestinal tract completes the maturation cycle.

Although individuals of any age can be infected by ascarides, children are more commonly heavily parasitized. The common manifestations in affected individuals are due to obstruction of the intestinal or biliary tracts, the pulmonary migration phase (Loeffler's syndrome), or nutritional deficiencies caused by the parasite. The diagnosis of ascariasis is based on microscopic fecal examination and is not difficult due to the prolific egg production in the intestinal tract by mature adult worms.

The treatment of choice is mebendazole, 100 milligrams twice a day for 3 days. Mebendazole is a broad-spectrum anthelmintic agent of the benzimidazole family, which is structurally related to thiabendazole. It is poorly absorbed from the gastrointestinal tract and thus has few systemic side effects except for diarrhea and abdominal pain. The latter symptom may be related to the worm burden and is infrequently observed in mild infections.

Mebendazole selectively and irreversibly blocks glucose uptake by the worm and leads to endogenous depletion of glycogen stores. In addition, cytoplasmic microtubular deterioration has been observed by electron microscopy and results in the accumulation of secretory granules, cytoplasmic lysis, and death of the organism.

Alternatives to mebendazole include a single dose of pyrantel pamoate (11 mgs/kg with a 1-gram maximum dose) or piperazine citrate (75 mgs/kg with a 3.5-gram maximum dose daily for 2 days). Pyrantel is a compound of the ami-

Table 18–1. Efficacy of broad-spectrum anthelminthics

Infection	Mebendazole	Pyrantel pamoate	Thiabendazole	Piperazine citrate
Ascaris	***	***	**	***
Hookworm	***	**	**	*
Strongyloides	*	—	**	—
Trichuris	**	—	*	—

— < 30% cured
* 30–60% cured
** 60–85% cured
*** > 85% cured

dine group and is minimally absorbed from the intestine. It inhibits neuromuscular transmission and results in spastic paralysis of the worm. This drug is well tolerated and has not been associated with toxic side effects. Piperazine citrate is one of the oldest anthelmintic drugs still in use. Unlike the other two drugs used in the treatment of ascariasis, piperazine is readily absorbed from the intestines and acts by blocking acetylcholine in the myoneural junctions of the helminths, producing a flaccid paralysis and facilitating the removal of the worm by normal peristalsis. Piperazine is especially useful in cases in which intestinal or biliary obstruction is suspected. Use of mebendazole under these circumstances has been associated with migration of the parasite and the onset of bothersome symptoms. Piperazine citrate is well tolerated and has been associated with few side effects. With accidental overdosages, however, ataxia, vertigo, confusion, muscular weakness and uncoordination, and myoclonic contractions have been observed. Piperazine is known to lower the seizure threshold in epileptic patients and should be used with caution in this setting. Current recommendations limit the use of this drug to nonpregnant patients as well as those with normal hepatic and renal function.

Trichuris trichiura

Humans are the principal hosts for this infection, which is directly transmitted by the ingestion of eggs. Larval forms hatch in the upper duodenum and attach to the intestinal villi. Following maturation, the worm migrates to the colon without a tissue invasion phase, embeds in the mucosa, and produces eggs.

Despite its highest prevalence in the humid tropics, trichuriasis remains an important public health problem in rural areas of the United States. Soil pollution is the determining factor in the prevalence and intensity of infection in a community and represents an important focus of disease control. As with ascariasis, children between five and 15 years of age are affected with the heaviest worm burdens.

Trichuriasis is typically a clinically silent disease. It has, however, been associated with anorexia, diarrhea, abdominal pain, and weight loss. Rectal prolapse, frequently a result of particularly heavy infestation, is also associated with this disease and is thought to be a result of prolonged colonic inflammation. Unlike infections with hookworm, blood loss due to *T. trichiura* is usually insignificant.

The preferred treatment of this disease combines the use of mebendazole (100 mgs twice daily for 3 days) and improved community sanitation. In some instances, compliance with this treatment schedule has been poor and is currently being replaced with a single dose of 500 milligrams, which has reported cure rates ranging from 93 to 100 percent. Side effects associated with single-dose therapy do not differ significantly from those of the traditional regimen.

Hookworm

Hookworm disease is an infection of the small intestine caused by either *Ancylostoma duodenale* or *Necator americanus*. The life cycle of both organisms is identical and involves penetration of the skin by a filariform larva following prolonged skin–soil contact (5–10 minutes is sufficient). The larvae are carried by the circulation to the lungs and, similar to *Ascaris,* penetrate the alveolar wall, migrate up the trachea, are swallowed, and attach to the intestinal mucosa where further maturation and egg production occur.

The primary geographic areas of hookworm infection are the tropical and subtropical zones. As a result of relatively effective eradication programs, it is not thought to be a major source of medical concern in the United States, even though it is known to persist in the rural Southeast. Unlike other intestinal parasites, hookworm affects adults as well as children. The main epidemiologic factor responsible for the transmission of the disease remains contact with soil contaminated by human feces.

Although the failure to reinfect oneself through repeated contact with contaminated soil may result in a cure over several years, treatment with either mebendazole or pyrantel pamoate produces a cure in 76 to 96 percent of cases. As with *Trichuris* infections, single-dose mebendazole (500 mgs) has been shown effective at producing high cure rates, although its use may be limited to less heavily parasitized individuals. Dosages for treatment and mechanisms of action of both mebendazole and pyrantel pamoate are the same for hookworm as for the intestinal nematodes described above.

Strongyloides stercoralis

The life cycle of *S. stercoralis* is similar to the hookworm in all respects but one: The rhabditiform larva in expelled feces can directly invade the skin of the host as well as penetrate the intestine or perianal skin, without maturation or additional developmental stages in the external environment. As a result, infection can persist in the absence of repeated exposure and need not be associated with direct contact with contaminated soil.

Strongyloidiasis occurs predominately in Southeast Asia and Africa. Host contact with infective feces and warm, moist soil providing an optimal environment for free-living larvae represent the two most important factors in the transmission of the disease. It occurs in hosts of any age, in a prevalence pattern similar to that of hookworm. Due to the organisms' ability to persist in the host, widespread dissemination of the disease to developed nations has been possible as well. In the United States, former prisoners of war of both Vietnam and World War II have been demonstrated to carry the organism undiagnosed for as long as 40 years. In the United States, the overall incidence of infection in the general population is 1 to 2 percent and as high as 5 percent in rural areas.

The drug of choice in the treatment of *S. stercoralis* is thiabendazole, a benzimidazole derivative that is rapidly absorbed and excreted in the urine. The mechanism of action is not well understood but may involve inhibition of the parasite-specific enzyme fumarate reductase. Standard treatment with 25 milligrams/kilogram twice a day (with a maximum of 3 gms/day) for 2 days is frequently complicated by the onset of side effects, which include dizziness, nausea, vomiting, anorexia, and diarrhea. Bradycardia, hypotension, erythema multiforme, and Stevens–Johnson syndrome have been reported but fortunately occur on a rare basis. Prolonged therapy is usually required in patients with hyperinfestations (generally those receiving immunosuppressives or those with debilitating disease) due to relatively larger parasite burdens. Alternatives to thiabendazole include mebendazole and pyrantel pamoate, but their use has been restricted due to reports of limited efficacy.

PEARLS AND PITFALLS

1. Hyperinfection with *S. Stercoralis* should be considered in any patient with polymicrobial sepsis. Ideally, patients from endemic areas should be screened for strongyloidiasis before receiving immunosuppressives.
2. Migration of *A. lumbricoides* has been reported following treatment with both mebendazole and thiabendazole but can be avoided by pretreatment with piperazine citrate.
3. It is important to monitor patients receiving theophylline for signs of toxicity while receiving thiabendazole because of altered pharmacodynamics due to competition for metabolism in the liver.

References

1. Berk SL, et al. Clinical and epidemiologic features of strongyloidiasis: A prospective study in rural Tennessee. Arch Intern Med 1987; 147:1257–1261.

    The incidence of *S. stercoralis* was studied in hospitalized and domiciliary patients (N = 575). Infected patients, composing 6.1% and 2.9%, respectively, were found to have a higher incidence of eosinophilia, heme positive stools, and complaints of abdominal bloating. A relapse rate of 15% was noted in patients treated with standard thiabendazole therapy.

2. Botero D. Chemotherapy of human intestinal parasitic diseases. Ann Rev Pharmacol Toxicol 1978; 18:1–15.

    The author outlines the nature of the public health problem represented by infection with gastrointestinal parasites, along with the rationale for therapy and the proposed mechanisms of action of each of the drugs.

3. Evans AC, Hollmann AW, DuPreez L. Mebendazole, 500 milligrams, for single-dose treatment of nematode infestation. So Afr Med J 1987; 72:665–667.

The results of a study using single-dose mebendazole in 217 children with mixed helminth infections are reported. The endpoints of therapy were reduction of egg production in the stool and total cure. The authors note the fact that the drug was well tolerated and that its use as a public health tool was enhanced by its acceptability.

4. Genta RM, et al. Strongyloidiasis in U.S. veterans of the Vietnam and other wars. JAMA 1987; 258:49–52.

The prevalence of strongyloidiasis among American veterans was evaluated by an ELISA method and correlated with stool specimen examination. The authors stress the importance of screening this population for *S. stercoralis* and initiating therapy with thiabendazole if positive results are obtained—before treatment with immunosuppressives.

5. Keystone JS, Murdoch JK. Mebendazole: Diagnosis and treatment drugs five years later. Ann Int Med 1979; 91:582–586.

This excellent review article outlines the history of mebendazole, its mechanism of action, pharmacology, application, and side effects.

19

Chemoprophylaxis of Traveler's Diarrhea

Lee R. Mandel

Diarrhea is the most common health problem encountered when traveling from low-risk parts of the world to developing countries. Chemoprophylaxis of traveler's diarrhea using antimicrobial agents dates back to studies published in the early 1960s. It was not until 1975, however, that it was demonstrated that a great proportion of cases of traveler's diarrhea are caused by enterotoxigenic *Escherichia coli* (ETEC). This organism has been isolated from 40 to 70 percent of cases of traveler's diarrhea. ETEC can produce a heat-stabile toxin, a heat-labile toxin, or both. Strains that contain both heat-labile and heat-stabile toxins are the most virulent ones, and they have been shown to possess colonization factor antigens. These colonization factor antigens have been identified as pili or fimbria that allow the organisms to adhere to the small bowel mucosa.

The next most frequent organism isolated is *Shigella,* followed by *Salmonella, Campylobacter,* rotaviruses, and *Giardia.* Overall, bacterial agents are responsible for about 80 percent of cases of traveler's diarrhea. Several agents have been found to be effective in preventing traveler's diarrhea and these agents are discussed below.

Trimethoprim-Sulfamethoxazole

Several studies have been done, involving students from the United States traveling to Mexico. They were enrolled in double-blinded, placebo-controlled trials shortly after arrival in Mexico. In one trial, study subjects were given trimethoprim-sulfamethoxazole (TMP/SMX), 160 milligrams/800 milligrams twice daily for 21 days, versus a group given placebo. Sixteen percent of the TMP/SMX group developed diarrhea, versus 55 percent of the placebo group. The percentage of protection, defined as [(percentage ill with placebo minus percentage ill with active drug) divided by percentage ill with placebo] times 100, was 71 percent in the study group.

In another trial using TMP-SMX, 160 milligrams/800 milligrams once daily for 14 days, versus placebo, only 2 percent of study patients developed diarrhea. Expressed as percent-protection, the study group achieved a rate of 95 percent.

MECHANISM OF ACTION AND PHARMACOLOGY

Trimethoprim-sulfamethoxazole works by blocking two steps in the biosynthesis of the nucleic acids and proteins essential to many bacteria. Trimethoprim inhibits the enzyme dihydrofolate reductase, and thus blocks the conversion of dihydrofolic acid to tetrahydrofolic acid. Sulfamethoxazole inhibits synthesis of dihydrofolic acid by competing with para-aminobenzoic acid. Most strains of enterotoxigenic *Escherichia coli,* including those producing both heat-stabile and heat-labile toxins, are susceptible to TMP/SMX. Although resistance to ETEC has occurred, it is rare. TMP/SMX is also active against other enteric pathogens such as *Shigella* and possibly *Salmonella*.

TMP/SMX is rapidly absorbed following oral administration, with peak blood levels for each component occurring after 1 to 4 hours. The mean serum half-life of each component is approximately 10 hours. Because TMP/SMX is excreted primarily by the kidneys, dosages must be decreased in cases of severe renal insufficiency.

DOSAGE AND ADMINISTRATION

The dosage for adequate chemoprophylaxis of traveler's diarrhea using TMP/SMX is 160 milligrams/800 milligrams (one double-strength tablet) daily. The drug must be continued, beyond the period of exposure, for 1 to 2 days after returning home.

SIDE EFFECTS

Up to 5 percent of people taking TMP/SMX prophylactically have developed generalized cutaneous eruptions. The gut flora of most people taking TMP/SMX prophylactically will develop resistance to TMP/SMX during the period of drug administration. More severe reactions, such as the Stevens-Johnson syndrome and antibiotic-associated colitis, may occur rarely.

Doxycycline

The efficacy of doxycycline in preventing traveler's diarrhea has been extensively studied in regions where most of the ETEC isolated were sensitive to antibiotics, and in regions of the world where antibiotic-resistant ETEC is known to be common. These studies involved U.S. Peace Corps volunteers who had recently arrived in endemic areas. They were treated with doxycycline, 100 milligrams daily for 21 days. The percent-protection achieved in areas where the ETEC were sensitive to antibiotics was approximately 85 percent. The percent-protection achieved in areas where antibiotic resistance to ETEC was known to be common was approximately 64 percent.

In all of the studies, the effect of the doxycycline lasted only as long as the drug was taken. At the end of the 3-week period of doxycycline prophylaxis, the study patients were as susceptible to traveler's diarrhea as were patients in the placebo groups at the beginning of the studies. It has been noted that for people taking doxycycline who developed diarrhea, episodes were less severe in terms of the number of stools per day and length of illness, when compared to people taking placebo.

MECHANISM OF ACTION AND PHARMACOLOGY

Doxycycline is synthetically derived from oxytetracycline. Its antimicrobial effect is believed to result from inhibition of protein synthesis. Most strains of ETEC are susceptible to doxycycline. High levels of doxycycline are secreted into the small bowel, where ETEC colonization occurs. After oral administration, doxycycline is virtually completely absorbed, and reaches peak serum levels in about 2 hours. The serum half-life of doxycycline is approximately 20 hours. There is no significant difference in serum half-life in people with normal and severely decreased renal function.

DOSAGE AND ADMINISTRATION

The dosage for adequate chemoprophylaxis of traveler's diarrhea using doxycycline is 100 milligrams daily. The drug must be continued, beyond the period of exposure, for 1 to 2 days after returning home.

SIDE EFFECTS

The incidence of side effects from doxycycline therapy is less than 1 percent. The side effects include candidial overgrowth, photosensitivity, and gastrointestinal symptoms such as nausea and vomiting. Doxycycline can interfere with tooth development during the last half of pregnancy, infancy, and early childhood; consequently, it is contraindicated in pregnant women and children below the age of eight.

Bismuth Subsalicylate

In 1980, DuPont et al. studied the effect of taking a liquid bismuth subsalicylate preparation prophylactically to prevent traveler's diarrhea in a group of U.S. students arriving in Mexico. The study group received 60 milliliters of a 1.75-percent bismuth subsalicylate solution orally 4 times a day (4.2 gms of active drug per day) for 21 days, as compared to a placebo group. Diarrhea illness developed in 23 percent of the study group, compared to 61 percent of the placebo group. Overall, the percent-protection afforded by bismuth subsalicylate in preventing traveler's diarrhea was 62 percent.

In 1987, DuPont et al. studied the efficacy of bismuth subsalicylate tablets in preventing traveler's diarrhea. They studied a similar subject population of U.S. students arriving in Mexico. One study group received two tablets of bismuth subsalicylate 4 times daily, another group received one tablet of bismuth subsalicylate 4 times daily, and the third group received placebo tablets 4 times daily. Each bismuth subsalicylate tablet contained 262 milligrams of active drug. The study period ran for 3 weeks. In the high-dose bismuth subsalicylate study group (who received 2.1 gms/day of active drug), the percent-protection afforded against traveler's diarrhea was 65 percent. In the low-dose bismuth subsalicylate group (who received 1.05 gms/day of active drug), the percent-protection was 40 percent.

MECHANISM OF ACTION AND PHARMACOLOGY

The mechanism of bismuth subsalicylate in preventing traveler's diarrhea is not exactly known. It has been demonstrated that the drug effectively neutralizes the diarrheagenic effects of crude toxins of *E. coli* and *V. cholerae*. This action is felt to be due to the subsalicylate moiety. Bismuth subsalicylate is thought to possibly interfere with the action of the colonization factor antigens of ETEC in facilitating adherence to the bowel epithelium.

DOSAGE AND ADMINISTRATION

Bismuth subsalicylate, which is most commonly marketed as Pepto-Bismol, has been shown to be effective in the dosage of 60 milligrams orally 4 times a day. The tablet formation has been shown to be effective in a dosage of two tablets orally 4 times a day.

SIDE EFFECTS

The most common side effects of bismuth subsalicylate are darkening of the tongue and stool. Mild tinnitus has been reported in study groups taking the medication. In addition, mild nausea and constipation have also been described.

Norfloxacin

Norfloxacin is the first fluoroquinolone antimicrobial agent released for clinical use in the United States. All known gastrointestinal bacterial pathogens have been shown to be susceptible to norfloxacin. It has been demonstrated to be extremely effective in eliminating the aerobic bacterial flora of the stool, without affecting the anaerobic flora or selecting resistant organisms. High concentrations of norfloxacin are obtained in the stool.

In a recent double-blinded study, norfloxacin was used prophylactically for traveler's diarrhea in U.S. subjects going to Mexico. Sixty-one percent of patients treated with placebo developed diarrhea, compared to only 7 percent of patients who received norfloxacin, 400 milligrams daily. The percent-protection afforded was 89 percent.

MECHANISM OF ACTION AND PHARMACOLOGY

Norfloxacin works by inhibiting bacterial DNA gyrase. The enzyme is necessary for DNA replication, gene transcription, and aspects of DNA repair and recombination. DNA gyrase is antagonized by nalidixic acid, norfloxacin, and other quinolone agents. Norfloxacin is rapidly absorbed after oral dosing, with peak serum concentrations reached in 1 to 2 hours. The effective half-life in serum and plasma is 3 to 4 hours. With severe renal impairment patients, the dosage of norfloxacin must be reduced.

DOSAGE AND ADMINISTRATION

There has been limited usage of norfloxacin for prophylaxis of traveler's diarrhea. However, an oral dosage of 400 milligrams daily has been shown to be effective in at least two studies.

SIDE EFFECTS

The incidence of side effects from norfloxacin appears to be low and the drug is well tolerated. The most frequent side effect described is nausea, and, less commonly, light-headedness. However, most reported studies citing side effects have involved norfloxacin in therapeutic doses of 400 milligrams twice daily.

Final Recommendations

Most experts do not recommend routine chemoprophylaxis against traveler's diarrhea for every traveler entering an endemic area. The risk of developing traveler's diarrhea when going from low- to high-risk areas (approximately 40%) must be weighed against the known risk of potential side effects when chemoprophylaxis is employed. Groups of travelers who should be considered for chemoprophylaxis when traveling to high-risk areas are

1. people on short, critical business trips;
2. people with underlying health problems that may increase their susceptibility to diarrhea (such as achlorhydria or known gastric resection);
3. people in whom there is the increased likelihood of complications secondary to dehydration from diarrhea;
4. military personnel; and
5. people who are taking much-needed and hard-earned vacations, honeymoon couples, and other people in similar situations.

Chemoprophylaxis against traveler's diarrhea is not recommended when the period of risk will exceed 2 weeks. If chemoprophylaxis is used, it should continue, beyond the period of exposure, for 1 or 2 days after leaving the high-risk area.

PEARLS AND PITFALLS

1. The mainstays of preventive therapy are careful attention to food and beverage selection in high-risk areas. The

traveler in these areas should avoid uncooked foods, unwashed salads, unpeeled fruits, and unboiled tap water, including ice.
2. Most experts recommend against routine prophylaxis. Instead, when mild symptoms of traveler's diarrhea develop (1–3 loose stools per 24 hours and no associated symptoms), oral rehydration is adequate. For more pronounced symptoms (3–5 loose stools per 24 hours and more notable but not disabling symptoms) the patient can be treated with bismuth subsalicylate, 30 mls every 30 minutes for eight doses, or an opiate drug such as loperamide, 4 mgs followed by 2 mgs after each unformed passed stool, up to 16 mgs/day. For severe traveler's diarrhea, TMP/SMX, one double-strength tablet twice daily for 3 to 5 days, is effective. Alternatives include doxycycline, 100 milligrams twice a day for 5 days; ciprofloxacin, 500 milligrams twice a day for 5 days; or furazolidone, 100 milligrams 4 times a day for adults, and 1.25 milligrams/kilogram for children. (See the furazolidone section under *Giardia* in Chapter 16 for further details).
3. The opiate derivatives diphenoxylate and loperamide hydrochloride are both effective antiperistaltic agents used in treating mild traveler's diarrhea. Loperamide is the preferred drug, as it does not cross the blood–brain barrier and has a lower incidence of side effects.
4. Because many areas of high risk for traveler's diarrhea are also areas of high risk for hepatitis A, travelers are recommended to receive immune serum globulin prior to arrival in these endemic areas.
5. Areas of high risk for traveler's diarrhea include Latin America, Africa, the Middle East, and Asia. Low-risk areas include Northern Europe, Canada, New Zealand, Puerto Rico, the Bahamas, and the Virgin Islands.

References

1. Consensus Conference. Travelers' diarrhea. JAMA 1985; 253:2700–2704.
   A review of the etiologies and therapies of traveler's diarrhea, and recommendations for prophylaxis by a panel of experts convened by the National Institutes of Health.
2. DuPont HL. Nonfluid therapy and selected chemoprophylaxis of acute diarrhea. Am J Med 1985; 79(suppl 6B):81–90.
   A detailed review of the etiologies, treatment, and prophylaxis of traveler's diarrhea.
3. DuPont HL, Ericsson CD, Johnson PC. Chemotherapy and chemoprophylaxis of traveler's diarrhea. Ann Intern Med 1985; 109:260–261.
   A brief review of chemoprophylaxis of traveler's diarrhea.
4. DuPont HL, et al. Prevention of traveler's diarrhea: Prophylactic administration of subsalicylate bismuth. JAMA 1980; 243:237–241.
   A study documenting the efficacy of bismuth subsalicylate solution in preventing traveler's diarrhea.

5. DuPont, et al. Antimicrobial agents in the prevention of traveler's diarrhea. Rev Infect Dis 1986; 8(suppl 2):167–171.

   A review of four major studies comparing the effects of trimethaprim-sulfa methoxazole, trimethoprim, norfloxacin, and bicozamycin in preventing traveler's diarrhea.

6. DuPont HL, et al. Prevention of traveler's diarrhea by the tablet formulation of bismuth subsalicylate. JAMA 1987; 257:1347–1350.

   A study of chemoprophylaxis of traveler's diarrhea that demonstrated the effectiveness of bismuth subsalicylate tablets.

7. Gorbach SL, et al. Traveler's diarrhea and toxigenic *Escherichia coli*. NEJM 1975; 292:933–936.

   The first study demonstrating that a high percentage of cases of traveler's diarrhea are caused by enterotoxigenic *E. coli*.

8. Johnson PC, et al. Lack of emergence of resistant fecal flora during successful prophylaxis of traveler's diarrhea with norfloxacin. Antimicrob Ag Chemo 1986; 30:671–674.

   A double-blind study demonstrating a percent-protection rate of 89 percent using norfloxacin, 400 mgs daily for 14 days.

9. Kean BH. The diarrhea of travelers to Mexico: Summary of five-year study. Ann Intern Med 1963; 59:605–614.

   An overview of a 5-year investigation that documented the effectiveness of phthalysulfathiazole and neomycin in preventing traveler's diarrhea.

10. Sack RB. Antimicrobial prophylaxis of traveler's diarrhea: A selected summary. Rev Infect Dis 1986; 8(suppl 2):160–166.

    A review of the major studies documenting the efficacy of doxycycline prophylaxis on traveler's diarrhea.

11. Wolfson JS, Hooper DC. Norfloxacin: A new targeted fluoroquinolone antimicrobial agent. Ann Intern Med 1988; 108:238–251.

    A comprehensive review of norfloxacin, including its potential use in preventing traveler's diarrhea.

20

Ciprofloxacin

John Malone

Fluoroquinolones, a new class of antibiotics related to nalidixic acid, have been developed through side chain modification of the basic 4-quinolone ring. Ciprofloxacin's cyclopropyl group on position-1 leads to increased tissue penetration and an enlarged bactericidal spectrum compared to norfloxacin, a related fluoroquinolone.

Due to excellent activity against many common aerobic gram-negative bacteria and high tissue levels in the gastrointestinal tract, ciprofloxacin is rapidly becoming recognized as a most effective agent against susceptible enteric pathogens.

MECHANISM OF ACTION

Ciprofloxacin's bactericidal action involves inhibition of bacterial DNA gyrase. This enzyme reduces the size of bacterial DNA by supercoiling and imposing a second reverse twist on the DNA helix. This compresses the DNA, allowing placement within the bacteria. Bacterial gyrase inhibition results in relaxation of the supercoiled DNA, with rapid cessation of cell division. Rupture and cell lysis are observed in gram-negative bacteria, while staphylococci become enlarged. Other antibacterial mechanisms are also possible.

PHARMACOLOGY

Besides possessing excellent bactericidal capability against many gram-negative bacteria, in vivo effectiveness in enteric infections is related to high drug levels in the gastrointestinal tract. Ciprofloxacin has a bioavailability of 71 percent. One third is excreted in the urine and fecal recovery accounts for 15 to 30 percent. Secretion may occur through the intestinal mucosa, since 15 percent of intravenously administered ciprofloxacin may be recovered in the feces. Hepatic degradation to four different metabolites also occurs.

Ciprofloxacin's bile concentration is several-fold higher than serum levels; specifically, common bile duct levels range from 2.5 to 20 micrograms/milliliter after a single 500-milligram dose.

Although the drug is not new, antimicrobial resistance to ciprofloxacin has not been a problem thus far. Fewer than four (excluding pseudomomas) of 24,000 strains of gram-negative rods studied from 1983 to 1986 were resistant to ciprofloxacin. Resistance mechanisms involve a mutation (frequency, 10^{11}) or acquisition of a foreign DNA, as in chromosome plasmid transferral. In fluoroquinolones, such a transference may be minimized due to an actual lethal effect of the drug on plasmid DNA.

INDICATIONS

Ciprofloxacin is FDA approved for use in bacterial diarrhea caused by Enterotoxigenic *E. coli, Campylobacter jejuni, Shigella sonnei,* and *Shigella flexneri.* Other enteric gram-negative rods causing diarrhea are also very susceptible. This includes *Salmonella* (including *Salmonella typhi*), *Yersinia enterocoliticus, Pleisomonas shigelloides, Aeromonas species,* and *Vibrio parahemolyticus.* Due to the ineffectiveness of trimthoprim/sulfamethoxazole against *Campylobacter* and the growing resistance of enteric pathogens, a large potential for appropriate usage of ciprofloxacin exists. Coverage does not include the intestinal protozoal pathogens such as *Giardia lamblia* and *Entameba histolytica.* Viral gastroenteritis (Norwalk agent, calicivirus, and enterovirus-cosackie and -echo) also do not respond to ciprofloxacin.

Clinical evidence for efficacy is good. A double-blind, randomized, placebo-controlled German study involved 85 adult patients with acute diarrhea. Individuals treated with ciprofloxacin, 500 milligrams twice a day for 5 days, had a shortened duration of fever and diarrhea, compared to placebo. Isolated pathogens included *Salmonella* species (16), *Campylobacter* (19), and *Shigella* (3). Relapse occurred in four patients with *Salmonellosis.* A Guatemala study cured 39 of 39 patients with *Salmonella typhi* infections, with a mean therapy duration of 14 days. Six of six *Shigella* patients were cleared, with a mean of 7 days of therapy. Thirty chronic carriers of *Salmonella typhi* in Peru were effectively cleared with ciprofloxacin, 750 milligrams twice a day for 1 month. Effectiveness has not been shown in AIDS patients with chronic *Salmonella typhi* carriage.

A double-blind, placebo-controlled U.S. study compared trimethoprim (160 mgs)/sulfamethoxazole (800 mgs) twice a day to ciprofloxacin (500 mgs bid) in 52 culture-positive diarrhea patients. By day 4 of treatment, stools were free of pathogens in 18 of 19 ciprofloxacin patients, seven of 16 TMP/SMX patients and six of 17 placebo patients. The conclusion was that ciprofloxacin eradicated most commonly isolated bacterial pathogens and should be useful for treatment of acute diarrheal illness.

Ciprofloxacin may offer an important option for treating traveler's diarrhea in TMP/SMX-allergic individuals and for use in TMP/SMX-resistant areas (Southeast Asia, Korea, and Mexico). In a study involving travelers to Mexico, of 24 ciprofloxacin-treated individuals, none shed a pathogen at the end of therapy, compared with eight of 61 TMP/SMX-treated and six of 28 TMP-treated.

Another approximate setting may include individuals with traveler's diarrhea undergoing tropical sun exposure, for whom doxycycline use is not desirable due to possible photosensitization.

In addition, a single 250-milligram ciprofloxacin tablet showed a 100 percent response against uncomplicated *Neisseria gonorrhea* urethritis. Chlamydial infection was only eradicated in 50 percent of cases.

CONTRAINDICATIONS AND SIDE EFFECTS

Ciprofloxacin is contraindicated during pregnancy and breast feeding, and in children younger than 18 years of age, due to arthropathy in immature animals given quinolones. Human breast milk data are not available; however, ciprofloxacin is excreted in lactating rats.

Side effects may include CNS stimulation after several days of therapy, resulting in insomnia, restlessness, dizziness, or headache. Ocular toxicity does not occur as with other quinolone compounds. Crystalluria due to drug precipitation is reported at higher doses (750 mgs bid); however, no decrease in renal function occurs. Maintaining a well-hydrated state is recommended. Transaminase elevation has been reported in 2 percent of patients, and nausea, vomiting, and diarrhea have also been described.

Drug interactions involve elevation of theophylline levels due to competition for hepatic enzymes, and diphenylhydantoin levels may also vary. Absorption is impaired by antacids.

In cases of renal failure, dosage should be decreased by 50 percent when creatinine clearance is less than 50 milliliters/minute. Individuals with creatinine clearances less than 30 milliliters/minute should receive half the dose on an 18-hour interval regimen.

DOSAGE

According to manufacturer's prescribing information, dosage for mild, moderate, or severe diarrhea is a 500-milligram tablet every 12 hours for at least 2 days after signs and symptoms of diarrhea have resolved. Traveler's diarrhea should respond symptomatically in 24 to 48 hours, especially if treated early, and probably will not require more than 5 days of therapy.

Length, dosage, and treatment indications for Salmonellosis is more controversial. Prolonged *Salmonella* stool excretion occurs in antibiotic-treated individuals, so routine treatment of these patients should be discouraged. If treatment is indicated in a particular patient, a long duration of therapy may be necessary.

PEARLS AND PITFALLS

1. Ciprofloxacin should be used only in adults. Arthropathy occurs when it is given to immature laboratory animals. Contraindications also exist for pregnancy and breast feeding.
2. Interference with theophylline metabolism occurs, therefore dosage adjustments may be necessary.
3. Ingestion of concomitant caffeinated beverages may cause increased central nervous system stimulation, since caffeine is metabolized via the same mechanism as theophylline.
4. Anaerobic coverage is poor, therefore use in perirectal abscesses would not be indicated.

5. When higher doses of ciprofloxacin are used, good hydration should be emphasized to avoid crystalluria.
6. Concomitant antacid administration interferes with ciprofloxacin absorption. Cimetidine slows hepatic metabolism of ciprofloxacin and increases serum levels.

References

1. Carlson JR, Thornton SA. Comparative in vitro activities of 10 antimicrobial agents against bacterial enteropathogens. Antimicrob Ag Chemo 1983; 24:509.

    Norfloxacin was one of the most active agents tested against multiple enteropathogenic bacteria isolated from worldwide sources.

2. Cohen PT, Neighbor M. Eradication of stool pathogens in patients with acute diarrhea—A comparison of ciprofloxacin, trimothoprim/sulfamethoxazole and placebo (abs 1125). Twenty-seventh interscience conference on antimicrobial agents and chemotherapy, New York, October 4–7, 1987.

    Ciprofloxacin effectively eradicated the most commonly isolated bacterial pathogens. Studies suggested that ciprofloxacin should be a useful antibiotic in acute diarrhea before culture results are known.

3. Eggleston M, Park SY. Review of the Y-quinolones. Infect Control 1987; 8:119.

    An excellent review, with a table of activity comparing ciprofloxacin against multiple pathogens.

4. Ericson CD, DuPont HL. Test of cure of stool cultures in traveler's diarrhea (abs 1123). Twenty-seventh interscience conference on antimicrobial agents and chemotherapy, New York, October 7, 1987.

    None of 24 ciprofloxacin-treated subjects shed a pathogen at the end of therapy, compared to eight of 61 treated with trimethoprim/sulfamethoxazole.

5. Fans RJ. The quinolones. Ann Intern Med 1985; 102:400.

    An editorial summarizing data and discussing useful therapeutic situations for quinolones.

6. Gasser JC, Ebert SC. Ciprofloxacin pharmacokinetics in patients with normal and improved renal function. Antimicrob Ag Chemo 1987; 31:709.

    A 50% dose reduction of ciprofloxacin is recommended for patients with less than 50 mls/min creatinine clearance.

7. Hooper DC, Wolfson JS. Mechanisms of action of and resistance to ciprofloxacin. Am J Med 1987; 82(suppl 4A):12.

    A subunit DNA gyrase is the target of ciprofloxacin. Resistance appears to occur both by mutation and drug penetration through the cell membrane.

8. Neu HC. Ciprofloxacin: An overview and prospective appraisal. Am J Med 1987; 82(Suppl 4A):395.

    A review discussing the drug's use in many different infectious settings.

9. Pichler JE. Clinical efficacy of ciprofloxacin compared with placebo in bacterial diarrhea. Am J Med 1987; 82(Suppl 4A):329.

Ciprofloxacin effectively eradicated *Salmonella* species, *Campylobacter,* and *Shigella* species, with duration of fever being 1.3 days.

10. Rubinstein E, Seger S. Drug interactions of ciprofloxacin with other nonantibiotic agents. Am J Med 1987; 82(Suppl 4A):119.

    Antacids significantly decreased absorption. Theophylline levels were raised and convulsions may be potentiated. Cimetidine antagonizes metabolism of ciprofloxacin.

11. Taylor DE, Courvelin P. Mechanisms of antibiotic resistance in *Campylobacter* species. Antimicrob Ag Chemo 1988; 32:1107.

    Resistance mechanisms in quinolones may involve the DNA gyrase or inability of the drug to penetrate.

12. Walker RC, Wright AJ. The quinolones. Mayo Clin Proc 1987; 67:1007.

    An excellent review article with comparative in vitro activity. Chemical structures of quinolones are also presented.

Acute Diverticulitis

Michael M. Van Ness

Diverticulosis was first described by Cruveilhier in 1849 and has been increasingly recognized since Beer's description in 1904. Several authors, including Rankin, Brown, and Young, estimate the incidence of asymptomatic diverticulosis in Western countries to be 5 percent at age 40, increasing linearly to 50 percent in the ninth decade.

Acute diverticulitis or bacteria-induced perforation and inflammation of colonic diverticuli may be mild and easily treated or serious and life-threatening. According to Horner, acute diverticulitis complicates asymptomatic diverticulosis with increasing frequency as the patient's age increases. Specifically, after 5 years of observation, he found that 10 percent of his cohort of 503 patients developed acute diverticulitis during a 5-year observation period. The incidence of acute diverticulitis increases to 35 percent after 20 years of observation.

Although medical therapy is sufficient in the majority of patients, Chappius and Cohn report that 20 percent of all patients with acute diverticulitis develop an abscess, fistula, or recurrent diverticulitis requiring surgical intervention.

PATHOGENESIS AND INCIDENCE

Microperforation of a single diverticulum is believed to be the initial event that causes peridiverticulitis, the initial stage of acute diverticulitis. Because diverticuli are pseudodiverticuli (they do not contain all the layers of the bowel wall but only mucosa and submucosa herniated through the circular muscle layer of the colon), peridiverticulitis may remain confined to the pericolic fat or may develop into a free macroperforation causing frank peritonitis.

Complications of acute diverticulitis include bacteremia and septicemia; abscess formation with extension into the mesentery, adjacent bowel, or bladder; and free perforation with peritonitis. Death is reported by Welch to occur in 5.9 percent of patients with diverticular abscess at the Massachusetts General Hospital. Fistulae may develop with communication into bowel, uterus, vagina, bladder, or skin. Transient colonic obstruction and bleeding may occur but rarely are serious or life-threatening.

Incidence figures for complicated diverticular disease are difficult to obtain. In a series of 140 cases of diverticulitis of the sigmoid colon, Frager found 10 small intestinal complications (5 colo-enteric fistulae, 3 small bowel obstructions, and 2 inflammatory changes of the small bowel from mesenteritis and the associated mass). Utilizing CT scanning of the abdomen in 68 patients with acute diverticulitis, Labs et al. found 13 cases of diverticular abscess and 12 cases of diverticular fistulae.

PRESENTATION AND DIAGNOSIS

The classic presentation for acute diverticulitis includes left-lower-quadrant pain, low-grade fever, leukocytosis, nausea and vomiting, and abdominal distention. Signs of acute diverticulitis reflect the degree of peritoneal inflammation, with variable degrees of abdominal tenderness, rebound, mass, or fullness.

The differential diagnosis includes acute appendicitis, sigmoid carcinoma, ischemic colitis and mesenteric venous thrombosis, pseudomembranous enterocolitis, and idiopathic inflammatory bowel disease.

Although much less prevalent than left-sided diverticulosis, right-sided diverticuli, both acquired and congenital, can perforate, with abscess and fistula formation. In the appropriate clinical setting, the signs and symptoms of right-sided diverticular disease can be easily confused with acute appendicitis as well as less common entities like Crohn's disease, carcinoid tumor, or ameboma.

Diagnosis of acute diverticulitis depends on the appropriate history, physical findings, and confirmatory studies. Plain abdominal radiographs may show an ileus pattern, mass effect in the left or right lower quadrant, or evidence of small bowel or colonic obstruction. Rarely, free abdominal air may be present. A water-soluble colonic enema (Hypaque-76, 66% diatriazole meglumine and 10% diatriazole sodium) is the best study to show "sawtooth" mucosa, fistulae, or perforation. Although difficult for most patients to tolerate during the initial phase of acute diverticulitis, flexible proctosigmoidoscopy may show peridiverticular erythema, edema, and exudate.

COMPLICATIONS OF DIVERTICULITIS

Abscess, perforation, and fistulae are the most common life-threatening complications of acute diverticulitis.

The presence of diverticular abscess should be suspected in the patient who fails to improve within 48 hours of initiation of antimicrobial therapy. High spiking temperatures, persistent leukocytosis, and a tender abdominal mass are clues to the diagnosis. Computed tomography is the diagnostic procedure of choice. In the appropriate patient, percutaneous drainage of diverticular abscess will allow stabilization of critically ill patients at high risk for surgical intervention.

Free perforation (Stage 3, generalized purulent peritonitis, or Stage 4, fecal peritonitis, Table 21–1) of an infected diverticulum is a surgical emergency and requires an aggressive surgical plan carried out in conjunction with intensive medical support. A combination of a primary resection of the involved areas, end colostomy, and Hartmann closure has the lowest morbidity and mortality and is the surgical procedure of choice.

Unlike abscess and perforation, fistula formation usually occurs between episodes of acute diverticular disease. Relative luminal stenosis and high-pressure segmental pres-

Table 21–1. Perforative diverticular disease

Stage 1: Contained pericolic abscess or phlegmonous diverticulitis
Stage 2: Walled-off pelvic abscess secondary to perforation of a pericolic abscess
Stage 3: Generalized purulent peritonitis resulting from rupture of a pericolic or pelvic abscess
Stage 4: Fecal peritonitis

Adapted from Hinchey EJ, Schaal PGH, Richards GK. Treatment of perforated diverticular disease of the colon. In Rob C (ed), Advances in surgery vol 12. Chicago: Yearbook, 1978, p. 85.

sures contribute to the development of fistulae to adjacent abdominal organs. Recurrent polymicrobial urinary tract infections, pneumoturia (spontaneous passage of gas in the urinary stream), and fecaluria are clues to the presence of a colovesical fistula, usually present in the posterior bladder wall.

Chronic diarrhea, steatorrhea, and small bowel overgrowth suggest the development of colo-enteric fistulae.

Feculent vaginal discharge or gas passage per vagina are supportive of the presence of colo-uterine or colovaginal fistulae.

Elective surgical fistulectomy and resection of the colon involved with diverticular disease is indicated in the presence of fistulae. Under these circumstances, a primary anastomosis should be possible.

Elective resection is also indicated for recurrent attacks of diverticulitis, to rule out malignancy, and for the patient under the age of 55 with his first attack of diverticulitis.

MEDICAL THERAPY

As shown in Table 21–2, a multitude of microorganisms are present in acute diverticulitis. Because diverticulitis is a polymicrobial infection, a broad spectrum of antimicrobial activity is required. In a rat model of secondary bacterial peritonitis and abscess formation, Onderdonk found that antibiotics need not be active against every and all organisms to treat diverticulitis and to prevent abscess formation. If the more virulent pathogens are controlled, the synergistic effect of the aerobes and anaerobes on abscess formation can be eliminated. For example, although gentamicin and clindamycin are known to have little or no activity against enterobacteriaceae and enterococcus, Bartlett et al. have shown this therapy to be effective in an experimental rat model of intraperitoneal infection, suggesting that the enterocoous is not a primary pathogen in secondary peritonitis. Following on this study, both Fass and Levison have treated patients with mixed aerobic and anaerobic infections with gentamicin and clindamycin, with good clinical results.

Table 21–2. Diverticulitis: organisms and antibiotics

1. Facultative aerobes
    Enterbacteriaceae
        Escherchia coli
        Klebsiella species
        Proteus species
        Enterobacter
        Citrobacter
    Enterococci
2. Obligate anaerobes
    Bacteroides fragilis
    Bacteroides melaninogenicus
    Peptococcus
    Peptostreptococcus
    Fusobacteriium
    Eubacterium species
    Clostridium species

Intravenous treatment regimens

1. Chloramphenical, 50–100 mgs/kg/day; and Gentamicin, 1.7 mgs/kg every 8 hours
2. Clindamycin, 600 mgs every 6–8 hours; and Gentamicin, 1.7 mgs/kg every 8 hours
3. Ceftizoxime (Cefizox), 2 gms every 12 hours (with dosage adjustment for patients with acute or chronic renal failure)
4. Imipenem-cilastatin (Primaxin), 500 mgs every 6–8 hours (with dosage adjustment for patients with acute or chronic renal failure)

Acceptable intravenous treatment regimens for patients with uncomplicated diverticulosis include:

1. Chloramphenical, 50 to 100 milligrams/kilogram/day; and Gentamicin, 1.7 milligrams/kilogram every 8 hours
2. Clindamycin, 600 milligrams every 6 to 8 hours; and Gentamicin, 1.7 milligrams/kilogram every 8 hours
3. Ceftizoxime (Cefizox), 2 grams every 12 hours (with dosage adjustment for patients with acute or chronic renal failure); or
4. Imipenem-cilastatin (Primaxin), 500 milligrams every 6 to 8 hours (with dosage adjustment for patients with acute or chronic renal failure).

PEARLS AND PITFALLS

1. The incidence of asymptomatic diverticulosis is estimated to be about 15 percent at age 50 and 35 percent at age 65.
2. The most common site for diverticulosis is the sigmoid colon, where herniation under pressures as high as 90 mm Hg occur. The locus minoris resistentiae is the pen-

etration site of small arterioles from the circumferential artery present on the antimesenteric side of the colon.
3. The most common cause of fistulae in diverticular disease is the colovesical fistula, while diverticulosis is the most common cause of this condition.
4. The second most common fistula associated with diverticular disease is the colocutaneous fistula. Failure to resect all the diseased sigmoid colon is felt to be the proximate cause in over two-thirds of the cases.
5. Percutaneous drainage of diverticular abscesses is a means of preventing urgent surgical intervention in unstable or frail patients. It may have a role in the long-term treatment of patients for whom surgical intervention is contraindicated.
6. Antibiotic therapy of uncomplicated acute diverticulosis should be tailored to cover the large number of pathogens present, keeping in mind the synergism between aerobic and anaerobic bacteria in the development of diverticular abscess.
7. Diverticular abscess and fistulae require surgical intervention.
8. Computerized tomography is more sensitive and specific than barium enema in the diagnosis of diverticular abscess.
9. Barium enema is more sensitive and specific than computerized tomography in the diagnosis of colovesical fistula.

CONCLUSION

The 20th century has seen many developments, including diverticulosis—now felt to be the result of a Western diet inadequate in terms of dietary fiber. Approximately 20 to 25 percent of all cases of chronic diverticulosis are complicated by acute diverticulitis, with surgical intervention in nearly 20 percent of these cases. Appropriate antibiotic therapy should cover a wide range of potential pathogens. A high index of suspicion is required for early detection of complications of acute diverticulitis, most commonly diverticular abscess and colovesical fistula. Coordination and cooperation between physicians and surgeons optimize patient care.

References

1. Bartlett JG, et al. Whither the enterococcus? (Abs 297) Fifteenth Interscience Conference on Antimicrobial Agents and Chemotherapy, September 24–26, 1975, Washington, DC.
2. Chappuis CW, Cohn I. Acute colonic diverticulitis. Surg Clin N Am 1988; 68:301–313.

    A complete and comprehensive review of the incidence (5% in the fifth decade to 50% in the ninth decade), pathogenesis (acquired pulsion-type pseudodiverticula, in that they do not contain all the layers of the bowel wall), diagnosis (LLQ pain, fever, leukocytosis), and management of acute diverticulitis.

3. Crist DW, et al. Acute diverticulitis of the cecum and ascending colon diagnosed by computed tomography. SGO 1988; 166:99–102.

   A report of seven patients presenting with right-sided abdominal pain of 2–7 days' duration, anorexia, fever, and guarding. Three of the seven had had previous appendectomy. Urgent CT scanning of the abdomen using 10-ml slice thickness after oral administration of 3% sodium diatrizoate showed extraluminal air suggestive of abscess in five of the seven, narrowing of the distal small bowel in three of the seven, and pericolic inflammation in all seven (eccentric in 5, concentric in 2). The authors conclude that CT scanning may be helpful in the evaluation of patients with a clinical history or physical findings atypical of acute appendicitis where right-sided diverticulosis may be present.

4. Eyer SD, Snover DC, Delaney JP. Diverticulitis in the multiple endocrine neoplasia type II B syndrome. Am J Gastro 1988; 83:183–186.

   As evidence that diffuse ganglioneuromatosis involves the entire gastrointestinal tract, the authors report a case of complicated diverticulitis (colovesical fistula) in a 37-year-old women and review the other three cases described in the medical literature. The authors emphasize that complications of diverticulosis tend to appear in patients with MEN II B earlier than in the general population.

5. Fass RJ, et al. Clindamycin in the treatment of serious anaerobic infections. AIM 1973; 78:853.

   Among 19 adults with anaerobic or mixed infections, 18 of the 19 were cured of their infections with clindamycin or clindamycin and gentamicin. Infections included actinomycosis (5), lung abscess (1), soft-tissue abscess (5), osteomylitis (3), and pneumonia with empyema (5). The only recurrence after therapy was one of the pneumonia with empyema patients.

6. Fazio VW, et al. Colocutaneous fistula complicating diverticulitis. Dis Colon Rectum 1987; 30:89–94.

   The authors emphasize the need to resect the sigmoid colon completely to prevent the development of postoperative colocutaneous fistulae.

7. Horner JL. Natural history of diverticulosis of the colon. Am J Dig Dis 1958; 3:343.

   A classic review and follow-up study providing the epidemiologic basis for current intervention and therapy.

8. Klein S, et al. Extraintestinal manifestations in patients with diverticulitis. AIM 1988; 108:700–702.

   An extraordinary series of three patients (2 males, 1 female, aged 54–67 years) who presented with sigmoid diverticulitis complicated by perforation (3 of 3), pericolic abscess (3 of 3), pyoderma gangrenosum (3 of 3), and lower extremity arthritis (3 of 3). All were treated for idiopathic inflammatory bowel disease with systemic corticosteroids, antibiotics, and local steroids without improvement in the extra-intestinal manifestations of their disease. All three patients went to sigmoid colon resection and experienced relief of pyoderma gangrenosum and lower extremity arthritis. Pathologic examination of the resected specimens showed no evidence of idiopathic inflammatory bowel disease.

9. Labs JD, et al. Complications of acute diverticulitis of the colon: Improved early diagnosis with computerized tomography. Am J Surg 1988; 155:331–335.

The authors review their experience in the early recognition of complications of diverticulitis in 68 patients hospitalized at the Johns Hopkins Hospital from 1982 to 1984. Uncomplicated diverticular disease occurred in 43 (63%), whereas complications occurred in 25 (13 of the 25 had diverticular abscesses, and 12 of the 25 had colovesical fistulae). Among the 43 with uncomplicated diverticulosis, CT scanning showed segmental and localized thickening of the colonic wall with luminal narrowing, pericolic reaction, and associated distant, scattered diverticulae without evidence of abscess or fistulae. Of the 13 patients with diverticular abscess, 10 underwent CT scanning, which confirmed the presence of a mass in all 10 (pericolic fluid collection). Colovesical fistulae were suspected in 12 patients. All 12 underwent CT scanning. Air was present in the bladder, with thickened segments of adjacent sigmoid colon in 11 of the 12. The authors advocate the early use of CT scanning in patients suspected of complicated diverticulosis.

10. Levison ME, et al. In vitro activity and clinical efficacy of clindamycin in the treatment of infections due to anaerobic bacteria. J Infect Dis 1977; 135:S79.

The clinical experience at the Medical College of Pennsylvania with clindamycin in anaerobic infections is reviewed.

11. Ludmerer KM and Kissane JM (eds.). Polymicrobial sepsis and jaundice in a 46-year-old man. Am J Med 1986; 81:649–654.

A case description of a 46-year-old white male presenting with polymicrobial bacteremia, bilateral lower abdominal pain, jaundice, and fever who had acute sigmoid diverticulitis complicated by perforation, peritonitis, and abscess formation. A very clear differential diagnosis is presented as well as speculation on the etiology of diverticulitis including abnormal vascular supply, incomplete diverticular emptying, or local ischemia and perforation. Last, the discussants emphasize that whereas bacteremia occurs regularly when aerobic organisms are inoculated intraperitoneally, abdominal abscess formation requires the presence of both aerobic and anaerobic organisms.

12. Neff CC, et al. Diverticular abscesses: Percutaneous drainage. Radiology 1987; 163:15–18.

Among 16 patients with known diverticular abscess, the placement of eight to twelve French gauge catheters percutaneously was used as a temporizing measure in 13 patients operated on 10 days to 6 weeks later and as definitive therapy in three high-risk patients. All three were asymptomatic 12 to 29 months later.

13. Onderdonk AB, et al. Microbial synergy in experimental intra-abdominal abscess. Infect Immuno 1976; 13:22.

    The authors injected rats with either combinations of facultative and anaerobic organisms, or each bacterial strain alone. Only those animals with both facultative and anaerobic infections formed abdominal abscesses, suggesting synergy.

14. Rankin FW, Brown PW. Diverticulitis of the colon. SGO 1930; 50:836.

    One of the first authoritative descriptions of the clinical entity of diverticulitis.

15. Welch CE. Computerized tomography scans for all patients with diverticulitis. Am J Surg 1988; 155:336.

    An editorial accompanying the article by Labs et al. Because of the high mortality associated with diverticular abscess (5.9%), Welch emphasizes that early CT scanning of patients with suspected diverticular abscess may prove beneficial in reducing mortality.

16. Young EL, Young EL III. Diverticulitis of the colon: A review of the literature and an analysis of ninety-one cases. NEJM 1944; 230:33.

    One of the first studies utilizing penicillin in the treatment of diverticulitis.

IV
Liver and Pancreatic Disease Drugs

Exciting advances in the pharmacologic therapy of liver, biliary, and pancreatic disease are few and far between. In 1988, we have advanced significantly in our knowledge of the identity and pathogenesis of acute and chronic liver disease compared to a generation ago. However, we have few agents—with notable exceptions detailed in this part—that were not available in the 1950s. General supportive measures and a vigilant search for infection and metabolic abnormalities continue to serve as the cornerstone for the treatment of most liver diseases. Careful application of immunosuppressive agents can be beneficial to selected patients. Widespread use of hepatitis B vaccine is possible.

Chronic Autoimmune Liver Disease and Wilson's Disease

Pharmacologic therapy of chronic autoimmune liver disease (CALD, or "lupoid" hepatitis) and Wilson's disease is of unquestioned benefit. Although neither condition is curable, the disease manifestations can be controlled with appropriate therapy.

Prednisone in CALD prolongs life, improves the patient's overall sense of well-being, and reverses abnormal histologic and laboratory findings. Many CALD patients require long-term prednisone therapy. Side effects of chronic, high-dose prednisone therapy can be lessened by dose reduction concurrent with initiation of azathioprine. Azathioprine alone is not effective for inducing a remission in severe, chronic autoimmune liver disease. However, Stellon has shown recently that azathioprine alone may be capable of maintaining a corticosteroid-induced remission.

Penicillamine remains the most effective and best-tolerated copper-chelation and cupruic agent. As much as 1000 to 3000 micrograms of copper are excreted per day with initiation of therapy. There is no place in the diagnosis of suspected Wilson's disease for a "penicillamine trial": Liver biopsy is required for diagnosis. Improvement in liver inflammation, dysarthria, intellectual capacity, and tremor may require 6 months of therapy. Penicillamine tolerance is usually very good in Wilson's disease patients. Only rarely is the lupuslike reaction seen. For severe, refractory penicillamine reactions, prednisone may provide temporary relief and trien (tetraethylene tetramine dihydrochloride) may be substituted for penicillamine. Penicillamine or trien therapy must be continued for life.

Primary Biliary Cirrhosis and Hepatitis B

Although new and exciting advances have been reported recently, the benefit of pharmacologic therapy for primary biliary cirrhosis (PBC) and hepatitis B remains unproven.

Both Kaplan and Bodenheimer have studied colchicine in PBC patients. Improvement in liver function and synthesis was apparent. Histology did not improve with therapy. After 4 years of therapy, Kaplan noted a trend toward a decrease in mortality in the colchicine-treated group.

Immunosuppressive therapy of PBC with either penicillamine, prednisone, or azathioprine appears to be of no benefit. On the other hand, Hoofnagle has published results demonstrating benefit from chlorambucil. Bichemical improvement was accompanied by decreases in inflammatory cell infiltrate in treated patients compared with controls. Whether chlorambucil will decrease mortality and improve survival is unknown.

Modification and manipulation of immune mechanisms by prednisone and interferon hold promise for the treatment of viral hepatitis. Perillo treated chronic hepatitis B patients with a steroid withdrawal followed by alpha-2b interferon. Nine of 18 patients cleared all markers of viral replication and remained clear for 9 months. Although longer periods of observation and larger numbers of subjects are needed, Aach believes that this type of immunomodulating therapy is most promising for these patients.

The hepatitis B vaccine (either plasma-derived or recombinant) is now widely available and is recognized to be safe and effective.

Alcoholic Liver Disease

Although there is renewed interest in the use of corticosteroids for acute alcoholic hepatitis, only abstinence, adequate nutrition, and supportive measures (vitamin K, lactulose) are widely accepted therapies.

Disulfiram may be useful in the treatment of chronic alcoholism.

Biliary and Pancreatic Disease

Pharmacologic therapy of cholelithiasis and choledocholithiasis with either monooctanoin or methyl tert-butyl ether remains at best a second- or third-line treatment for stone disease. As of this writing, surgical or endoscopic intervention methods are the preferred treatment modalities, with monooctanoin or methyl tert-butyl ether reserved for patients with severe systemic illnesses precluding more traditional therapy.

Pancreatic enzyme replacement benefits patients with pancreatic insufficiency and chronic pancreatic pain. Alkalinization of gastric contents preserves lipase, colipase, and trypsin activity as much as possible.

Michael M. Van Ness

References

1. Aach RD. The treatment of chronic type B viral hepatitis. AIM 1988; 109:89–91.
   The author reviews the rationale behind the current efforts to induce remission of hepatitis B by manipulation of immune processes.
2. Bodenheimer H, Schaffner F, Pezzullo F. Evaluation of colchicine therapy in primary biliary cirrhosis. Gastroenterology 1988; 95:124–129.
   Biochemical, but not histologic, improvement was noted with colchicine therapy.
3. Hoofnagle JH, et al. Randomized trial of chlorambucil for primary biliary cirrhosis. Gastroenterology 1986; 91:1327–1334.

Chlorambucil improved biochemical and inflammatory parameters, but not the degree of fibrosis or histologic stage of the disease.

4. Kaplan MM, et al. A prospective trial of colchicine for primary biliary cirrhosis. NEJM 1986; 315:1448–1454.

    Biochemical improvement in liver function was apparent in the colchicine-treated PBC patients. Side effects were few.

5. Maddrey WC, et al. Prednisolone therapy in patients with severe alcoholic hepatitis: Results of a multicenter trial. Hepatology 1986; 6:1202.

    Prednisolone benefitted patients with acute alcoholic hepatitis. Only two of 35 prednisolone-treated patients died, compared to 11 of 31 placebo-treated patients.

6. Perrillo RP, et al. Prednisone withdrawal followed by recombinant alpha interferon in the treatment of chronic type B hepatitis. AIM 1988; 109:95–100.

    Immunologic priming with prednisone followed by interferon may prove an effective treatment for selected hepatitis B patients.

7. Stellon AJ, et al. Maintenance of remission in autoimmune chronic active hepatitis with azathioprine after corticosteroid withdrawal. Hepatology 1988; 8:781–784.

    Two mgs/kg of azathioprine maintained corticosteroid-induced remission in CALD.

22
Corticosteroids
Michael M. Van Ness

Because many hepatic diseases are believed to occur because of immunologic abnormalities, corticosteroids have been utilized in their treatment. Close analysis of the results of numerous clinical trials of a wide variety of hepatic diseases has shown benefit in only a few, carefully circumscribed situations such as acute attacks of chronic autoimmune liver disease (lupoid hepatitis) and severe alcoholic liver disease. Newer, unproven, but intriguing applications of corticosteroids in conjunction with antiviral therapy await further study and analysis.

MECHANISM OF ACTION

Corticosteroids act by reducing inflammation, inhibiting fibrosis, and minimizing immunologic processes. More specifically, corticosteroids stabilize lyzosomes, reduce the damaging effects of antigen–antibody interactions, increase albumin synthesis, and retard production of type I collagen. In lymphocytes, the corticosteroid–cell membrane receptor complex appears to act by stimulation of transcription of mRNA coding for an inhibitory protein, resulting in an overall catabolic response.

INDICATIONS

Chronic Autoimmune Liver Disease

Patients with chronic autoimmune liver disease, as defined by Waldenstrom in the 1950s and modified by Mistilis in 1970, require appropriate, aggressive immunosuppressive therapy. These patients are systemically ill, with fatigue, anorexia, and weight loss. They may exhibit jaundice and splenomegaly as well as spider angiomas, palmar erythema, acne, and right upper-quadrant tenderness. Severely ill patients may present with bleeding, ascites, and encephalopathy. Characteristic laboratory findings include antinuclear antibodies of the IgG class (50–70% of patients) and antibodies to double-stranded or native DNA (42% of patients). A marked and broad-banded, polyclonal elevation of gamma globulins is characteristic. Associated organ system involvement includes pulmonary diffusion defects, fibrosing alveolitis, pericarditis, glomerulonephritis, arthritis, urticaria, thyroiditis, and hemolytic anemia. The cumulative survival of untreated patients at 5 years is 65 percent, with few survivors in the group with an abrupt and severe onset of disease. Results from the Royal Free Hospital, the King's College Hospital, and the Mayo Clinic all clearly show benefit from corticosteroid therapy. Azathioprine alone is not effective therapy for chronic autoimmune liver disease. The goal of therapy is to reduce inflammation without causing side effects. Asymptomatic patients with only mild transaminase elevations should not be treated.

Alcoholic Liver Disease

In mild to moderate alcoholic liver disease, corticosteroids are of no benefit. In the treatment of severe alcoholic hepatitis complicated by encephalopathy, marked icterus, elevated prothrombin time, and ascites, three clinical trials show survival benefit from corticosteroid therapy. In the first study, published by Helman in 1971, 14 patients with severe alcoholic hepatitis and hepatic encephalopathy were treated with either prednisolone (40 mgs/day) or placebo over a 4-week interval. All six who received placebo died, compared to only one death in the group of eight receiving prednisolone.

In a second study, published by Maddrey in 1978, 55 patients were treated in a double-blind manner with either prednisolone (40 mgs/day) or placebo. After 32 days of therapy, six of the 31 patients receiving placebo died, compared to only one of the 24 receiving prednisolone.

To confirm these results, a multicenter, double-blind, placebo-controlled trial of methylprednisolone (32 mgs/day) was conducted. Sixty-six patients meeting the criteria for severe alcoholic hepatitis, as defined by the discriminant function formula (DF equal to 32 or more defined severe disease and was calculated as follows; DF = 4.6 × [prothrombin time of the patient minus the control) + serum bilirubin]) were involved. Eleven of the 31 placebo-treated patients died within the 28-day study period, compared to only two of the 35 patients treated with methylprednisolone ($p = 0.006$).

Therefore, in addition to alcohol abstinence, resumption of a nutritious diet, management of alcohol withdrawal phenomena, and treatment of bleeding, infection, and metabolic complications, management of the alcoholic patient with severe disease (DF > 32) might well include corticosteroid therapy.

Viral Hepatitis

Corticosteroids alone have no role in the treatment of acute or chronic hepatitis B or non-A, non-B hepatitis.

Corticosteroids in conjunction with alpha and gamma interferon may be beneficial in the treatment of chronic hepatitis B characterized by active viral replication (positive e antigen). A short course of prednisone (40–60 mgs/day for 6 weeks), with an abrupt taper prior to therapy with alpha and gamma interferon for 4 months, resulted in a greater than 40 percent clearance of the e antigen with concomitant production of e antibody. At this time, although promising, this type of therapy remains experimental and should only be used in clinical trials under the auspices of experienced researchers.

Corticosteroids are of no benefit when used for the treatment of acute viral hepatitis. Liver necrosis, healing, antibody formation, and recovery are not improved by corticosteroid therapy. The steroid "whitewash," as described by Shaldon and Sherlock (prednisolone, 30, 20, 15, 10, and 5 mgs orally, each dose given for 5 days) is inadvisable for even the nonhepatitis B patient with prolonged cholestasis,

Table 22–1. Results of controlled trials of corticosteroids in fulminant hepatic failure

	Ware (1974)	Redeker (1976)	European trial (1979)	Rakela (1979)
1. Treated with corticosteroids				
Number	4	17	26	37
Number of survivors	0	6	3	9
2. Treated with placebo				
Number	11	16	14	20
Number of survivors	7	6	2	5

From Jones EA, Schafer DF. Fulminant hepatic failure. In D Zakim, TD Boyer (eds.), *Hepatology, a Textbook of Liver Disease.* Philadelphia: Saunders, 1982, p. 434. Adapted and reproduced with permission of the authors.

despite its proven beneficial effect on both patient and physician morale. Subsequent studies by DeRitis, Blum, and Dudley fail to demonstrate any real benefit from corticosteroids in acute viral hepatitis and suggest interference with the normal immune response, resulting in higher relapse rates and a propensity for development of chronic hepatitis. The use of corticosteroids for uncomplicated viral hepatitis is unjustifiable.

The rationale for use of corticosteroids in fulminant hepatic failure regardless of cause was based on the assumption that the anti-inflammatory action of corticosteroids would reduce hepatocellular necrosis. As depicted in Table 22–1, no benefit is realized by the use of corticosteroids in fulminant hepatic failure; in fact, there is strong evidence of an adverse effect. Corticosteroids should not be used in the treatment of fulminant hepatic failure.

The use of corticosteroids for the chronic, active hepatitis associated with inflammatory bowel disease is controversial. Several authors (Gray, Read, and Harris) have described the benefits of corticosteroids (decreased symptoms and decreased transaminase values). Czaja and Wolf compared the results of corticosteroid therapy in eight patients with ulcerative colitis and chronic active hepatitis with the results of corticosteroid therapy in 141 patients with active hepatitis (25 of whom had chronic autoimmune liver disease; i.e., lupoid hepatitis). As expected, corticosteroids alleviated the symptoms in the eight patients with ulcerative colitis and active hepatitis but had no effect on the chronic active hepatitis. Therefore, chronic active hepatitis associated with inflammatory bowel disease is not an indication for corticosteroid therapy.

Primary Biliary Cirrhosis

Although corticosteroids relieve pruritus and might be expected to reduce inflammation in patients with primary biliary cirrhosis, bone thinning precludes their use, except in the very early anicteric phase when patients may experience intense pruritus.

ADMINISTRATION

In patients with chronic autoimmune liver disease (lupoid hepatitis), liver biopsy must precede the commencement of corticosteroid therapy—unless severe coagulopathy precludes biopsy, in which case a biopsy must be performed as soon as possible after a remission is obtained. Sherlock recommends 30 milligrams of prednisolone for 1 week, reducing the dose to a maintenance level of 10 to 20 milligrams as quickly as possible. Tong has found that higher initial doses are often required, 40 to 60 milligrams of prednisone per day, to induce a remission. Regardless of the initial dose, tapering of the dosage of the corticosteroid used should be based on improvement of the serum transaminase values. Some authors prefer prednisolone over prednisone, since the 11-hydroxylation conversion of prednisone to prednisolone must occur in the liver before prednisone can exert its glucocorticoid effect. In practice, there seems to be little advantage of one agent over the other. A suggested regimen for steroid therapy in autoimmune liver disease is presented in Table 22–2.

SIDE EFFECTS

The side effects of chronic corticosteroid therapy are well recognized and include the development of cushingoid or moon facies, diabetes, hypertension, acne, obesity, hirsutism, and striae. Growth retardation in children, diabetes, bone thinning (osteoporosis), and serious infection (fungal infections or reactivation of tuberculosis) are particularly troublesome. In patients with chronic autoimmune liver disease, the addition of azathioprine (50–100 mgs/day) may allow reduction in the corticosteroid dose and amelioration of these side effects.

PEARLS AND PITFALLS

1. The only well-studied and justifiable uses of corticosteroids alone in the treatment of liver disease are in patients with acute or chronic autoimmune liver disease and severe alcoholic liver disease with or without encephalopathy.
2. In patients with autoimmune liver disease, azathioprine may allow a reduction in corticosteroid dose so as to ease the complications of long-term corticosteroid use. Azathioprine alone or during pregnancy is contraindicated for the treatment of autoimmune liver disease.
3. Long-term use of corticosteroids in patients with primary biliary cirrhosis may lead to serious and severe osteoporosis.
4. Corticosteroids in combination with antiviral (ara A) or immunomodulating agents (alpha and gamma inter-

Table 22–2. Corticosteroids in autoimmune liver disease

First week: 10–15 mgs of prednisolone 3 times a day, or 15–20 mgs of prednisone 3 times a day

Second week: Clinical and liver test check; if marked improvement is noted, then reduce corticosteroids by two-and-a-half mg increments.

Third week: Clinical and liver test check; if stable, continue dose reduction to maintenance (10–15 mgs prednisolone a day, or 20 mgs prednisone a day).

Every month: Clinical and liver test check

At six months: Liver biopsy

Full remission: Complete corticosteroid withdrawal, slowly (decrease by 2.5 mgs/week); restart at full dose if relapse occurs.

No remission: Continue maintenance dose for 6 more months, consider the addition of azathioprine (50–100 mgs/day); maximum dose, 20–30 mgs prednisolone, or 40–60 mgs prednisone with 100 mgs azathioprine

---

feron) may prove ultimately to be of benefit in the treatment of patients with chronic hepatitis B.
5. Although a more consistent dose-response might be expected from the use of prednisolone instead of prednisone for the treatment of severe liver disease, the advantage of prednisolone over prednisone appears to be theoretical only.

References

1. Acute Hepatic Failure Study Group (rep J Rakella). A double-blinded, randomized trial of hydrocortisone in acute hepatic failure. Gastroenterology 1979; 76:1297.

    Among patients treated with corticosteroids for acute hepatic failure, the mortality was equivalent (9 of 37 or 24%) to the mortality among a group treated with placebo (5 of 20 or 25%).

2. Blum AL, et al. A fortuitously controlled study of steroid therapy in acute viral hepatitis I: Acute disease. Am J Med 1969; 47:82.

    Steroid treatment was associated with more rapid resolution of elevated serum levels of bilirubin throughout hospitalization, and of transaminases and alkaline phosphatase during the first 2 weeks. The frequency of intercurrent illness, chiefly peptic ulcer and pyogenic infections, was twice as high at the hospital using steroids routinely.

3. Czaja AJ, Wolf AM. Immunopathic disease associated with severe chronic active liver disease: Determinants of treatment response? (abs) Gastroenterology 1980; 78:1152.

    A delay longer than 2 weeks, or slow resolution of abnormalities noted prior to treatment, is a poor prognostic sign.

4. Czaja AJ, Rakela J, Ludwig J. Features reflective of early prognosis in corticosteroid-treated severe autoimmune chronic active hepatitis. Gastroenterology 1988; 95:448.

   Patients who resolved at least one pretreatment laboratory abnormality, improved a pretreatment hyperbilirubinemia, or did not experience biochemical deterioration after 2 weeks of therapy survived at least 6 months in 98% of cases.

5. DeRitis R, et al. Negative results of prednisone therapy in viral hepatitis. *Lancet* 1964; 1:533.

   Sixty-five patients with viral hepatitis received either prednisone, 30 mgs/day (N = 34), or placebo (N = 31). No statistically significant differences were observed in the biochemical data, and the disease was not shortened in the treated group of patients.

6. Dudley FJ, Scheuer PJ, Sherlock S. Natural history of hepatitis-associated antigen-positive chronic liver disease. *Lancet* 1972; 2:1388.

   Corticosteroid treatment in the acute phase of disease appears, in this clinical and pathological study of 59 hepatitis B patients, to predispose to relapse and chronicity.

7. EASL Study Group. Randomized trial of steroid therapy in acute liver failure. Gut 1979; 20:620.

   Corticosteroids are of little or no benefit in acute (fulminant) hepatic failure (usually hepatitis B in the U.S.). Complications of therapy include systemic fungal infections, gastric erosions, and pancreatitis.

8. Gray N, et al. Hepatitis, colitis, and lupus manifestations. Am J Dig Dis 1958; 3:481.

   A classic description of lupoid hepatitis.

9. Gregory PB, et al. Steroid therapy in severe viral hepatitis: A double-blind, randomized trial of methyl-prednisolone versus placebo. NEJM 1976; 294:681.

   Seven of 15 randomized to methylprednisolone and 2 of 15 randomized to placebo died during the 16-week study period.

10. Harris AI, Newgarten J. Chronic active hepatitis and ulcerative colitis associated with eosinophilia, nonthrombocytopenic hypergammaglobulinemia, purpura, and serological abnormalities. Am J Gastro 1978; 69:191.

    Ulcerative colitis, but not the liver disease, improves with corticosteroid therapy.

11. Howat AT, et al. The late results of long-term treatment of primary biliary cirrhosis by corticosteroids. Rev Int Hepatol 1966; 16:227.

    Corticosteroids had no beneficial effect on the progression of primary biliary cirrhosis, but they did promote the development of osteoporosis in the majority of patients.

12. Lesesne HR, Bozymicki E, Fallon H. Treatment of alcoholic hepatitis with encephalopathy: Comparison of prednisolone with caloric supplements. Gastroenterology 1978; 79:169.

    North Carolina females with severe alcoholic liver disease appear to benefit from corticosteroid therapy.

13. Maddrey W, et al. Corticosteroid therapy of alcoholic hepatitis. Gastroenterology 1978; 75:193.

An early study suggesting the benefit of corticosteroid therapy in patients with severe alcoholic liver disease complicated by encephalopathy.

14. Maddrey WC, et al. Prednisolone therapy in patients with severe alcoholic hepatitis: Results of a multicenter trial. Hepatology 1986; 6:1202.

    Eleven of the 31 placebo recipients died within the 28-day study period, compared with only 2 of 35 methylprednisolone-treated patients.

15. Madsbad S, et al. Impaired conversion of prednisone to prednisolone in patients with liver cirrhosis. Gut 1980; 21:52.

    Mean serum prednisolone concentration was only 53% ($p < 0.05$) of that observed in the seven patients with only slightly impaired liver function.

16. Mistilis SP, Blackburn CRB. Active chronic hepatitis. Am J Med 1970; 48:484.

    Enthusiasm for corticosteroid therapy was exhibited by the authors of this retrospective review.

17. Perrillo RP, et al. Prednisone withdrawal followed by recombinant alpha interferon in the treatment of chronic type B hepatitis: A randomized, controlled trial. Ann Int Med 1988; 109:95.

    A study of 39 patients with chronic hepatitis B in which one group received combination therapy ($N = 18$) and the other received placebo ($N = 21$). A statistically significant difference in the rate of clearance of HBV-DNA and DNA polymerase was seen, in favor of the treatment group.

18. Read AE, Sherlock S, Harrison CV. Active "juvenile" cirrhosis considered as part of a systemic disease and the effect of corticosteroid therapy. Gut 1963; 4:378.

    The authors find utility for corticosteroid therapy early in the course of viral hepatitis.

19. Shaldon S, Sherlock S. Virus hepatitis with features of prolonged bile retention. BJM 1957; 2:734.

    Persistent jaundice, high serum globulins, and elevated transaminases can be improved with prednisolone therapy, although the real benefit is more to morale than to histology, healing, or survival.

20. Ware A, et al. Controlled trial of corticosteroid therapy in severe acute viral hepatitis. Gastroenterology 1978; 75:992.

    From the study of 74 patients, the authors concluded that therapy with prednisolone does not influence the outcome of severe acute viral hepatitis.

23
Azathioprine
Michael M. Van Ness

Azathioprine was once thought to have great potential in the treatment of acute and chronic liver disease. It has been studied in a number of conditions, including primary biliary cirrhosis, acute and chronic autoimmune liver disease, and chronic active hepatitis (non-A, non-B). Despite widespread hopes, the use of azathioprine appears limited to the long-term treatment of patients with chronic autoimmune liver disease and the rare primary biliary cirrhosis patient unable to tolerate colchicine therapy. The side effects of azathioprine are potentially formidable and require a careful follow-up plan.

MECHANISM OF ACTION

Azathioprine is an imidazole derivative of 6-mercaptopurine with antimetabolite and immunosuppressive actions that result in inhibition of purine-ring biosynthesis and thus cellular division.

INDICATIONS

Azathioprine is approved by the Food and Drug Administration for the treatment of severe, active rheumatoid arthritis and acute leukemia, and as an adjunct for the prevention of orthotopic renal transplant rejection. Its use in chronic autoimmune liver disease (CALD) is well established. Efficacy of azathioprine in chronic liver diseases like primary biliary cirrhosis and chronic hepatitis B is by no means proven.

Primary Biliary Cirrhosis

In 1976, Heathcote published the results of the first prospective, controlled trial of azathioprine in primary biliary cirrhosis (chronic, intrahepatic, nonsuppurative cholangitis). Forty-five patients (stage I, II, or III) were studied from 1968 until 1974. Of the 45, 22 received 2 milligrams of azathioprine per kilogram body weight a day. Although subjective improvement in pruritis and objective improvement in serum aspartate transaminase levels were noted, it was not until the sixth year of the trial that survival benefit could be demonstrated. The statistical power of that survival benefit was low.

Crowe published the preliminary results of a multicenter, double-blind, randomized, placebo-controlled trial of azathioprine in 1980. Azathioprine, 1 milligram/kilogam body weight, up to a maximum of 100 milligrams/day, was given, with the drug suspended temporarily if leukocyte counts dropped below 2000 cells per microliter or platelet counts dropped below 20,000 cells per microliter. Annual liver biopsies were performed.

At the time of the report, 236 patients (all stages of the

disease were included) had been entered, with 124 receiving azathioprine and 112 receiving placebo.

Patients at prefibrotic and precirrhotic stages of the disease (stages I and II) were expected to receive the greatest benefit from azathioprine. Unfortunately, survival, progression to cirrhosis, and symptoms (pruritus, need for cholestyramine treatment, jaundice, edema, and xanthoma formation) were not improved by azathioprine.

The follow-up, final report of this international trial was published in 1985 and concluded that the 1980 preliminary report contained some random imbalance between the two treatment groups that might have obscured benefit of azathioprine therapy in primary biliary cirrhosis. This final report was produced using multivariate Cox regression analysis. Five variables with independent prognostic influence were noted, and a modest benefit of azathioprine was established. The authors conclude that although the benefit of azathioprine on survival is not dramatic, the agent should be considered a valuable medical treatment for primary biliary cirrhosis.

Chronic Autoimmune Liver Disease

Soloway and his colleagues published a prospective, double-blind, randomized trial of prednisone alone (20 mgs), prednisone (10 mgs) and azathioprine (50 mgs) in combination, and azathioprine alone (100 mgs) in the treatment of chronic autoimmune liver disease. Life expectancy, survival, liver function, serologic abnormalities, and hepatic histology improved on immunosuppressive therapy with prednisone alone and prednisone in combination with azathioprine. Toxicity from prednisone alone (osteoporosis, diabetes, Cushingoid features) and azathioprine alone (leukopenia, thrombocytopenia) were common (21% and 53%, respectively). Only one patient (7%) receiving combination therapy had a serious side effect (leukopenia and thrombocytopenia) requiring drug discontinuation. The authors conclude that the benefits of prednisone alone or prednisone in combination with azathioprine in the treatment of patients with CALD far outweigh the potential complications and side effects.

Stellon has published a study recently documenting maintenance of remission in CALD with azathioprine after corticosteroid withdrawal. Azathioprine, 2 milligrams/kilogram, was required. After 1 year of therapy, there was no significant difference with respect to liver function or histology between the "control" group (N = 22) treated with prednisolone and azathioprine (1 mg/kg) and the group of 25 treated with higher doses of azathioprine.

Chronic Hepatitis (non-A, non-B)

Stellon published an intriguing abstract in 1984 comparing the results of azathioprine withdrawal and azathioprine maintenance in a group of 50 patients with prednisone- and azathioprine-induced remission of chronic active hepatitis. Over a median follow-up period of 20 months, reactivation of disease occurred significantly more often in the azathioprine withdrawal group (7 of 27), compared to the azathioprine maintenance group (1 of 23). Further studies are needed in this area.

ADMINISTRATION

Azathioprine, 1 milligram/kilogram body weight/day, is given as a single daily oral dose as the initial treatment for chronic autoimmune liver disease and primary biliary cirrhosis. If necessary, the dose can be increased in one-half milligram/kilogram/day increments every 4 weeks up to a maximum dose of 2 milligrams/kilogram/day.

For treatment of acute flares of chronic autoimmune liver disease, azathioprine should be given in combination with corticosteroids, not as a single agent.

For maintenance of remission of chronic autoimmune liver disease, azathioprine in combination with corticosteroids or alone may be efficacious.

Allopurinol interferes with the enzymatic oxidation of azathioprine by xanthine oxidase. Concomitant azathioprine and allopurinol therapy can result in elevated blood levels of azathioprine and increased frequency and severity of side effects. A marked reduction in azathioprine dose (25% of a normal dose) prevents dose-related side effects.

Monitoring of complete blood counts, including platelet counts, during the first months of therapy is required. During the first month of therapy and after incremental dose increases, weekly blood counts should be obtained and will give prompt warning of bone marrow suppression. If either leukocyte, red blood cell, or platelet counts drop significantly, a reduction in dosage or temporary withdrawal of azathioprine is prudent.

SIDE EFFECTS

Azathioprine must be used carefully and the patient followed conscientiously to minimize the side effects known to occur with this agent. Hematologic, gastrointestinal, and oncologic complications are well described.

Azathioprine has a dose-related effect on all blood elements. Leukopenia, thrombocytopenia, and anemia are well described and occur in 10 to 20 percent of cases receiving as little as 50 to 100 milligrams of oral azathioprine a day. Weekly monitoring of blood counts starting at initiation of therapy and after incremental increases in dosage is necessary for early detection of bone marrow suppression. Dose reduction or temporary cessation of therapy is required if the white blood cell count drops below 2000 cells per microliter, if the platelet count drops below 20,000 cells per microliter, or if the hematocrit decreases to 30 percent or less.

Azathioprine has been implicated on rare occasions as causing a mixed cholestatic, hepatocellular injury. With the high-dose therapy required in the treatment of renal transplant patients, veno-occlusive disease can be seen. Hypersensitivity pancreatitis and vasculitis is well described and is fortunately rare (<1% of recipients).

The oncogenicity of azathioprine has long been suspected but never proved. Tage-Jensen et al. reviewed their group's experience with 154 patients with nonalcoholic chronic liver disease, randomized to treatment with either azathioprine or prednisone. Tage-Jensen found that 13 of 39 (33%) azathioprine-treated patients died from malignant neoplasia, compared to only 4 of 32 (13%) prednisone-treated patients, and thus urged caution in the long-term use of azathioprine. In an accompanying editorial, Schaffner refuted their conclusion by noting the lack of statistical evidence implicating azathioprine oncogenicity. Schaffner concludes that "nothing so far reported should prevent us from using a drug that appears to be both potent and remarkably safe."

Aplastic anemia has been noted in a liver-transplant patient receiving azathioprine. Only one of the nine patients reviewed by the Pittsburgh group received azathioprine. The authors conclude that the high incidence of aplastic anemia in the group relates more to the underlying liver disease (non-A, non-B hepatitis) than to any particular drug therapy.

PEARLS AND PITFALLS

1. The most clear indication for azathioprine in the treatment of chronic liver disease is the steroid-sparing effect (and possibly additive efficacy) of azathioprine in patients with chronic autoimmune liver disease.
2. Allopurinol markedly increases the risk of azathioprine toxicity by blocking azathioprine degradation by xanthine oxidase.
3. The utility of azathioprine for the treatment of primary biliary cirrhosis has, by and large, been superseded by colchicine.
4. The use of azathioprine during pregnancy is relatively contraindicated unless potential benefits far outweigh the potential fetal risks. Azathioprine is mutagenic in humans, teratogenic in rodents, crosses the placental barrier, and is known to cause limited immunologic abnormalities in infants born to renal homograft recipients.

References

1. Bergman SM, et al. Azathioprine and hypersensitivity vasculitis. Ann Int Med 1988; 109:83–84.

    Two patients with end-stage renal disease received azathioprine and developed vasculitis within 8–14 days of initiation of drug therapy. Rechallenge precipitated the symptoms of fever, headache, malaise, purpura, and bullae.

2. Christensen E, et al. Beneficial effect of azathioprine and prediction of prognosis in primary biliary cirrhosis. Gastroenterology 1985; 89:1084–1091.

    Using Cox multiple-regression analysis and adjusting for the slight imbalance between the two treatment groups, the therapeutic effect of azathioprine was statistically significant, with azathioprine reducing the risk of dying to 59 percent of that observed during placebo treatment, and improving survival by 20 months in the average patient.

3. Crowe J, et al. Azathioprine in primary biliary cirrhosis: A preliminary report of an international trial. Gastroenterology 1980; 78:1005–1010.

    Although most of the trends observed were in favor of azathioprine, no significant effects were seen on survival, clinical course, hepatic histology, liver tests, or immunologic abnormalities among 124 patients treated with azathioprine, compared to 112 treated with placebo.

4. DePinho RA, Goldberg CS, Lefkowitch JH. Azathioprine and the liver: Evidence favoring idiosyncratic, mixed cholestatic-hepatocellular injury in humans. Gastroenterology 1984; 86:162.

    Azathioprine has been implicated on rare occasions in causing a mixed cholestatic-hepatocellular injury.

5. Heathcote J, Ross A, Sherlock S. A prospective controlled trial of azathioprine in primary biliary cirrhosis. Gastroenterology 1976; 70:656–660.

    Survival was similar for the first 5 years of the trial, with a significant difference in favor of the treated group in the sixth year.

6. Lawson DH, et al. Adverse effects of azathioprine. Adv Drug React Ac Pois Rev 1984; 3:161–171.

    A thorough review of the pharmacology and side effects of azathioprine. A must prior to initiation of this type of immunosuppressive therapy.

7. Schaffner F. The oncogenicity of azathioprine? Hepatology 1988; 8:693.

    The author maintains a healthy skepticism over the issue of azathioprine-induced neoplasms.

8. Soloway RD, et al. Clinical, biochemical, and histological remission of severe chronic active liver disease: A controlled study of treatments and early prognosis. Gastroenterology 1972; 63:820.

    Prednisone or a combination of prednisone (10 mgs) and azathioprine (50 mgs) significantly improved life expectancy; resolution to normal of clinical, biochemical, and immunological abnormalities; and histological resolution from chronic active hepatitis to nonspecific hepatitis. By contrast, deterioration usually occurred with azathioprine alone.

9. Stellon AJ, et al. Maintenance of remission in autoimmune chronic active hepatitis with azathioprine after corticosteroid withdrawal. Hepatology 1988; 8:781–784.

    The authors show that azathioprine alone is sufficient to maintain a remission of chronic autoimmune liver disease induced by azathioprine and prednisone.

10. Stellon AJ, et al. Controlled trial of azathioprine withdrawal in autoimmune chronic active hepatitis. Lancet 1985; 1:668–670.

    A beneficial effect of azathioprine (50 to 100 mgs) was demonstrated by the authors. This dose, in combination with corticosteroids, resulted in a relapse rate of only 6 percent in 3 years. Corticosteroid therapy alone resulted in a 33 percent relapse rate.

11. Tage-Jensen U. Copenhagen Study Group for Liver Diseases. Malignancies following long-term azathioprine treatment in chronic liver disease. Liver 1987; 7:81–83.

Among 154 patients with histologically proven nonalcoholic liver disease, randomized to treatment with either azathioprine or prednisone, the cause of death after a median follow-up period of 91 months was from a malignant neoplasm in 33 percent of the azathioprine group and 13 percent in the prednisone group.

Heavy Metal Antagonists

Michael M. Van Ness

Penicillamine is a useful agent in the treatment of one disease of the gastrointestinal system and may yet prove efficacious in two others. For years it was hoped that the efficacy of penicillamine would be demonstrable in a wide variety of conditions, including all stages of primary biliary cirrhosis. At this time, penicillamine is indicated for the acute and chronic management of Wilson's disease and is justified for the palliative treatment of late-stage primary biliary cirrhosis in patients unable to receive a liver transplant.

MECHANISM OF ACTION

Penicillamine is an anti-inflammatory agent with antifibrotic actions capable of chelating copper. While the antiinflammatory and antifibrotic actions remain of unproved benefit, copper chelation has been proved valuable in the treatment of Wilson's disease.

Penicillamine chelation therapy induces urinary copper excretion of 2 to 5 milligrams/24 hours. With the initiation of therapy and cupriuria, active hepatic inflammation and hemolysis often subside dramatically, although mild elevation of liver-associated enzymes may persist for months. Hepatic fibrosis and portal hypertension are less responsive to penicillamine therapy.

Penicillamine combines with free aldehyde groups in collagen, preventing cross-linking and thereby interfering with collagen formation and collagen tensile strength. It does not prevent collagen synthesis.

Penicillamine has several immune-system effects. Serum immunoglobulin synthesis, polymorphonuclear leukocyte chemotaxis, and Ciq binding protein are all reduced by penicillamine. D-penicillamine also inhibits T-lymphocyte function by suppressing T-cell mitogen response.

INDICATIONS

Wilson's Disease

Penicillamine is the treatment of choice for patients with Wilson's disease. In 1956, Walshe published the first report of penicillamine use in Wilson's disease patients. Most published series of penicillamine therapy for Wilson's disease show good drug efficacy with reversal of psychiatric, neurologic, and hepatic abnormalities. For example, 16 of 22 symptomatic and all 16 asymptomatic Wilson's disease patients treated by Strickland were asymptomatic after 2 years of therapy.

The drug may be less efficacious in patients who present with liver disease. Scott reported that nine of 17 adolescent patients presenting with active hepatitis died despite penicillamine treatment.

Table 24–1. The effect of D-penicillamine on primary biliary cirrhosis

	European (1985)	Mayo Clinic (1985)	Boston (1982)
Number of patients	189	227	52
Dose (gms)	1.2	1.0	1.0
Adverse effects (%)	36	22	31
Histology	NS	ND	ND
Mortality (%; 2-year)	18	12	27
Survival	ND	ND	ND
Length of study (mos)	60	120	28

NS, not stated
ND, no difference in progression between treatment and placebo
Adapted and reprinted with permission of the authors, Cramer GL, et al. Bile excretory function, cholestasis, and hyperbilirubinemia. In G Gitrick, ed, Current hepatology. Chicago: Yearbook, 1987, p. 266.

Clinical improvement may require 1 to 3 months of therapy. On occasion, a deterioration in neurologic symptoms precedes the gradual long-term amelioration induced by chelation therapy. If such a deterioration is noted, temporary dose reduction or cessation of therapy is *not* suggested, as the risk of a sensitivity reaction is increased with resumption of penicillamine. If therapy must be stopped, an attempt at desensitization with gradually increasing daily doses with steroid coverage is preferable to the alternative chelating agent triethylene tetramine dehydrochloride (trien 2 HCL). Likewise, avoidance of foods high in copper content (shellfish, organ meats like liver and kidney, nuts and mushrooms) and domestically softened water is advisable. Although promising, zinc therapy remains of unproven value.

Several other diseases of the liver are characterized by elevated hepatic copper content (greater than 250 mg/dry weight), including primary biliary cirrhosis, extrahepatic biliary obstruction or atresia, intrahepatic cholestasis of childhood, Indian childhood cirrhosis, and vineyard workers spraying and inhaling copper salts. Of these conditions, only patients with primary biliary cirrhosis may benefit from penicillamine therapy. Penicillamine would be expected to reduce hepatic copper content and decrease hepatic inflammation. Despite several authors' initial enthusiasm, consistent improvement in liver function and patient survival has not been demonstrated (see Table 24–1). In the Mayo Clinic study, Dickson did find a favorable influence on histologic progression of disease with six of seven subjects receiving 1 gram of D-penicillamine a day, a low copper diet, and pyridoxine supplements showing no progression from stage I to stage II disease over twelve months compared to progression seen in seven of ten receiving placebo. Side effects may limit the use of penicillamine to poor prognosis patients (pruritis, jaundice, rising bilirubin greater than 7 mg/dl, ascites, and splenomegaly), who are not candidates for liver transplantation. In this group of stage III or IV patients, Epstein has shown improvement in survival—but only after eighteen months of therapy. Improvement in liver function, a fall in serum immunoglobulins, and decreased liver copper content were seen.

D-penicillamine should not be given to asymptomatic patients in whom colchicine (see Chapter 25) may prove a more satisfactory alternative.

The use of penicillamine has been studied in noncirrhotic alcoholic liver disease. Although a suggestion of decreased fibrosis was made for patients receiving one gram of penicillamine a day, neither survival nor rates of recovery from acute alcoholic liver injury were altered by penicillamine therapy. Given its narrow toxic/therapeutic index, penicillamine cannot be recommended for use in patients with noncirrhotic alcoholic liver disease.

SIDE EFFECTS

Hematologic, gastrointestinal, allergic, and renal abnormalities occur in 5 to 25 percent of patients treated with penicillamine.

Thrombocytopenia (4%), leukopenia (2%), and aplastic anemia (<1%) usually occur early in the treatment course (first 3 months) and necessitate complete blood cell and platelet counts every two weeks during this period.

Altered or diminished taste (10%) and epigastric pain, nausea, and diarrhea (15%) are common. Rare (<1%) gastrointestinal side effects include hepatitis, pancreatitis, and intrahepatic cholestasis.

A systemic lupus erythematosus–like syndrome (<1%) with rash, fever, anemia, leukopenia, and proteinuria is well described with penicillamine. For patients with Wilson's disease, this syndrome is best treated with a 50-percent dose reduction—*not* cessation—an antihistamine such as diphenhydramine (50 mgs orally every 6 hours), and prednisone (20 mgs orally every 12 hours). With resolution of the lupuslike syndrome, small incremental increases in the daily penicillamine dosage, with continued steroid coverage, allow restoration of full-dose therapy.

Proteinuria as an early sign of membranous glomerulonephropathy is common enough (6%) to mandate performance of a urinalysis every 2 weeks during the first 6 months of therapy. Proteinuria exceeding 1 gram every 24 hours necessitates progressive dose reduction. If significant proteinuria persists then complete cessation of therapy is required.

Pyridoxine, 25 milligrams a day, is necessary for Wilson's disease patients receiving penicillamine therapy, to prevent the development of cheilosis, glossitis, seborrhea, neuropathy, and anemia.

Since penicillamine can inhibit iron absorption, menstruating women and children benefit from short courses of iron supplementation (3 months, 325 mgs 3 times a day) given 2 hours after penicillamine. Continuous oral iron therapy is inadvisable since iron can inhibit penicillamine absorption.

Successful pregnancies are reported in Wilson's disease patients receiving 1 gram of penicillamine daily, with no untoward fetal effects. Discontinuation of the drug has deleterious effects on the mother and should be avoided. Scheinberg and Sternlieb have used penicillamine to preserve hepatic and renal function in over 150 pregnant patients without untoward fetal or maternal side effects. Dose reduction to 250 milligrams/day for the 6 weeks prior to a scheduled caesarian section is advisable to restore wound healing to near normal. Breast feeding by mothers receiving penicillamine should be very strongly discouraged.

ADMINISTRATION

For Wilson's disease, penicillamine, 250 milligrams 4 times a day 1 hour before meals, is an appropriate starting regimen. If tolerated, then incremental increases of 250 milligrams/day every 3 to 4 days, to a daily dose of 2 grams/day are suggested. Cupriuresis of more than 2 milligrams/day is desirable. After 3 months of therapy, the daily dose can be modified to keep the serum copper level lower than 10 micrograms/deciliter and the hepatic copper content lower than 55 micrograms/gram dry liver weight. (Concentrations > 250 µgs/gm dry liver weight are usual in homozygous Wilson's disease patients.)

Maintenance therapy of Wilson's disease usually requires 1500 to 2000 milligrams of penicillamine a day for life.

For treatment of poor-prognosis, primary biliary cirrhosis patients, the initial daily dose of 125 milligrams is increased by 125 milligrams every 2 weeks until the maintenance dose of 500 milligrams daily is reached. As with patients with Wilson's disease, monitering of hematologic (complete blood cell and platelet count) and renal function (urinalysis) every week is required during the first weeks of therapy.

PEARLS AND PITFALLS

1. Once penicillamine is initiated for the treatment of Wilson's disease, it should not be stopped unless serious side effects occur, as reinstitution of therapy after a delay of even a few days is associated with potentially severe hypersensitivity side effects.
2. There is no place in the evaluation of a patient suspected of having Wilson's disease for a penicillamine trial.
3. Penicillamine therapy should continue through pregnancy to protect the mother from the hepatic and renal complications of Wilson's disease.
4. Liver transplantation is a real therapeutic option for the

younger patient with severe hepatic disease unresponsive to penicillamine therapy.
5. Penicillamine may benefit stage III or IV primary biliary cirrhosis patients who are not candidates for hepatic transplantation.
6. Indications for D-penicillamine therapy in nongastrointestinal diseases include cystinuria and severe active rheumatoid arthritis unresponsive to conventional therapy.
7. Penicillamine should be given at least 1 hour before or 2 hours after meals and at least 1 hour apart from snacks or other drugs.

References

1. Berry WR, et al. Effects of penicillamine therapy and low copper diet on dysarthria in Wilson's disease (hepatolenticular degeneration). Mayo Clin Proc 1974; 49:405–408.

    Improvement in general neurologic status by penicillamine, 750–1500 mgs/day, was graded by voice recordings, intention tremor, and rigidity.

2. Brewer GJ, et al. Oral zinc therapy for Wilson's disease. Ann Int Med 1983; 99:314–320.

    Although not approved for maintenance therapy for Wilson's disease, oral zinc (150 mgs/day in divided doses) is shown in this article to maintain a neutral or negative copper balance in five of five patients.

3. Cossack ZT. The efficacy of oral zinc therapy as an alternative to penicillamine for Wilson's disease. NEJM 1988; 318:322.

    In a letter, the author proposes zinc as an effective alternative therapy for Wilson's disease patients who (1) develop renal failure, (2) are pregnant, (3) need adjunctive therapy to prevent zinc deficiency, (4) require penicillamine dose reduction, and (5) face intolerable toxicities. A response refuting these suggestions is given by Scheinberg and Sternlieb.

4. Deiss A. Treatment of Wilson's disease. Ann Int Med 1983; 99:398–400.

    Penicillamine (dimethylcysteine), a degradation product of penicillin, promotes copper excretion as well as dimercaprol but may require 3–6 months to achieve a sustained benefit. Children and adolescents with severe liver disease are particularly susceptible to further deterioration during this time. Oral zinc is not an effective treatment alternative during this time of tenuous liver function.

5. Dickson ER, Fleming CR, Ludwig J. Primary biliary cirrhosis. In H Popper, F Schaffner (eds), *Progress in Liver Disease* vol 6. New York: Grune and Stratton, 1978, p. 487.

    The initial report of the efficacy of penicillamine benefiting early-stage PBC has not stood the test of time.

6. Epstein O, et al. D-Penicillamine treatment improves survival in primary biliary cirrhosis. *Lancet* 1981; 1:1275–1277.

In a randomized trial of penicillamine treatment among 55 patients with primary biliary cirrhosis, drug reactions occurred in 16 (29%). In those able to tolerate the drug, death occurred in only 14 percent of the penicillamine treatment group, compared to 43 percent of the placebo-treated cohort.

7. Epstein O, et al. Reduction of immune complexes and immunoglobulins induced by D-penicillamine in primary biliary cirrhosis. NEJM 1979; 300:274–278.

    Twenty-eight patients randomly allocated to receive either penicillamine, 600–900 mgs/day, or placebo for 24 months demonstrated significant reductions in IgA, IgM, and IgG concentrations, bilirubin values, and serum aspartate transaminase levels. The authors conclude that penicillamine may favorably change the course of primary biliary cirrhosis by these immunologic manipulations, in addition to the drug's copper-chelating action.

8. Matloff DS, et al. A prospective trial of D-penicillamine in primary biliary cirrhosis. NEJM 1982; 306:319–326.

    In a prospective, double-blind study, 26 patients received 1 gm of penicillamine a day and were compared to a group of 26 placebo-treated patients. There was no improvement in survival, liver-associated enzymes, or histology despite adequate urinary excretion of copper. Serious side effects occurred in 31% of patients, with an additional 46% suffering less serious complications.

9. Resnick R, et al. Preliminary observations of D-penicillamine therapy in acute alcoholic liver disease. Digestion 1974; 11:257.

    Despite a modest improvement in liver histology ascribable to penicillamine therapy, the drug cannot be recommended in this patient population.

10. Scheinberg IH, Sternlieb I. Letter. NEJM 1988; 318:323.

    A response to the letter of Cossack cited previously, emphasizing that (1) in more than 400 patients with Wilson's disease, only one has suffered renal failure (secondary to nephrocalcinosis), (2) penicillamine-induced proteinuria occurs in only about 4% of patients, (3) penicillamine has been given to more than 150 pregnant women without untoward effect, (4) no zinc deficiency has ever been observed during penicillamine therapy, and (5) trientine is the only other drug approved by the U.S. Food and Drug Administration for treatment of Wilson's disease.

11. Scheinberg IH, Sternlieb I. Wilson's disease. In LH Smith (ed.), *Major Problems in Internal Medicine* vol 23. Philadelphia: Saunders, 1984.

    A comprehensive review of the use of penicillamine in Wilson's disease. No better single resource exists for those interested in its treatment.

12. Scott J. Wilson's disease presenting as chronic active hepatitis. Gastroenterology 1978; 74:645–651.

    A series of 17 teenage patients presenting with chronic hepatitis, emphasizing the serious nature of this form of the disease. Nine of the 17 died of liver failure within weeks of the initiation of treatment with penicillamine.

25
Colchicine

Michael M. Van Ness

Therapeutic options for patients with primary biliary cirrhosis (PBC) and non-PBC cirrhosis have been limited by the effectiveness of the available agents and the toxicities of potential therapeutic candidates. Recently, the anti-inflammatory and antifibrotic agent colchicine has shown promise in decreasing the morbidity and mortality associated with both primary and non-PBC cirrhosis. These preliminary studies found little toxicity with colchicine and offer hope that an effective and well-tolerated therapy may soon be available.

MECHANISM OF ACTION

Although many of the actions of colchicine are well characterized, its mechanism of action in liver disease is unknown. Colchicine is derived from the autumn crocus and was first isolated in 1820. Among its many actions, it binds to tubulin, blocks mitosis, and inhibits polymorphonuclear leukocyte function. Colchicine accumulates intracellularly in human lymphocytes (16 times the serum concentration).

With respect to primary biliary cirrhosis, colchicine corrects the deficiency of concanavalin A–induced suppressor cell function characteristic of these patients. It decreases elevated levels of interleukin-1 in monocytes. For example, colchicine decreases interleukin-1 levels in monocytes from patients with primary biliary cirrhosis by 50 percent.

In patients with cirrhosis, colchicine increases the level of cathepsin B and D and hydroxyproline in hepatic tissue. Colchicine also increases liver blood flow as measured by an indirect, noninvasive method. It interferes with transcellular movement of collagen, reduces the activity of hepatic collagen-processing enzymes in rats, and stimulates collanenase production in vitro.

PHARMACODYNAMICS

Colchicine is well absorbed after oral ingestion and is excreted in bile, stool, and urine. The drug half-life is 24 to 36 hours. Intracellular drug concentrations are significantly higher than serum concentrations and are maintained for several days after cessation of drug therapy.

INDICATIONS

Primary Biliary Cirrhosis

Colchicine may have a useful role in the treatment of primary biliary cirrhosis. (See Table 25-1.) The first uncontrolled clinical trial of colchicine was reported in 1980 by Koldinger. He found significant decreases in hepatic enzymes in five patients with primary biliary cirrhosis treated

Table 25–1. Controlled trials of colchicine in cirrhosis

Author	Number	Follow-up (mos)	Dose (mgs)	Improved?
Primary biliary cirrhosis				
Koldinger (1980)	5	40	0.6 bid	Biochemically
Warnes (1987)	64	23	1 mg/day 5 days a wk	Biochemically; Pathologically? Survival?
Kaplan (1986)	60	24	0.6 bid	Biochemically; Not survival
Bodenheimer (1988)	57	33	0.6 bid	Biochemically; Not pathologically
Nonprimary biliary cirrhosis				
Kershenobich (1988)	100	14	1 mg/day 5 days a wk	Biochemically; Pathologically; Survival
Kershenobich (1979)	43	—	1 mg/day 5 days a wk	Biochemically; Pathologically; Survival
Bahgat (1985)	96	—	—	No benefit

with 0.6 milligrams twice a day for up to 40 months. After 12 months of therapy, the serum alkaline phosphatase levels decreased an average of 2.7 times the upper limit of normal (from a mean of 8.6 times the upper limit of normal, to 4.9 times the upper limit of normal).

This encouraging preliminary report was followed by Warnes's report. In a group of 64 patients, half treated with colchicine (1 mg/day) and half treated with placebo, significant improvement in serum albumin, immunoglobulin, and bilirubin levels were accompanied by a decreasing trend in mortality in the colchicine-treated group. One fourth of the colchicine-treated patients developed diarrhea.

Kaplan's group reported the results of their double-blind, randomized, placebo-controlled trial of colchicine (0.6 mg twice a day) in 1986. They found improvement in serum enzymes (alkaline phosphatase and serum alanine aminotransferase) and liver function (bilirubin, cholesterol, and albumin), as well as a statistically significant improvement in mortality. Interestingly, there was no accompanying improvement in liver histology (inflammation or fibrosis) in those colchicine-treated patients who underwent serial liver biopsy.

A second placebo-controlled trial of colchicine confirmed Kaplan's findings. Bodenheimer gave 57 patients either placebo or colchicine, 0.6 milligrams twice a day, for 4 years. Patients were evaluated every 3 months and underwent liver biopsy annually. Apparent were decreases in both alkaline phosphatase (mean alkaline phosphatase pretreatment was 281 IU/liter and post-treatment, 112 IU/liter and serum alanine aminotransferase (last-first ratio in the colchicine cohort was 0.68, compared to 0.94 in the placebo cohort; p<0.0001). The mean rise in serum bilirubin levels was slowed (0.54 mg/dl/year in the colchicine group, versus 1.77 mg/dl/year in the placebo group). Like Kaplan, Bodenheimer noted no improvement in the histologic progression of the disease. Few side effects were encountered except diarrhea, which responded to colchicine dose reduction.

In a recent review of the subject of colchicine therapy for primary biliary cirrhosis, Wiesner concludes that treatment with colchicine appears to be associated with hepatic biochemical and functional improvement and a trend toward increased survival. The failure of colchicine to ameliorate clinical symptoms or to halt histologic progression of the disease precludes an enthusiastic endorsement of colchicine therapy for primary biliary cirrhosis.

Cirrhosis (Nonprimary Biliary Cirrhosis)

In 1979, Kershenobich published the preliminary results of a double-blind, randomized, placebo-controlled study of colchicine, 1 milligram orally 5 days a week, in the treatment of cirrhosis. Improvement in hepatic biochemical function (albumin), histology, and survival created considerable interest in the utility of colchicine as an antifibrotic and antiinflammatory drug for cirrhosis.

A follow-up study by Bahgat in Egypt was less enthusiastic. Despite Kershenobich's initial results, Bahgat noted no improvement clinically, biochemically, or histopathologically in 96 patients with biopsy-proved, chronic, active hepatitis treated with either corticosteroids, azathioprine, corticosteroids and azathioprine, chlorambucil, 5-fluorouracil, isoprinosine, or colchicine, compared to placebo. Given the number of treatment options in this study and the small number of patients enrolled in each arm, the possibility of a type II error encourages further work in the area.

In 1988, Kershenobich reported the final results of 100 Mexican patients (45 with alcoholic cirrhosis, 41 with posthepatic cirrhosis, and 14 with cirrhosis of various etiologies) treated with either placebo or colchicine, 1 milligram/day 5 days a week. The cumulative 5-year survival rate for the colchicine group was 75 percent, compared to a 34-percent survival rate in the placebo group. Improvement in the hepatic histology was apparent in 60 percent of the 30 colchicine-treated patients undergoing repeat biopsy. No improvement in liver histology was apparent in the 14 placebo-treated patients who underwent repeat biopsy.

Enthusiasm generated by Kershenobich's article must be tempered by Boyer and Ransohoff's accompanying editorial. They note a higher mean serum albumin level in the colchicine group at the start of the study, a high rate of patients lost to follow-up—20 percent in both treatment groups—and a lack of nutritional or compliance data. Because of these study deficiencies, Boyer and Ransohoff do not yet endorse colchicine as a treatment for nonprimary biliary cirrhosis liver disease.

SIDE EFFECTS AND CONTRAINDICATIONS

From the experience of using colchicine in the treatment of acute gout, it is well known that diarrhea, nausea, and abdominal pain occur frequently with doses of 4 to 6 milligrams in a 24-hour period. With the doses used for chronic liver disease, 0.6 milligrams twice a day or 1 milligram once a day, as many as one-third of patients experience an increase in bowel frequency and liquidity. Dose reduction to 0.6 milligrams once a day is appropriate in this situation. If diarrhea persists, then cessation of therapy may be necessary.

Rarely reported side effects include alopecia, aplastic anemia, myopathy, angioneurotic edema, epistaxis, and azoospermia. A recent case report by Finklestein of profound granulocytopenia in a 76-year-old woman with primary biliary cirrhosis receiving colchicine, 0.6 milligrams twice a day for 2 months, emphasizes the potential for agranulocytosis with this agent. Bone marrow examination revealed moderate hypocellularity of all cell lines. With cessation of colchicine therapy, the patient recovered.

PEARLS AND PITFALLS

1. Although not approved by the Food and Drug Administration for the treatment of primary biliary cirrhosis, col-

chicine, 0.6 milligrams twice a day, may have benefit in terms of mortality and liver function in these patients.
2. Overdoses of colchicine (as little as 7 milligrams orally) have been associated with death.
3. Diarrhea from colchicine usually responds to a 50-percent dose reduction.

References

1. Bahgat MH, et al. Comparative study of different types of treatments in chronic active hepatitis. Chemioterapia 1985; 4:227–235.

   A study of 96 patients with biopsy-proved chronic active hepatitis treated with either corticosteroids, azathioprine, corticosteroids and azathioprine, chlorambucil, 5-fluorouracil, colchicine, or isoprinosine, with no significant improvement in hepatic function, histology, or biochemistries. There was no difference in response to treatment between HBsAg-positive and HBsAg-negative patients.

2. Bodenheimer H, Schaffner F, Pezzullo J. Evaluation of colchicine therapy in primary biliary cirrhosis. Gastroenterology 1988; 95:124–129.

   A double-blind, placebo-controlled trial of colchicine, 0.6 mg orally twice a day, in 57 patients with various stages of primary biliary cirrhosis, demonstrating significant improvement in serum alkaline phosphatase levels (mean AP pretreatment, 281 IU/L; post-treatment, 112 IU/liter); mean annual rise in bilirubin levels (0.54 mg/dl/year in the colchicine group, versus 1.77 mg/dl/year in the placebo group); and serum alanine aminotransferase values (last-first ratio in the colchicine cohort, 0.68, compared to 0.94 in the placebo cohort; $p<0.0001$). No difference in histologic progression was demonstrable. In contrast to penicillamine (an antifibrotic, immunosuppressive drug with the potential for severe and frequent side effects), no serious side effects were experienced in this trial. Diarrhea responded to colchicine dose reduction.

3. Boyer JL, Ransohoff DF. Is colchicine effective therapy for cirrhosis? NEJM 1988; 318:1751–1752.

   An editorial critical of the Kershenobich article pointing out that chance, bias, and biologic factors may have unintentionally improved survival in the colchicine treatment group. The authors note that a higher mean serum albumin level in the colchicine group (567 versus 510 μ/liter) a high rate of patients lost to follow-up (20% in both groups), and a lack of nutritional or compliance data weaken the endorsement of colchicine as treatment for cirrhosis.

4. Finklestein M, et al. Granulocytopenia complicating colchicine therapy for primary biliary cirrhosis. Gastroenterology 1987; 93:1231–1235.

   A 76-year-old woman with primary biliary cirrhosis and adult polycystic liver disease developed granulocytopenia 2 months after starting colchicine therapy (0.6 mg bid po). Granulocytopenia reversed 4 days after the drug was stopped. Bone marrow examination revealed moderate hypocellularity of all cell lines and striking dysplastic changes in the late myeloid and erythroid series. There was no apparent toxicity of other organ systems, and the patient recovered fully.

5. Ilfeld D, et al. In vitro correction of a deficiency of con A–induced suppressor cell function in primary biliary cirrhosis by a pharmacological concentration of colchicine. Clin Exper Immun 1984; 57:438–442.

Primary biliary cirrhosis patients' mononuclear cells were cultured for 44 hours with concanavalin A, with and without colchicine at a pharmacological concentration or at a suprapharmacological concentration, and then tested for their ability to suppress proliferation of phyohemagglutinin-stimulated healthy volunteers' mononuclear cells. Eleven PBC patients had significantly decreased suppressor cell function, as compared to 37 healthy volunteers. In the nine PBC patients tested with the pharmacological concentration of colchicine, suppressor cell function was increased 40%, an increase significantly different than without colchicine but not significantly different than healthy volunteers. In other words, in vitro colchicine at a pharmacological concentration corrected PBC patients' deficiency of con A–induced suppressor cell function, raising the possibility that oral colchicine might be clinically useful as an immunomodulating drug in PBC.

6. Kaplan MM. Another treatment for primary biliary cirrhosis. Gastroenterology 1987; 92:255–257.

An editorial accompanying the Hoofnagle chlorambucil article reviewing the role of immunosuppressive therapy in the treatment of PBC, which helps to put in perspective the potential utility of colchicine in the treatment of PBC.

7. Kaplan MM, et al. A prospective trial of colchicine for primary biliary cirrhosis. NEJM 1986; 315:1448–1454.

Sixty patients with primary biliary cirrhosis were entered in a double-blind, randomized, controlled trial. Thirty patients had early disease (stages 1 and 2) and 30 had advanced disease (stages 3 and 4). Fifteen patients with early disease and 15 with advanced disease received colchicine (0.6 mg bid) and the remainder received placebo. Patients were studied every 2 months, and at 2 years underwent repeat liver biopsy. During the 2-year study period the colchicine-treated patients had improvement in levels of serum albumin, serum bilirubin, alkaline phosphatase cholesterol, and aminotransferase. However, there was no such improvement in the severity of symptoms or physical findings; moreover, there was no significant difference in the histologic changes noted at liver biopsy in the two treatment groups. At 4 years after entry, the cumulative mortality from liver disease was 21% in patients given colchicine and 47% in those given placebo.

8. Kershenobich D, et al. Treatment of cirrhosis with colchicine: A double-blind, randomized trial. Gastroenterology 1979; 77:532–536.

An early report of the efficacy of colchicine in improving hepatic tests (albumin), survival, and histology in patients with non-PBC cirrhosis.

9. Kershenobich D, et al. Colchicine in the treatment of cirrhosis of the liver. NEJM 1988; 318:1709–1713.

   A randomized, double-blind, placebo-controlled trial of 100 Mexican patients, 45 with alcoholic cirrhosis, 41 with posthepatitic cirrhosis, and 14 with cirrhosis of various etiologies, treated with either placebo or colchicine, 1 mg/day 5 days a week. All patients but one were Childs's class A or B. Analysis of mortality utilizing the intent-to-treat rule showed marked improvement in the colchicine group, with cumulative 5-year survival rates of 75%, compared to a 34-percent survival rate in the placebo group. On repeat liver biopsy of 30 colchicine-treated patients, improvement in histology was apparent in nine (30%), was normal in two (7%), and showed only minimal portal fibrosis in seven (23%). No improvement in liver histology was apparent in 14 placebo-treated patients who underwent repeat liver biopsy.

10. Koldinger RE. Treatment of primary biliary cirrhosis with colchicine. Gastroenterology 1980; 78:1309.

    The first published report documenting improvement in liver function in PBC patients receiving colchicine.

11. Stancikova M, Frysak Z, Trnavsky K. Effect of colchicine on the activity of cathepsin B and D in human liver cirrhosis. Acta Medica Hungarica 1987; 44:181–188.

    The activity of cathepsin B and D in and the hydroxyproline content of human liver biopsy specimens from normals and cirrhotic patients before and after 1 year of colchicine treatment were studied. Cathepsin B activity was higher in cirrhotic liver samples as compared with the controls, whereas the increased activity of cathepsin D was not significant. The hydroxyproline content in the liver samples was two- or threefold that of the control group. After colchicine, it remained unchanged or in some patients decreased. The ratio of cathepsin B and D activity to hepatic hydroxyproline content was significantly reduced in cirrhotic livers. Colchicine treatment was followed by an increase in the levels of the enzymes investigated as well as a significant rise in the ratio of cathepsin B and D activity to hepatic hydroxyproline content. Further studies of this type may shed light on the mechanism of cirrhosis and potential means of intervention.

12. Tapalaga D, et al. Colchicine treatment effects on liver cirrhosis assessed by liver blood flow measurements. Med Interne 1986; 24:69–73.

    In a group of 22 patients with liver cirrhosis, the hemodynamic changes associated with cirrhosis were studied before and after 24 months of antifibrotic treatment with colchicine (1 mg daily, 5 days a week). The liver blood flow was estimated every year by a noninvasive radioisotopic method. A significant improvement of the liver blood supply was noted. The simultaneous and favorable changes of liver chemistries and hemodynamic parameters suggest that the perfusion improvement might explain the tendency of the biochemical data to improve.

13. Warnes TW, et al. A controlled trial of colchicine in primary biliary cirrhosis. J Hepatol 1987; 5:1–7.

Colchicine (1 mg/day) was given to 64 patients with PBC in a double-blind, placebo-controlled trial. In comparison with placebo, colchicine produced a beneficial effect on serum albumin and bilirubin levels at 3 months in patients who had abnormal liver function (bilirubin >20 μmol/liter) at entry. In patients with normal liver function at entry, beneficial effects were noted on total globulin levels at 3 months and on immunoglobulin G levels at 3 and 6 months. At 18 months, survival estimates in the colchicine and placebo groups were 84% and 69%, respectively.

14. Wiesner RH, et al. Clinical and statistical analyses of new and evolving therapies for primary biliary cirrhosis. Hepatology 1988; 8:668–676.

A rigorous analysis and critique of the therapeutic trials in PBC, with special attention to colchicine. In light of the intent-to-treat rule, the authors conclude that there currently is no effective therapy for PBC.

26

Vitamin K

Margaret Andrea and Michael M. Van Ness

Vitamin K is one of four fat-soluble vitamins required by the liver for synthesis of clotting factors. It was first recovered from hog liver fat and alfalfa. Two forms of vitamin K are known. Vitamin K_1 (phytonadione), 2 methyl, 3-phytyl 1, 4-naphthoquinone, is found in vegetable products such as broccoli, cabbage, lettuce, spinach, and kale. Vitamin K_2 (menaquinone) is synthesized by intestinal gram-positive bacteria, has as its side chain two to 13 phenyl units, and is about 60 percent as potent as vitamin K. *Koagulation vitamin* is the name Dam gave vitamin K while studying bleeding tendencies in chickens fed fat-free diets back in 1929. Subsequent studies in animals and humans showed a correlation between hemorrhage and decreased prothrombin level. Thirty years passed before it was determined that vitamin K is required for production of the prothrombin precursor of active prothrombin.

MECHANISM OF ACTION

Vitamin K is essential for the production of prothrombin. It acts to convert glutamic acid residues on the precursor protein of prothrombin to γ-carboxyglutamic acid residues, a conversion required for the activation of prothrombin. This conversion allows the peptide to build calcium, a step essential for phospholipid surface-building and initiation of the clotting cascade.

Bile salts are necessary for the absorption of vitamin K. From the small intestine, it is carried by lipoproteins in the lymph and stored in the liver.

In the absence of vitamin K, the vitamin K–dependent blood clotting factors—prothrombin (II), proconvertin (VII), plasma thromboplastin (Christmas factor, IX), and the Stuart factor (X)—are biologically inactive.

Anticoagulant drugs such as warfarin sodium act as antagonists to vitamin K by disrupting hepatic production of prothrombin and the other vitamin K–dependent clotting factors, by inhibiting conversion of glutamic acid residues on the precursor protein to γ-carboxyglutamic acid residues. Acarboxyprothrombin, an inactive prothrombin precursor, accumulates in the blood during coumadin therapy and lacks the calcium-binding capacity necessary to bind to phospholipid surfaces and initiate the clotting cascade.

INDICATIONS

Vitamin K is indicated for treatment of hypoprothrombinemia as a result of inadequate vitamin K intake, absorption, or utilization.

Infants may have a low prothrombin level immediately after birth as a result of a sterile gut. Because dietary deficiency is rare and hepatic stores are quickly filled, vitamin

K supplementation after the perinatal period is rarely necessary.

Impaired bile salt production may occur in serious liver disease. Cirrhosis and hepatitis may be accompanied by decreased production of vitamin K–dependent clotting factors despite adequate dietary levels of vitamin K. Since bile is needed for the absorption of vitamin K_1, hepatic or biliary obstruction may limit its uptake.

It is useful to antagonize the effects of anticoagulant therapy with coumadin.

DOSAGE AND ADMINISTRATION

Vitamin K_1 (phytonadione) is available as Mephyton in 5-milligram tablets for oral administration; as ampules of Konakion, either 2 or 10 milligrams/milliliter, for intramuscular administration; or as Aquamephyton, 2 or 10 milligrams/milliliter, for intravenous therapy.

A single intramuscular dose of 0.5 to 1 milligram is recommended for the normal newborn infant.

Generally, vitamin K, 10 milligrams/day orally or intravenously, is recommended in patients with biliary tract obstructive disease from either congenital defects (extrahepatic biliary atresia), tumors (Klatskin tumor, cholangiocarcinoma, or pancreatic carcinoma), or stone (choledocholithiasis).

In children with hypoprothrombinemia from intestinal malabsorption or drug therapy, dosages range from 2 milligrams for infants to 5 to 10 milligrams for older children, either orally or parenterally. If the deficiency is due to prolonged hyperalimentation, the proper child's dose is 2 to 5 milligrams intramuscularly on a weekly basis.

Vitamin K may be useful in overcoagulated patients. Depending on the clinical manifestations, overdose may be treated by complete withdrawal of the anticoagulant agent, by a decrease in anticoagulant dosage, or by a single (1–5 milligram) dose of vitamin K. With massive bleeding, 20 to 40 milligrams of vitamin K is indicated, with repeated dosing every 4 hours until hypoprothrombinemia is reversed.

There is no recommended daily allowance for vitamin K. Although the total amount needed appears to be small, what is obtained from the diet is supplemented by vitamin K_2 manufactured by the intestinal flora. There is little vitamin K stored in the liver or elsewhere in the body. If a patient is receiving oral vitamin K replacement due to obstruction of bile flow, the bile salts (ox bile, 250–500 mgs 3 times a day; Bilenzyme, one to two tablets 3 times a day; or Digepepsin, two tablets 3 times a day) must be given concurrently.

SIDE EFFECTS

Phytonadione (vitamin K_1) and menaquinone (vitamin K_2) are nontoxic even in large doses. Parenteral administration should be slow (5–10 minutes) to avoid flushing, dyspnea, chest pain, and cardiovascular collapse (rarely seen).

PEARLS AND PITFALLS

1. Vitamin K is essential for the activation of precursors of the vitamin K–dependent factors II, VII, IX, and X.
2. Vitamin K promotes the conversion of protein glutamic acid side-chain moieties to the carboxyglutamic acid required for calcium building, surface phospholipid binding, and initiation of the clotting cascade.
3. Rapid infusion of vitamin K can cause flushing, chest pain, dyspnea, and, rarely, death.
4. There is no recommended daily allowance for vitamin K.
5. Hypoprothrombinemia can occur in patients receiving antibiotics, by inhibiting production of vitamin K_2 by intestinal flora.
6. Oral vitamin K should be supplemented by bile salts in patients with a completely obstructed extrahepatic biliary tree. Either drinking bile collected from percutaneous drainage or exogenous bile salt replacement are satisfactory options.

References

1. Friedman P. Vitamin K. In M Irwin Arias, et al. (eds), *The Liver Biology and Pathobiology*. New York: Raven Press, 1982. Pp. 359–365.

   A commentary on the history and pharmacology of vitamin K in humans, in health and disease.

2. Hardman RH. Metabolism of vitamins by the liver in normal and pathologic conditions. In D Zakim, TD Boyer (eds), *Hepatology: A Textbook of Liver Disease*. Philadelphia: Saunders, 1982. Pp. 185–189.

   A discussion of the pharmacokinetics of vitamin K.

3. Hull RD, Raskah GE, Hirsh J. Thrombosis and anticoagulation. In JH Stein (ed), *Internal Medicine* (2nd ed.) Boston: Little, Brown, 1987. Pp. 1026–1027.

   A discussion of vitamin K in anticoagulant therapy.

4. Mandel HG, Cohn VH. Fat-soluble vitamins—Vitamins A, K, E. In A Goodman, et al. (eds), *Goodman and Gilman's The Pharmacological Basis of Therapeutics* (6th ed). New York: Macmillan, 1980. Pp. 1592–1596.

   A complete description of the pharmacology and mechanism of action of vitamin K.

5. McEvoy GK, Pharm D (eds). American Hospital Formulary Service Drug Information. Bethesda, MD: American Society of Hospital Pharmacists, 1988. P. 2122.

   A discussion of the uses and dosages of vitamin K.

6. Shiau YF. Lipid digestion and absorption. In LR Johnson (ed), *Physiology of the Gastrointestinal Tract* vol. 2 (2nd ed.). New York: Raven Press, 1987. Pp. 1546–1547.

   A synopsis of the absorption of fat-soluble vitamins.

7. White GC II, Levin J. Disorders of blood coagulations. In JH Stein (ed), *Internal Medicine* (2nd ed.). Boston: Little, Brown, 1987. Pp. 1018–1023.

   A discussion of vitamin K in blood dyscrasias.

27

Vaccination Agents

Ira Knepp

The incidence of reported hepatitis B has increased steadily over the last decade and is now the most commonly reported cause of infectious hepatitis in the United States. The estimated lifetime risk of hepatitis B varies as a function of lifestyle. Virtually 100 percent of intravenous drug users in New York City and promiscuous homosexuals in San Francisco are infected. At the other end of the spectrum, less than 5 percent of the general population are affected in their lifetime. The incidence of the infection is estimated to be in excess of 300,000 cases per year in the United States. Twenty-five percent of these patients become clinically ill with malaise, jaundice, and right upper quadrant tenderness. More than 10,000 require hospitalization, and approximately 250 die of fulminant disease each year. Between 6 and 10 percent become chronic carriers of hepatitis B.

Currently there is an estimated pool of 1 million carriers in the United States. Chronic active hepatitis occurs in over 25 percent of these carriers. It is estimated that 4000 persons die from hepatitis B–related cirrhosis each year in this country, and that more than 800 die from hepatitis B–related liver cancer. With widespread application of the currently available vaccines against hepatitis B, the incidence of infection and its attendant morbidity and mortality should be reduced substantially.

VACCINE DEVELOPMENT

Currently there are two hepatitis B vaccines available. The plasma-derived hepatitis B vaccine, Heptavax (Merck, Sharpe, and Dohme), is a suspension of inactivated, alum absorbed, 22-nanomole surface antigen particles purified from the plasma of homosexual patients with chronic hepatitis B. A combination of ultracentrifugation and biochemical inactivation (a threefold process using eight-molar urea, pepsin at pH 2 for 18 hours, and incubation in a 1:10,000 dilution of formalin at 37 degrees C for 72 hours) kills representatives of all classes of viruses found in human blood, including HTLV III/LAV. Special attention has been given to the potential for transmitted AIDS-related virus. Sensitive dot-blot hybridization assays did not detect any human immunodeficiency virus–related nucleic acid in the product. No evidence of AIDS or anti–human immunodeficiency virus seroconversion has been observed among the estimated 1 million nonhomosexual, nonintravenous drug user vaccinees. This vaccine contains 20 micrograms/milliliter of hepatitis B surface antigen protein.

In July, 1986, a second vaccine, a genetically engineered hepatitis B vaccine was licensed: Recombivax HB (Merck, Sharp, and Dohme). The yeast *Saccharomyces cerevisias* (common baker's yeast) was genetically altered by the addition to its genome of a plasmid containing the DNA coding for the hepatitis B surface antigen. Hepatitis B surface antigen is then prepared by lysing yeast cells, separating the yeast component from antigen by hydrophobic interaction, purifying the hepatitis B surface antigen by sterile filtration, and sterilizing with formalin. The vaccine contains 10 micrograms of hepatitis B surface antigen per milliliter.

Hepatitis B immune globulin is a sterile solution of antibodies from human plasma containing high titers of hepatitis B surface antibody (usually in excess of 1:100,000). It provides temporary passive protection and is indicated only after acute intense exposure to hepatitis B virus such as (1) needle sticks, mucous membrane contact, or swallowing hepatitis surface antigen positive blood or secretions; (2) sexual contact with people with active hepatitis B replication; or (3) contact of infants of mothers with acute or chronic hepatitis B. The dose is 0.06 milliliters/kilogram intramuscularly. The perinatal dose is 0.5 milliliter intramuscularly. All these situations require the simultaneous administration of hepatitis B vaccine. There is no evidence that acquired immunodeficiency syndrome has been transmitted by hepatitis B immune globulin, and it is not contraindicated in pregnancy. The cost of one injection is approximately 150 dollars.

CLINICAL TRIALS

Hepatitis surface antigen is the sole constituent of both vaccines. The immune response elicited is the hepatitis B surface antibody. No hepatitis B core antibody is produced.

Studies comparing antibody response in healthy adults to the plasma-derived vaccine and the recombinant vaccine show equal rates of seroconversion following three doses of either the recombinant vaccine (10 µg/dose) or the plasma-derived vaccine (20 µg/dose). The mean titers of antibody developed by the recipient of plasma-derived vaccine have ranged from 100 percent to 300 percent, as high as the recombinant vaccine. It appears that the antibody persists for at least 5 years at detectable but slowly declining levels. Current data do not allow determination of the risk of infection following a decline in antibody concentration below a specific level, nor what minimal protective antibody levels may be.

INDICATIONS

The vaccine is recommended for (1) health care workers having a significant risk of exposure to blood or needle sticks, including (2) residents and staff of institutions for the developmentally disabled, (3) hemodialysis patients, (4) recipients of multiple units of blood products or component products, such as hemophiliac patients, (5) homosexual men, (6) intravenous drug users, (7) household members and sexual contacts of hepatitis B virus carriers, (8) infants born to hepatitis B virus–positive mothers, and (9) all non-immunized people after exposure to hepatitis B virus from needle sticks. It is also important to consider the vaccine for

(1) prison inmates, (2) heterosexuals with multiple partners, and (3) international travelers to areas where hepatitis B virus is endemic.

When administered properly, hepatitis vaccine produces hepatitis surface antigen in more than 90 percent of healthy people. The plasma-derived hepatitis B vaccine is given in a series of three doses over a 6-month period. The second dose is 1 month after the first, the third dose 6 months after the second. For normal adults and children over 10 years of age, the recommended dose is 20 micrograms (1 ml) intramuscularly for each of the three inoculations. Children less than 10 years old should receive a 10-microgram dose (0.5 ml) on the same schedule.

Newborns of mothers positive for hepatitis B surface antigen should receive the three-dose series on the same schedule (10 μg/dose); however, the first dose should be given as soon as possible after birth (usually within the first 24 hours of life), with a single dose of hepatitis B immune globulin (0.5 ml) given intramuscularly at a second site. To reiterate, the vaccine and immune globulin should not be given in the same muscle group.

For hemodialysis and immunosuppressed patients, a 2-milliliter dose (40 μgs) should be used for each of the three injections.

The recombinant vaccine should be given as a series of three intramuscular injections of 1.0 milliliter (10 μg/ml) each. The second and third doses are given 1 and 6 months, respectively, after the first. The recommendations stated above about newborns of mothers positive for hepatitis B surface antigen apply to the recombinant vaccine as well.

Seroconversion occurs in 30 to 60 percent of normal recipients 1 month after the first dose; and in 90 percent of patients having circulating hepatitis surface antibody at 3 and 6 months. Despite the fact that only an additional 5 to 10 percent more people have seroconversion after the third booster, this final injection leads to a substantial increase in hepatitis surface antibody titer in seroconverters.

The response rates of immunocompromised patients are lower (50–60%), even with the 40-microgram vaccine dose studied in hemodialysis patients. Unfortunately, in hemodialysis patients, hepatitis B may occur even when patients demonstrate an antibody response to the vaccine. However, in most recipients who produce hepatitis surface antigen the protective efficiency reaches 100 percent. Vaccine failures occur in approximately 5 percent of normal individuals. People who do not complete the full complement of vaccine doses or who are already incubating hepatitis B at the time of vaccination are also less likely to have a satisfactory response to the vaccine.

Five-year booster doses of vaccine in the patient with normal immune status are not routinely recommended, nor is routine serologic testing to assess antibody levels. Testing for immunity following vaccination is recommended only for persons in whom suboptimal response to the vaccine is anticipated, such as those patients on hemodialysis.

In the vaccinated person who experiences percutaneous

or needle exposure to hepatitis surface antigen–positive blood, serologic testing to assess immune status is recommended—unless testing within the previous 12 months has indicated adequate levels of antibody. If the exposed person is tested and found to have an inadequate antibody level (<10 million iu/ml), treatment with hepatitis B immune globulin and a booster-dose of vaccine is indicated.

Semiannual antibody testing should be employed in hemodialysis patients, with a booster dose given when antibody levels decline below 10 million international units/milliliter.

Booster doses are 40 micrograms of the plasma-derived vaccine in hemodialysis patients, 20 micrograms plasma-derived vaccine, or 10 micrograms recombinant vaccine for normal adults. Half the adult dose is appropriate for children.

SIDE EFFECTS AND CONTRAINDICATIONS

Both vaccines are safe, with minor side effects occurring with equal frequency after vaccine and placebo injections. Soreness at injection site occurs in 25 percent. Mild systemic reactions (fever, headache, fatigue, or nausea) are seen in 15 percent. These side effects are seen with equal frequency after plasma-derived and recombinant vaccines and placebo injections. To date, no severe adverse effect and no transmission of the acquired immunodeficiency syndrome have been suspected or documented. Since both vaccines contain only noninfectious hepatitis B surface antigen particles, vaccination of a pregnant woman entails no additional risk to either the woman or the fetus.

PEARLS AND PITFALLS

1. Intramuscular injection is preferable to injection into subcutaneous fat, as a measurable increase in seroconversion rates and serum titers is seen with intramuscular injections. Therefore, deltoid muscle injection is strongly preferred over buttock injection.
2. The plasma-derived vaccine should be stored at 2 to 8 degrees C, but not frozen. Freezing destroys the potency of the vaccine.
3. Inadvertent immunization of hepatitis B carriers produces neither therapeutic nor adverse effects.
4. The only population in whom prevaccination serologic screening is cost effective are those groups at high risk for hepatitis B, i.e., homosexual males and intravenous drug users.
5. Preventive measures provide the only realistic approach to hepatitis control. In hospitals with hepatitis B vaccine programs, only 36 percent of the people at high risk have actually received the vaccine. The incidence of hepatitis B infection continues to rise, presumably because vaccination programs fail to reach the major risk groups.

References

1. Alter H. The evolution, implication, and applications of the hepatitis B vaccine. JAMA 1982; 247:2272–2275.

    An in-depth account of the evolution of and indications for hepatitis B vaccine.

2. Centers for Disease Control. Recommendations for protection against viral hepatitis. Ann Int Med 1985; 103:391–402.

    Detailed, specific indications for the use of immune globulin, hepatitis B vaccine, and screening.

3. Centers for Disease Control. Recommendations of the immunization practices advisory committee: Update on hepatitis B prevention. Ann Int Med 1987; 107:353–357.

    A discussion of the immunogenicity, safety, efficacy, and precautions in the recombinant vaccine and the indications for booster injections.

4. Dienstag J, et al. Hepatitis B vaccine in health care personnel: Safety, immunogenicity, and indicators of efficacy. Ann Int Med 1984; 101:34–40.

    A double-blind trial of 1330 high-risk health care personnel, which confirmed the plasma vaccine's safety and efficacy.

5. Friedman L, Dienstag J. Recent developments in viral hepatitis. Disease a Month 1986; 6:331–363.

    An excellent, detailed summary of hepatitis B epidemiology, clinicopathology, and prevention.

6. Hollinger F. Hepatitis B vaccines—to switch or not to switch? JAMA 1987; 257:2634–2636.

    An excellent comparison of plasma-derived and recombinant hepatitis B vaccines pointing out the superior antigenicity of the plasma-derived vaccine.

7. Kumar M, et al. Should all pregnant women be screened for hepatitis B? Ann Int Med 1987; 107:273–277.

    Routine maternal hepatitis B surface antigen screening may be needed if the transmission of hepatitis B from mother to infant is to be prevented.

8. Zuckerman A. Appraisal of intradermal immunization against hepatitis B. *Lancet* 1987; 435:435–436.

    An article urging further controlled trials before intradermal injection is used widely.

28

Disulfiram

Galen Grayson

Disulfiram (antabuse) is used as an adjunctive therapy in the treatment of chronic alcoholism. Some clinical trials support the short-term effectiveness of disulfiram when employed with behavioral and psychological counseling; however, there is no evidence that the drug is effective in sustaining continuous abstinence or delaying the resumption of drinking. Nevertheless, disulfiram is utilized by many alcohol rehabilitation programs in the United States and abroad.

Originally used as a rubber antioxidant during the late-1800s, disulfiram was first used clinically as a scabicide in the 1930s. Thirty-nine years ago, two Danish physicians, Wald and Jacobsen, accidentally and subjectively experienced the "antabuse–alcohol" reaction while attending a cocktail party. At the time, they were investigating the potential use of disulfiram as an antihelminic. Subsequent investigations suggested promise for the use of disulfiram in the treatment of alcoholism.

MECHANISM OF ACTION

Disulfiram blocks the oxidation of alcohol by interfering with the conversion of acetaldehyde to acetic acid by aldehyde dehydrogenose. This blockade results in an increase of blood acetaldehyde levels that is 5 to 10 times higher than controls who ingest no alcohol alone. The increased acetaldehyde level is responsible for what is called *acetaldehyde syndrome* or the *antabuse–ethanol reaction*. Table 28–1 lists signs and symptoms associated with this chemical interaction.

The onset of symptoms usually occurs within 5 to 10 minutes and the duration of the reaction ranges from 30 minutes to several hours. The severity of the reaction is individually specific and dependent on the amount of ethanol and disulfiram ingested.

SIDE EFFECTS

Adverse reactions in the absence of alcohol include allergic reactions, acneform eruptions, dermatitis, urticaria, optic neuritis, peripheral neuritis, polyneuritis, fatigue, tremor, restlessness, decreased sexual potency, garliclike or metallic taste, psychotic reactions, and mild gastrointestinal disturbances. Cases of reversible hypertension have been reported, as well as cholestatic and fulminant hepatitis.

INDICATIONS AND ADMINISTRATION

Disulfiram is indicated for use in selected patients in the treatment of chronic alcoholism. Individuals who are highly motivated to abstain from ethanol may benefit from the

Table 28–1. Common and severe signs and symptoms associated with the simultaneous ingestion of disulfiram and ethanol

Warmth	Chest pain
Flushing	Palpitation
Throbbing (head and neck)	Dyspnea
Nausea	Hyperventilation
Copious vomiting	Tachycardia
Hyperhidrosis	Hypotension
Confusion	Syncope
Thirst	Marked uneasiness
Blurred vision	Vertigo

Severe reactions include:
Respiratory depression
Cardiovascular collapse
Arrhythmias
Myocardial infarct
Acute CHF
Convulsions
Death

ethanol-sensitizing effects of disulfiram. Such an individual should abstain from ethanol for at least 12 hours before receiving an initial dose of 500 milligrams daily, given in a single dose for 1 to 2 weeks. A maintenance regimen follows, with an average amount of 250 milligrams daily (range, 125–500 mg) and should not exceed 500 milligrams. The preferred mode of delivery is crushed tablets, well mixed with liquid.

PEARLS AND PITFALLS

1. Disulfiram inhibits the drug-metabolizing enzymes of the microsomal system, which can result in toxic levels of a second drug taken in usual doses concurrently (Table 28–2).
2. There are certain drugs that are known to exhibit a disulfiramlike reaction in the presence of ethanol (Table 28–3).
3. Marijuana has been reported to interact adversely with disulfiram.
4. Because of the disulfiram–ethanol reaction, extreme caution is necessary for patients with such disorders as diabetes mellitus, epilepsy, hypothyroidism, cerebral damage, nephritis, and liver disease.
5. Patients allergic to rubber should be evaluated for hypersensitivity to disulfiram, which is a thiuram derivative. Also, there is a reported case of disulfiram intoxication in a child, characterized by lethargy or somnolence, weak-

Table 28–2. Drugs with biotransformation inhibited by disulfiram

Chlordiazeposide (Librium)
Clorazepate Dipotassium (Tranxene)
Diazepam (Valium)
Flurazepam (Dalmane)
Halazepam (Paxipam)
Isoniazid (INH, Nydrazid)
Phenytoin (Dilantin)
Prazepam (Centrax)
Rifampin (Rifadin, Rimactane)
Thiopental (Pentathal)
Tranylcypromine (Parnate)
Warfarin (Athrombin-K, Coumadin, Panwarfin)

From Oettingen W. F. von. The diphabic alcohols: Their toxicity and potential dangers in relation to their chemical constitution and their fate in metabolism. Public Health Bulletin N. 281, U.S. Government Printing Office, Washington, D.C., 1943, p. 185.

Table 28–3. Drugs exhibiting a disulfiramlike action

Acetohexamide (Dymelor)
Chloramphenicol (Chloromycetin)
Chlorpropamide (Diabinese)
Furazolidone (Furoxone)
Griseofulvin (Grifulvin V, Fulvicin, etc.)
Tolazamide (Tolinase)
Tolbutamide (Orinase)
Phentolamine (Regitine)
Quinacrine (Atabrine)
Metronidazole
Cefmenoxime

ness, hypotonia, and vomiting, which began 12 hours after ingestion and progressed to stupor and coma.
6. The former practice of inducing the first disulfiram–ethanol reaction in a patient being started on disulfiram no longer holds the popularity of previous years. Disulfiram should never be used as the sole therapy for alcoholism without supportive counseling or psychotherapy; success is unlikely. Never administer disulfiram to an intoxicated patient.
7. Finally, the patient must be fully informed of the objectives, potential adverse effects, and rationale of treatment.

References

1. Benitz WE, et al. Disulfiram intoxication in a child. I Pediat 1984; 3:487–488.

   A case study of the unique features associated with disulfiram intoxication in a child.

2. Brown CG, et al. Delirium with phenytoin and disulfiram administration. Ann Emerg Med 1983; 12:25.

   A case study of delirium secondary to drug toxicity in a patient taking maintenance doses of both phenytoin (Dilantin) and disulfiram (antabuse).

3. Eneanya OI, et al. The actions and metabolic fate of disulfiram. Ann Rev Pharmacol 1981; 21:525–596.

   An extensive review of many pharmacologic aspects of disulfiram.

4. Ferko AP. Present status of disulfiram. Am Fam Phys 1983; 6:183–185.

   A pharmacologic review and the clinical use of disulfiram.

5. Fuller RK. Disulfiram treatment of alcoholism. JAMA 1986; 11:1449–1455.

   A Veterans Administration cooperative study.

6. Kannangara DW, et al. Disulfiramlike reactions with newer cephalosporins: Cefmenoxime. Am J Med Sci 1948; 2:45–47.

   A case report of a disulfiramlike reaction with cefmenoxime.

7. Kitson TM. The disulfiram–ethanol reaction. J Stud Alc 1977; 1:96–113.

   A detailed review of the disulfiram–ethanol reaction.

8. Lacoursiere RB, Swatek R. Adverse interaction between disulfiram and marijuana. Am J Psychiat 1983; 140:2.

   A case report of a hypomaniclike reaction in a patient taking disulfiram and marijuana simultaneously.

9. Rothrock JF, et al. Fulminant polyneuritis after overdose of disulfiram and ethanol. Neurology 1984; 34:357–359.

   A case report of severe sensorimotor polyneuritis after simultaneous ingestion of ethanol and disulfiram in high doses.

10. Schade RR, et al. Fulminant hepatitis associated with disulfiram. Arch Intern Med 1983; 6:1271–1273.

    A case study of disulfiram's causing hepatitis in a man with previously normal hepatocellular function.

11. Volicer L, Nelson KL. Development of reversible hypertension during disulfiram therapy. Arch Intern Med 1984; 6:1294–1296.

    A case study of an alcoholic patient who had a gradual increase in blood pressure while he was treated with disulfiram.

12. Wald J, Jacobsen E. A drug sensitizing the organism to ethyl alcohol. *Lancet* 1948; 2:1001–1004.

    The original article revealing the potential use of disulfiram in the treatment of alcoholism.

29

Lactulose

Frank A. Hamilton

Lactulose is a synthetic disaccharide analog of lactose, which acts as a laxative by stimulating colonic peristalsis. Unlike the other laxatives described in this book, lactulose has the unique property of being an effective ammonia detoxifying agent and is therefore an ideal agent for therapy in portal-systemic encephalopathy. The clinical diagnosis of hepatic encephalopathy or portal-systemic encephalopathy is suggested by the insidious development of mental changes, asterixis, elevated blood ammonia levels, and fetor hepaticus in patients with cirrhosis of the liver. In contrast, portal-systemic encephalopathy can occur abruptly in patients with previously normal livers that have sustained an acute injury, such as fulminant viral hepatitis or a toxin-induced liver injury.

One critical factor that has been shown to be responsible for inducing hepatic coma is ammonia, an important intermediate in the metabolism of nitrogen. In the gut, ammonia production is attributed to the action of bacterial ureases on ingested protein and blood entering into the gastrointestinal tract. In the normal setting, ammonia is generally brought to the liver via the portal vein and converted to urea. However, when the liver is significantly impaired, absorbed ammonia circulates to the brain, bypassing the liver unchanged, with resultant neuropsychiatric changes.

Perhaps the most important measures in the management of hepatic encephalopathy are eliminating exogenous sources of ammonia by restricting dietary protein, controlling gastrointestinal bleeding, and reducing the number of ammonia-producing bacteria. For many years, the antibiotic neomycin was commonly used to suppress ammonia-producing colonic bacteria. This form of treatment is and has been shown to be effective in reducing ammonia levels and improving the neurologic status of the patient. Although very effective, neomycin has the untoward side effects of ototoxicity, which is usually irreversible, and nephrotoxicity. Over the past 10 to 15 years, clinical studies have clearly demonstrated the effectiveness of lactulose in reducing ammonia levels in most patients with portal-systemic encephalopathy, with fewer side effects.

MECHANISM OF ACTION

The exact mechanism of action of lactulose is not clear. When lactulose is administered it passes unabsorbed and unchanged to the ileum and the colon, where it is hydrolyzed by bacterial action to lactic acid, acetic acid, and formic acid. These acids stimulate colonic motility, with resultant catharsis, and thereby inhibit coliform growth and ammonia production. Vince et al. showed that lactulose exerted its beneficial effect by lowering the colonic pH, thereby creating a pH gradient favoring non-ionic diffusion of ammonia and reducing its absorption.

DOSAGE AND ADMINISTRATION

In the adult, therapy with lactulose is usually begun with an oral dose of 30 to 45 milliliters 3 times a day. After 2 days, this dosage may be adjusted so that the patient produces two or three soft stools per day. However, in infants and children, the dosage and efficacy have not been established.

In a double-blind trial, Atterbury demonstrated that the hourly administration of 30 to 45 milliliters of lactulose syrup was as effective and rapid in action as was neomycin in the acute setting of portal-systemic encephalopathy.

An alternate route of administration of lactulose is as a retention enema. This route of administration is indicated when the danger of aspiration exists during impending coma or advanced stages of portal-systemic encephalopathy. It is administered as a mixture of 300 milliliters of lactulose with 700 milliliters of water or normal saline. Studies by Kersh demonstrated the effectiveness of the rectal route, with improvement in mental status within 2 hours after the administration of the lactulose enema in patients with portal-systemic encephalopathy.

Since lactulose contains galactose (<2.2 gm/15 ml) and lactose (<1.2 gm/15 ml), its administration should be used cautiously in the diabetic. In addition, when lactulose therapy is instituted, care should be taken not to use other laxatives because the appearance of loose stools may give the clinician a false sense that a therapeutic effect of lactulose has been achieved.

In a minority of patients lactulose alone may not be effective in portal-systemic encephalopathy. Supporting studies from several investigators demonstrate that the concomitant use of neomycin and lactulose is additive in reducing ammonia levels, with subsequent improvement in mental status. In a more recent study, Weber demonstrated that the combined use of neomycin and lactulose reduced urea production in cirrhotic patients. Since lactulose is effective in the long-term management of chronic portal-systemic encephalopathy, it is prudent that the clinician follow the serum electrolytes in elderly patients to monitor for potential complications such as hypokalemia and hypernatremia.

SIDE EFFECTS

Although lactulose has been proved effective in the therapy of acute and chronic portal-systemic encephalopathy, it has some side effects. The commonly encountered side effects are gaseousness, abdominal distension, flatulence, belching, and abdominal cramping. Nausea and vomiting occur on rare occasions.

PEARLS AND PITFALLS

1. Lactulose, a synthetic disaccharide analog of lactose, is metabolized by colonic bacteria and traps in the gastrointestinal lumen ammonia in an ionized form.
2. In addition to lactulose, adjunctive measures in the management of hepatic encephalopathy include dietary protein restriction, cessation of gastrointestinal bleeding, and reduction of ammonia producing colonic bacteria.
3. Lactulose works not only by trapping ammonia in the colonic lumen by converting it to an ionized form, it also decreases colonic bacteria by stimulating colonic motility and by stimulating laxation.
4. In addition to oral therapy sufficient to produce two to four soft, liquidy bowel movements a day, lactulose can be given as a retention enema for patients at risk for aspiration from central nervous system abnormalities. A mixture of 300 mls of lactulose and 700 mls of water should be given per rectum and held for at least 20 minutes.
5. The addition of neomycin to lactulose may be of benefit to patients who continue to manifest CNS changes.
6. Chronic use of lactulose is associated with hypokalemia and hypernatremia. Serial electrolyte determinations are required with chronic use of lactulose.

References

1. Atterbury CE, Maddrey WC, Conn HO. Neomycin-sorbitol and lactulose in the treatment of acute portal-systemic encephalopathy: A controlled, double-blind clinical trial. Am J Dig Dis 1978; 28:398–406.

   Neomycin-sorbital (1.5 g neomycin and 50 ml of sorbital syrup q.i.d.) and lactulose (50 ml every 1–2 hours orally) were comparable in improving mental status in patients with acute nitrogenous portal-systemic encephalopathy and underlying cirrhosis.

2. Breen KJ, et al. Neomycin absorption in man: Studies of oral and enema administration and effect of intestinal ulceration. Ann Intern Med 1972; 76:211–218.

   The authors studied neomycin absorption in patients with normal intestinal mucosa and patients with ulcerated upper and lower gastrointestinal mucosa (peptic ulcer disease, Crohn's disease, ulcerative colitis). They found no significant differences in urine or serum neomycin levels between the two groups.

3. Conn HO, et al. Comparison of lactulose and neomycin in the treatment of chronic portal-systemic encephalopathy. Gastroenterology 1977; 72:573–583.

   A randomized, double-blind clinical comparison of neomycin and lactulose in 33 cirrhotic patients with chronic portal-systemic encephalopathy. Both are effective in the majority of patients (83% and 90%, respectively) in improv-

ing mental state, trail making test results, electroencephalograms, and arterial ammonia levels.
4. Conn HO, Lieberthal MM. *The Hepatic Coma Syndromes and Lactulose.* Baltimore: Williams and Wilkins, 1979. Pp. 317–319.

    A comprehensive and detailed monograph by the pioneer author and researcher in this field.
5. Demeulenaere L, Van Waes L, Van Egmond J. Emergency treatment of acute portal-systemic encephalopathy (PSE) with lactulose enemas: A controlled study. Gastroenterology 1977; 72:A-151/1174.

    Lactulose enemas (lactulose 300 ml—tap water 700 ml; retention 20 minutes) produce a rapid decrease in blood ammonia levels with a rapid reversal of mental status abnormalities. By contrast, cleansing tap water enemas do not produce any colonic acidification nor do they result in decreased blood ammonia levels or mental status improvement.
6. Fessel JM, Conn HO. Lactulose in the treatment of acute hepatic encephalopathy. Am J Med Sci 1973; 266:103–110.

    Another series demonstrating efficacy of lactulose and neomycin in the treatment of hepatic encephalopathy. The mean duration of encephalopathy after initiation of therapy was 2.2 days in the lactulose group and 3.7 days in the neomycin group—an advantage of lactulose therapy.
7. Kersh ES, Rifkin H. Lactulose enema. Ann Intern Med 1973; 78:81–84.

    An early report of efficacy of lactulose (4-O-β-D-galactopyranosyl-D-fructose) in the treatment of hepatic encephalopathy in 4 patients.
8. Nelson DC, McGrew WRG, Hoyumpa AM. Hypernatremia and lactulose therapy. JAMA 1983; 249:1295–1298.

    The authors note that in 20 of 75 courses of lactulose treatment of portal-systemic encephalopathy, serum sodium level exceeded 145 mEq/l. In the group with hypernatremia, mortality was 41% compared with 14% in those who remained eunatremic. The proposed mechanism of lactulose-induced hypernatremia is excess fecal water loss with resulting contraction of extracellular fluid volume.
9. Orlandi F, et al. Comparison between neomycin and lactulose in 1973 patients with hepatic encephalopathy: A randomized clinical study. Dig Dis Sci 1981; 26:498–506.

    A large study complementing the work of Conn. Both studies conclude that lactulose and neomycin are efficacious in the treatment of hepatic encephalopathy.
10. Simmons I, Goldstein H, Boyle JD. A controlled clinical trial of lactulose in hepatic encephalopathy. Gastroenterology 1970; 59:827–832.

    An early VA trial suggesting benefit of oral lactulose therapy in patients with hepatic encephalopathy.
11. Vince A, Killingby M, Wong OM. Effect of lactulose on ammonia production in a fecal incubation system. Gastroenterology 1978; 74:544–549.

    An in vitro fecal incubation system was used to demonstrate that lactulose decreases fecal ammonia concentrations by (1) increasing bacterial assimilation of ammonia, (2) reducing deamination of nitrogenous compounds, and (3) reducing bacterial metabolism in general by decreasing colonic pH.

12. Weber FL Jr, et al. Nitrogen in fecal bacterial, fiber, and soluble fractions of patients with cirrhosis: Effects of lactulose and lactulose plus neomycin. J Lab Clin Med 1987; 3:259–263.

    Lactulose administration increased fecal nitrogen content by 165% and decreased fecal urea production by 23%.

30

Gallstone Therapeutic Agents

Michael S. Gurney

Cholelithiasis is a major health problem in America today. Gallstones afflict 15 to 20 million Americans, and approximately 500,000 cholecystectomies are performed each year. The cost of medical and surgical management of cholelithiasis is probably over 1 billion dollars annually.

The high prevalence of cholelithiasis with its complications has led physicians for many years to search for a safe, easy method to dissolve the stones. The first successful report on a patient was in 1891, by John Walker, an English surgeon who dripped ether onto an impacted cystic duct stone through a cholecystocutaneous fistula. Since then, many have dreamed of duplicating his feat by the use of oral medications.

In the early 1970s, gallstone dissolution by chenodeoxycholic acid, an oral bile salt, was reported. Amid much excitement, the National Cooperative Gallstone Study was launched to examine the efficacy, safety, and optimal dose of the medication. The discouraging results amplified the difficulties facing medical dissolution therapy: Only 14 percent of patients had complete dissolution after 2 years, and a significant number experienced side effects. Furthermore, advances in anesthesia and surgery have made cholecystectomy—the standard by which medical therapy must be measured—a safe and effective procedure. Elective cholecystectomy in a low-risk patient provides a permanent remedy for the problem, with a mortality rate in most series.

Chenodiol

Chenodeoxycholic acid (Chenix) is currently the only approved oral dissolution agent. It is a naturally occurring bile acid, comprising 20 to 30 percent of the total bile salt pool. Unlike cholic acid, the predominant bile salt, chenodeoxycholate is effective in decreasing bile cholesterol saturation and can dissolve cholesterol gallstones. However, because of a slow dissolution rate and the high incidence of side effects, chenodiol therapy requires a considerable commitment by both physician and patient.

PHARMACOLOGY

Chenodiol decreases cholesterol bile saturation by several mechanisms. It impairs endogenous cholesterol synthesis by decreasing the activity of HMG Co-A reductase, the rate-limiting enzyme of cholesterol synthesis. It also suppresses bile acid synthesis. The decreased synthesis, along with the additional chenodiol in the bile from oral administration, lead to a significant increase in the chenodiol percentage of the bile and expansion of the total bile salt pool. Physiochemically, chenodiol transports biliary cholesterol in micelles. These changes all favor the removal of cholesterol from the solid form of a gallstone into the bile solution, thus gradually dissolving the stone.

A portion of chenodiol, whether given orally or synthesized by the liver, is 7-dehydroxylated by intestinal bacteria to lithocholic acid. Lithocholic acid is poorly absorbed and is largely excreted in the feces. Lithocholate is hepatotoxic and the small amount reabsorbed may account for the hepatotoxicity often seen with chenodiol administration.

INDICATIONS

The majority of gallstones are asymptomatic and never cause clinical symptoms. Most authorities believe such silent stones do not require therapy of any type. For patients who do have true biliary colic, the pain is usually severe enough that a rapid, reliable, and permanent solution is needed—cholecystectomy. Thus, oral dissolution therapy is reserved mainly for those patients who have symptomatic cholelithiasis and medical problems severe enough to make them a high operative risk. There are patients who have an irreconcilable fear of surgery and will not consent to the procedure under any circumstances. Chenodiol therapy may be indicated in such patients, but only after the physician has carefully reassured and educated them about the safety of surgery and the limitations and side effects of dissolution therapy. Table 30–1 summarizes important issues the physician should consider when counseling patients about the choice of therapy.

Table 30–1. Issues to consider before deciding on medical dissolution therapy

1. The presence, frequency, and severity of biliary symptoms
2. The size and location of stones
3. The probability that the stones are primarily composed of cholesterol
4. Concomitant problems caused by the stones, such as pancreatitis, jaundice, and cholangitis
5. The patient's age and operative risk
6. The patient's future accessibility to medical and surgical care of good quality
7. The presence of hepatic or intestinal problems that might be exacerbated by medical therapy
8. The patient's emotional set toward surgery (versus taking long-term medications) and repeated laboratory or radiographic studies to monitor drug toxicity, stone dissolution, or recurrence
9. The patient's feeling about living with the unpredictability of gallstones for several years
10. The need for repeat therapy should the stones dissolve and recur

Table 30-2. Radiographic criteria favoring stone dissolution

1. Radiolucent stones
2. Patent cystic duct
3. Stones <2 cm in diameter
4. Floating stones (with Telepague)

The success of chenodiol therapy is dependent on patient selection. Factors favoring dissolution are listed in Table 30-2. Those who have nonfunctioning gallbladders (nonvisualization on oral cholecystogram) or calcium detectable in the stones on radiographs do not have successful dissolution and are not candidates for medical therapy. When gallstones are larger than 2 centimeters, or when multiple stones nearly fill the gallbladder, dissolution therapy is unlikely to be successful and the indications for medical therapy should be reexamined. Overall, 40 to 80 percent of appropriately selected patients have at least partial dissolution within 2 years of treatment; about one half of these (20–40% overall) will have full dissolution. Complete dissolution is more common in women, in patients with high-normal serum cholesterol concentrations, in thin patients, and in those with cholesterol gallstones less than 15 millimeters in diameter. Carefully selected patients with small, "floating" (on oral cholecystogram), radiolucent stones who are able to take a full dose of chenodiol for 2 years have an 80-percent chance of complete dissolution. Unfortunately, only 10 to 15 percent of patients meet these criteria. Patients who have existing hepatitis or hyperlipidemia are likely to have these problems exacerbated by chenodiol and are not candidates for the drug. Pregnant women or those likely to become pregnant during the 2 years of therapy should not be treated with chenodiol, since its safety during gestation has not been studied.

SIDE EFFECTS

The most common side effect is diarrhea, which occurs in as many as 40 percent of patients on a full dose of chenodiol. The diarrhea is usually mild, improves with a decreased dose, and is rarely a threat to the patient or enough to cause cessation of the therapy.

Of more concern is the elevation in liver aminotransferases seen in as many as 25 percent of patients, with significant elevation seen in 5 to 10 percent. The elevations are generally reversible, but the enzymes should be carefully followed to avoid significant damage to the liver. A suggested monitoring schedule for chenodiol toxicity is presented in Table 30-3.

Chenodiol also raises low density lipoprotein cholesterol by 10 percent. High density lipoprotein cholesterol levels are unaffected. The significance of this elevation for the 2 years of therapy is unknown.

Table 30–3. Suggested monitoring schedule for chenodiol toxicity

1. Measure serum aminotransferase levels:
   a. Before and after 2 and 4 weeks of therapy
   b. If normal, at 3 and 6 months into therapy and every 6 months thereafter
   c. If aminotransferases rise less than threefold above the upper limits of normal, repeat in 1 week. If stable, check the level monthly as long as the test is elevated.
   d. If the rise is more than threefold above normal, stop the drug and repeat in 1 week. Consider other etiologies.
   e. When the enzyme levels return to normal, consider the risks and benefits of a rechallenge. If rechallenged, the patient should be closely monitored.
2. Measure total serum cholesterol before and after 3 to 6 months of therapy. If the level rises, advise dietary therapy and recheck after 3 to 6 months.

Dyspepsia is an uncommon complaint and usually diminishes or disappears after 2 to 4 weeks of therapy.

DOSAGE

The keys to initiating chenodiol therapy are to start at a low dose and increase it gradually to the full dose of approximately 15 milligrams/kilogram/day. If therapy is begun with the full dose, side effects are likely and the patient may be hesitant to take that dose at a later date. If the patient is unable to tolerate a full dose, then the chance for a successful dissolution is significantly reduced.

Begin therapy by giving the patient 500 milligrams at night for 1 week, then increase to 750 milligrams nightly. If a higher dose is required to reach 15 milligrams/kilogram/day, add 250 milligrams at breakfast each week, to a total dose of 1250 milligrams (500 mg in the morning, 750 mg at night). Further increments should be given with the evening dose. If mild diarrhea occurs, withhold the drug for 1 day and then return to the same dose. If it is more severe, decrease the dose by 250 milligrams for 1 week, then reinstitute the higher dose only on alternate days, followed by full dose 1 to 2 weeks later. Lomotil or Imodium may help manage the diarrhea during therapy.

Efficacy of dissolution should be monitored during therapy. Cholecystograms at 6 and 12 months are useful to look for partial dissolution. Partial dissolution is indicative of ultimate success if therapy is continued and helps with patient compliance. If partial dissolution is not evident at 12 months, success is unlikely and treatment should be abandoned. However, if the patient still has biliary symptoms and surgery is not possible, treatment may be continued. In addition, if the patient is obese (>150% of ideal body weight), the dose may be increased to 18 to 20 milligrams/

kilogram/day if tolerated and if the liver enzymes do not rise to an unacceptable level.

Once full dissolution is achieved, this should be confirmed by ultrasound and therapy continued for an additional 3 months.

A significant problem is recurrence of the gallstones. Five years after therapy, 25 to 50 percent of patients again have cholelithiasis. Ultrasonography every 1 to 2 years is recommended to look for recurrences. These stones usually dissolve after another course of therapy if a cholecystogram again demonstrates good gallbladder function, a patent cystic duct, and radiolucent stones. A low maintenance dose of 375 milligrams/day of chenodiol is not effective in preventing recurrence. A higher dose for prophylaxis has not been studied and is not advisable at this time. A better alternative is to alter the risk factors for gallstones, i.e., obesity, diet, clofibrate therapy, or exogenous estrogens.

Ursodeoxycholic Acid (Ursodiol)

Ursodeoxycholate is the 7-beta-hydroxy epimer of chenodeoxycholate and is normally present in only trace amounts in human bile. A Japanese drug manufacturer had marketed a combination of ursodeoxycholate and B vitamins as a general hepatic tonic for over 2 decades when, in 1974, reports of gallstone dissolution in patients medicating themselves with the combination drug appeared in the Japanese literature. Subsequent therapeutic trials in Japan and Europe demonstrated efficacy in gallstone dissolution, without the diarrhea or liver enzyme elevations seen with chenodiol therapy. Ursodiol is now the leading dissolution agent in Japan and Western Europe, but only recently was approved for use in the United States.

PHARMACOLOGY

Ursodiol is well absorbed after ingestion and passes into the portal circulation. Extraction by the liver is so efficient that only a small amount reaches the circulation. It is then conjugated with either glycine or taurine and excreted into the bile. Enterohepatic recirculation of ursodeoxycholate is quite efficient, yielding a prolonged half-life of 3.5 to 5.8 days.

On a full dose of the drug, ursodiol constitutes 50 to 60 percent of the total bile salt pool. This is a lower percentage than in chenodiol therapy, probably because bile salt synthesis is not suppressed by ursodiol. Nonetheless, the net effect is the production of bile unsaturated in cholesterol.

Stone dissolution by ursodiol is a complex physiochemical process. The drug surrounds stones with a cholesterol and phospholipid ionophase, which enhances cholesterol solubilization from the stone. Cholesterol is not transported in micelles, as with chenodiol therapy, but in a liquid crystalline form. Cholesterol in lipid membranes is less disrupted by ursodiol; this may explain its lack of both hepatotoxicity and diarrhea.

INDICATIONS

Ursodeoxycholic acid is indicated for the dissolution of cholesterol gallstones. It is limited by the same selection requirements in terms of stone size and composition as is chenodiol. In clinical trials it does not appear to be significantly more effective than chenodiol. The advantage of ursodiol is the significantly lower incidence of side effects. Diarrhea and hepatotoxicity are extremely rare, serum cholesterol is unaffected, and triglycerides may fall. The chief disadvantage is expense: The cost of therapy is almost 5 times that of chenodiol.

Several trials have studied the combination of lower doses of ursodiol and chenodiol together in an effort to avoid the side effects of chenodiol and the expense of ursodiol. Preliminary results show the combination to be as efficacious as either drug alone and without adverse effects on transaminases, lipids, or bowel habits. Many lithotripsy centers are using the combination successfully to solubilize the debris remaining after lithotriptic destruction of gallstones.

SIDE EFFECTS

Diarrhea is only a rare problem with ursodiol, and liver enzyme or cholesterol elevations do not occur. Calcification of the gallstone surface occurs in 10 percent of patients during therapy and may interfere with further dissolution. This incidence may not be significantly greater than the native calcification rate.

DOSAGE

The drug should be taken with meals or milk since it dissolves more rapidly in the presence of bile and pancreatic juice. The total daily dose is 8 to 10 milligrams/kilogram/day divided into morning and evening doses (usually a 300-mg capsule with breakfast and dinner). Alternatively, a single nighttime dose may be given and is considered more effective by some investigators.

Monooctanoin (Moctanin)

Monooctanoin is a semisynthetic vegetable oil that has been shown in vivo to dissolve common cholesterol bile duct stones.

PHARMACOLOGY

Thistle demonstrated the ability of monooctanoin to act as a cholesterol solvent and to dissolve gallstones in vitro. It can solubilize 12 grams of cholesterol per 100 milliliters of solution. Monooctanoin must be administered directly into the biliary tract via indwelling T tube, nasobiliary tube, percutaneous transhepatic catheter, or cholecystostomy tube. The solution is viscous and must be warmed above 70 degrees F, preferably to body temperature, to maintain its liquid state and allow easy administration. Monooctanoin is bacteriostatic itself, and contamination has not proved to be a problem. It can be diluted by the addition of a 10% volume of sterile water. This dilution decreases viscosity and does not significantly affect cholesterol solubility.

INDICATIONS

Monooctanoin is indicated as a dissolution agent for radiolucent gallstones retained in the biliary tract following cholecystectomy. It is usually not effective for pigment stones or recurrent bile duct stones. Because of the significant incidence of side effects and the lower rate of efficacy, monooctanoin therapy is best reserved for those cases where surgical, endoscopic, or radiographic methods of stone removal are unsuccessful or unable to be undertaken.

Complete dissolution is achieved in one-fourth to one-third of patients, and another one-fourth may have enough of a reduction in size to allow extraction by another means. Dissolution is less successful for multiple stones and in diabetics.

CONTRAINDICATIONS AND SIDE EFFECTS

Side effects are common, occurring in two-thirds of patients, and life-threatening complications occur in 5 percent. Gastrointestinal complaints are the most common, with abdominal pain reported in 40 percent, nausea or vomiting in 30 percent, and diarrhea in 20 percent. Anorexia, fever, and lethargy are seen less commonly. Serious complications include respiratory distress, severe acidosis, pancreatitis, sepsis, and anaphylaxis.

Monooctanoin is contraindicated in patients with preexisting jaundice or liver disease, duodenal ulcer, inflammation of the jejunum, or ischemic bowel. Monooctanoin should *never* be given intramuscularly or intravenously.

The drug is administered by continuous perfusion through a catheter placed above the stones in the bile duct. Perfusion pressures higher than 15 centimeters of water may result in back diffusion into the hepatic veins and systemic circulation. Pulmonary edema and severe respiratory distress can then occur. Therefore, an overflow manometer (such as a central venous pressure manometer broken at the 15-cm mark), peristaltic pump, or similar device to assure a pressure less than 15 centimeters of water must be used. The rate should not exceed 3 to 5 millimeters/hour at a pressure less than 10 centimeters of water. The solution should be warmed to 70 to 80 degrees F prior to perfusion and should not fall below 65 degrees F during administration. A suggested apparatus for administration is shown in Fig. 30–1.

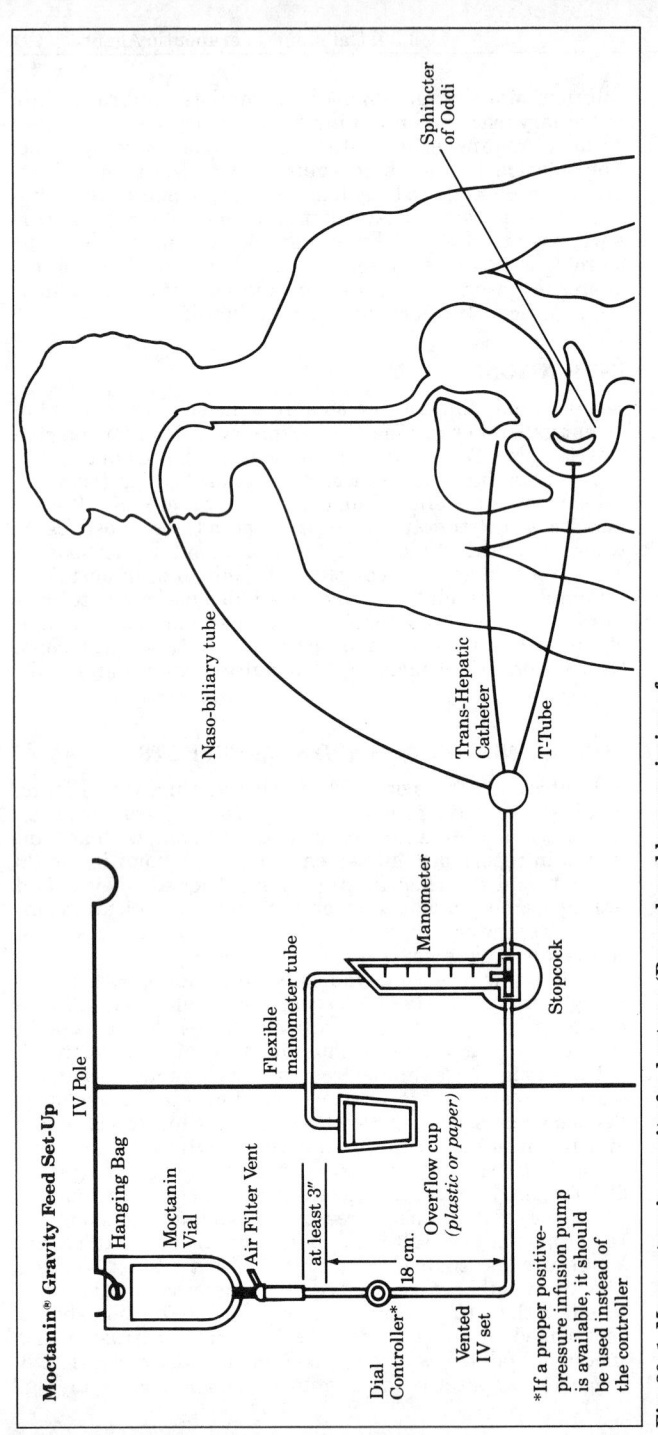

Fig. 30–1. Monooctanoin gravity feed set-up. (Reproduced by permission of Ascot Pharmaceuticals Inc., 8104 Lawndale Ave., Skokie, IL 60076.)

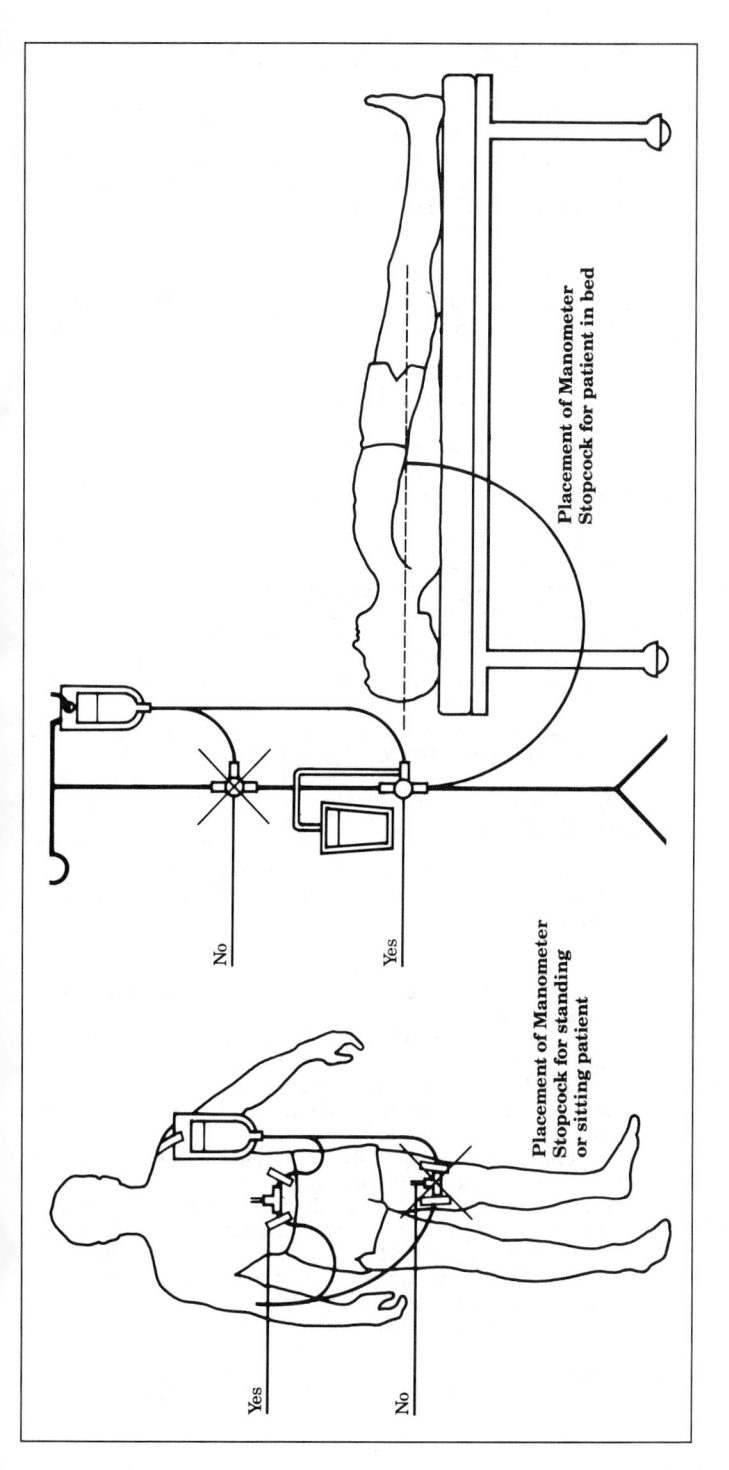

Placement of Manometer Stopcock for patient in bed

Placement of Manometer Stopcock for standing or sitting patient

Yes

No

Yes

No

The duration of perfusion is 7 to 21 days. Serial cholangiograms should be done every 3 to 4 days to monitor the effectiveness of treatment. If a reduction in the size or number of stones is not seen after 7 days, success is unlikely and the therapy should be stopped.

PEARLS AND PITFALLS

1. Concomitant use of aluminum-based antacids, colestipol, or psyllium agents interferes with chenodiol or ursodiol absorption.
2. Chenodiol, because of its effect on bowel habits, is an ideal choice for the gallstone patient with chronic constipation.
3. Lomotil or Imodium are often enough to manage the increase in stool frequency caused by chenodiol.
4. A low-cholesterol diet improves the efficacy of dissolution agents.
5. Bile cholesterol content increases during rapid weight loss, reducing the effectiveness of drug therapy for gallstones. If weight loss is recommended during treatment it should be slow and gradual.
6. Although transaminase elevation and diarrhea are common with chenodiol therapy, the possibility of viral hepatitis or an infectious diarrhea should also be considered if these problems occur during therapy.
7. During monooctanoin infusion, the catheter tips should always be above the most proximal stone.

References

1. Bachrach WH, Hofmann, AF. Ursodeoxycholic acid in the treatment of cholesterol cholelithiasis. Dig Dis Sci 1982; 27: 737, 833.

    An exhaustive review, in two parts, of ursodeoxycholic acid pharmacology, efficacy, and side effects.
2. Fromm H. Gallstone dissolution therapy. Gastroenterology 1986; 91:1560.

    An excellent review of the physiology of dissolution therapy.
3. Marks JW, et al. Low-dose chenodiol to prevent gallstone recurrence after dissolution therapy. Ann Intern Med 1984; 100:376.

    Three hundred seventy-five mg of chenodiol daily is no better than placebo in preventing gallstone recurrence.
4. Marks JW, et al. Additional chenodiol therapy after partial dissolution of gallstones with 2 years of treatment. Ann Intern Med 1984; 100:382.

    Seven hundred fifty mg of chenodiol daily for another 2 years completely dissolved an additional 23% of the stones that were partially dissolved during the first 2 years of therapy.
5. Palmer HC, Carey MC. An optimistic view of the National Cooperative Gallstone Study. NEJM 1982; 306:1171.

An opinion professing just what the title promises, for a study that could use an optimistic outlook.
6. Palmer KR, Hoffman AF. Introductal monooctanoin for the direct dissolution of bile duct stones: Experience in 343 patients. Gut 1986; 27:196.

   A summary of US experience between 1977 and 1983. A good discussion of the efficacy and complications of Moctanin.
7. Pitt HA, McFadden DW, Gadacz TR. Agents for gallstone dissolution. Am J Surg 1987; 153:233.

   An excellent and well-written summary of the medical management of gallstones.
8. Roehrkasse R, et al. Gallstone dissolution treatment with a combination of chenodeoxycholic acid and ursodeoxycholic acids. Dig Dis Sci 1986; 31:1032.

   A combination of the two agents in lower doses is as efficacious as a full dose of either; and avoids the side effects of chenodiol and reduces the expense of ursodiol.
9. Thistle JL. Monooctanoin, a dissolution agent for retained cholesterol bile duct stones: Physical properties and clinical application. Gastroenterology 1980; 78:1016.

   A good summary of monooctanoin's cholesterol solubility properties and clinical application.

31

Pancrealipase

Michael S. Gurney

Malabsorption from pancreatic disease begins to occur when pancreatic function falls below 10 percent of normal secretory capacity. Patients then experience weight loss, a decreased sense of well-being, and steatorrhea. The most common causes of exocrine pancreatic insufficiency in the adult are chronic pancreatitis (usually due to alcohol), pancreatic resection, and pancreatic carcinoma. In children, cystic fibrosis or Schwachman's syndrome (congenital exocrine pancreatic insufficiency and neutropenia) are the usual causes. The therapy for exocrine insufficiency is simple, in theory: replace the missing pancreatic enzymes with oral supplements. In practice, unless therapy follows several principles of intestinal physiology, treatment can be less than rewarding for both the patient and physician.

PHARMACOLOGY

All pancreatic enzyme products are derived from hog pancreas and contain standardized enzyme activity, which varies in amount from product to product. Most products now are pancrealipase, an enzyme preparation with high lipase activity—the most important enzyme for the relief of steatorrhea. The various products' potencies are best judged on the basis of their lipase content. Table 31–1 shows a list of various available preparations and their lipase activity.

The primary problem in enzyme replacement therapy is irreversible inactivation of the lipase by gastric acid at a pH of 4. Concomitant antacid therapy with sodium bicarbonate is usually enough to prevent this inactivation, but in gastric hypersecretors, this can still be a problem. Histamine 2-receptor antagonists have not been as effective as sodium bicarbonate, but the combination of the two may be helpful.

Enteric-coated tablets and coated microspheres in a capsule are also available. The enteric coating is designed to dissolve at pH 6, protecting the enzymes from acid degradation in the stomach. However, the enteric-coated tablets have been shown to have poor bioavailability and are not advised. The microsphere preparations can be useful but are plagued by questions of gastric emptying of the spheres, premature release of the enzyme in the stomach if concomitant bicarbonate is given, and lack of release in the duodenum due to poor duodenal alkalinization from the diseased pancreas. The microspheres are best reserved as a second-line medication.

INDICATIONS

Pancreatic enzyme replacement is indicated for the treatment of malabsorption due to pancreatic insufficiency. Enzyme replacement therapy does not help malabsorption from other causes, such as gluten sensitive enteropathy or

Table 31-1. Lipase content of available enzyme preparations

Medication	Lipase content per tablet (units)
8 × Pancreatin, 900 mg	22,500
Cotazyme	8000
Ku-zyme	8000
Viokase	8000
Viokase powder (per ¼ tsp)	16,800
Cotazyme (S)*	5000
Pancrease MT 4*	4000
Pancrease MT 10*	10,000
Pancrease MT 16*	16,000

*Enteric-coated microspheres

small bowel overgrowth. Thus, a firm diagnosis of pancreatic insufficiency should be made before therapy is begun.

Toskes has shown that enzyme replacement therapy is also effective in alleviating the pain of chronic pancreatitis. This beneficial effect is believed to be due to feedback inhibition of the pancreas, chiefly through sufficient administered trypsin and chymotrypsin activity to suppress CCK. The patients who seem to gain the most pain relief are those with mild to moderate nonalcoholic pancreatitis.

In patients with both pancreatic exocrine insufficiency and diabetes, the steatorrhea must be controlled before glucose control is attempted. Without control of the steatorrhea, such patients are very sensitive to any changes in insulin dose and often have a decreased glucagon reserve as well, making their response to hypoglycemia inadequate.

Pancreatic enzyme replacement is not indicated as a digestive aid, alone or in combination with bile salts, sedatives, or antiflatulents. Bile salts or proteolytic enzymes of plant origin (Papase) are of no benefit in pancreatic insufficiency.

CONTRAINDICATIONS AND SIDE EFFECTS

There are no absolute contraindications to enzyme replacement therapy, although it should be given with caution to patients allergic to pork. Large doses of pancreatic enzymes may cause nausea, bloating, or cramps. Large doses in children have also been associated with elevated serum uric acid levels and uricosuria.

DOSAGE

Table 31-2 is a suggested regimen for pancreatic enzyme replacement. Lipase activity of at least 20,000 units is suggested as a starting dose, with further benefit often seen

Table 31–2. Pancreatic enzyme replacement therapy regimen

1. Give a nonenteric-coated medication with a total lipase content of 20,000 to 40,000 units with each meal.
2. Give an additional dose at bedtime if attempting relief of chronic pancreatic pain.
3. Enzyme replacements should be taken at the beginning of the meal, or may be spread throughout the meal.
4. If no improvement occurs, add 650 mg of sodium bicarbonate (one tablet) before and after meals.
5. If there is still no improvement, consider—
   a. Adding another tablet of bicarbonate before and after meals, or
   b. Adding a potent histamine 2-receptor antagonist 30 minutes before the meal, or
   c. Changing to an enteric-coated preparation.

with up to 40,000 Units per meal. Increases above this are less likely to be of benefit, are difficult for patients to comply with, and may cause side effects.

If no significant improvement occurs with the extract alone, acid inactivation of lipase may be the problem and bicarbonate should be added. If there is still no benefit seen, the patient may be a hypersecretor and a histamine 2-receptor antagonist may be added. An H_2-receptor antagonist without bicarbonate is not as effective as bicarbonate alone. Occasionally, a combination of enzyme tablets and enteric-coated microspheres yields improvement when either preparation alone is ineffective.

In children, microspheres may be mixed with food, and activity is maintained as long as the food is ingested within 30 minutes. Enzyme powder (Viokase) can be mixed with food, but low-pH foods such as applesauce should be avoided since the lipase will be inactivated.

Response to enzyme replacement should be measured by fecal-fat determination; patients' subjective impressions are often unreliable.

PEARLS AND PITFALLS

1. Postgastrectomy patients have rapid gastric emptying, making the bioavailability of enteric-coated microspheres uncertain and often less than optimal.
2. Patients with cystic fibrosis are often acid hypersecretors. This, combined with poor bicarbonate secretion from the diseased pancreas, makes acid neutralization especially important in these patients.
3. Small bowel overgrowth is a frequent concomitant problem in patients with pancreatic insufficiency and is usually due to previous surgery or hypomotility from narcotics. If pancreatic enzyme replacement is not efficacious, a course of antibiotic treatment may result in significant improvement.

4. In patients with severe pancreatic insufficiency, enzyme replacement may not completely reverse steatorrhea. A low-fat diet is then often enough to give symptomatic improvement. Supplemental MCT oil (not dependent on lipase for absorption) can be given, if then needed, for caloric supplementation.
5. Do not routinely give bicarbonate to patients on enteric-coated microspheres. The bicarbonate may make the enteric coat dissolve prematurely, subjecting the enzymes to subsequent inactivation.
6. A high-fiber diet makes enzyme replacement therapy less effective and should be avoided if possible.
7. Wait for 3 to 4 weeks before measuring the response to therapy. Steatorrhea often gradually improves as malnutrition is corrected.
8. Remember that whatever regimen is arrived at, it is a regimen for the rest of the patient's life. Therefore, the number of tablets, the ease of compliance, and the cost are all important issues.
9. Do *not* give magnesium- or calcium-containing antacids or other products to patients with pancreatic insufficiency. The magnesium or calcium forms soaps with free fatty acids, worsening steatorrhea.

References

1. Dutta SK, Rubin J, Harvey J. Comparative evaluation of the therapeutic efficacy of a pH-sensitive enteric-coated pancreatic enzyme preparation with conventional pancreatic enzyme therapy in the treatment of exocrine pancreatic insufficiency. Gastroenterology 1983; 84:476.

    The improvement of steatorrhea and the actual amount of enzymes delivered to the duodenum was studied with enteric-coated and standard enzyme preparations. There was no significant difference between the two.
2. Graham DY. Pancreatic enzyme replacement: The effect of antacids or cimetidine. Dig Dis Sci 1982; 27:485.

    The effect of supplemental sodium bicarbonate, aluminum hydroxide, magnesium hydroxide, calcium carbonate, or cimetidine on the efficacy of enzyme replacement was studied. Only sodium bicarbonate or aluminum hydroxide increased effectiveness. Magnesium hydroxide and calcium carbonate actually worsened the steatorrhea.
3. Graham DY. Treatment of steatorrhea in chronic pancreatitis. Hosp Prac 1986; 21:125.

    An excellent overview of pancreatic enzyme replacement therapy.
4. Regan PT, et al. Comparative effects of antacids, cimetidine, and enteric coating on the therapeutic response to oral enzymes in severe pancreatic insufficiency. NEJM 1977; 297:854.

    In contrast to Graham's study, this report from the Mayo Clinic showed greater improvement with adjunctive cimetidine than with bicarbonate. However, the bicarbonate was given 30 minutes after the meal, rather than before and after the meal, as Graham prescribed.

5. Stapleton FB, et al. Hyperuricosuria due to high-dose pancreatic extract therapy in cystic fibrosis. NEJM 1976; 295:246.

   Very high levels of enzyme replacements were associated with impressive uricosuria. The pancreatic enzymes were analyzed, and nucleic acids comprised 10% of the medication.

6. Toskes PP. Chronic pancreatitis: Exocrine and endocrine insufficiencies. In TM Bayless (ed), *Current Therapy in Gastroenterology and Liver Disease II*. Toronto: BC Decker, 1986.

   An excellent guide to enzyme replacement from one of the leaders of the field. The chapter contains a good discussion of enzyme replacement therapy for pancreatic pain.

7. Worning H. Exocrine pancreatic substitution: Facts and controversies. Scand J Gastro 1986; 126 (Suppl):49.

   The measurement of intestinal enzymes from various enzyme preparations correlated poorly with improvement in steatorrhea. Cimetidine pretreatment did not improve steatorrhea or enzyme delivery.

V

Motility Disorder Drugs

The modern study of gastrointestinal motility began in earnest with the work of Cannon in the early 1900s. His classic monograph, entitled "The Mechanical Factors of Digestion," closes its introduction with the opinion that "some who think that nothing of importance happened the day before yesterday may be surprised by it." The ensuing 4 score years have supported that statement. The expansion of the study of gut motility since that time has been inexorable. We are now confronted monthly with a large and often bewildering or contradictory volume of data on gastrointestinal motility. Despite this, we are seemingly no closer today to a unifying theory of motility than we were in Cannon's time. Indeed, only now are we understanding the effects on normal emptying and transit of various hormones, neuropeptides, luminal elements, and the intrinsic and extrinsic nervous systems of the gut. When one considers the multiple endogenous regulators of gut motility, and the emotional, physical, and dietary stresses to which we subject our systems daily, it is a wonder that the majority of the population is able to maintain the regularity of bowel movements that it does.

The difficulty in understanding the physiology of normal subjects as well as the pathophysiology of abnormal conditions has slowed the development of drugs to treat gastrointestinal motility disorders. Clinicians and pharmacologists have had no other choice but to use drugs empirically, to relieve symptoms or alter definable abnormalities toward normal. Thus, the most significant progress in drugs for motility disorders has been in the discovery of the mechanism of action of drugs that have been in clinical use for years. For example, it used to be thought that most contact laxatives exerted their effect by irritating the intestinal mucosa, thereby stimulating contraction. We now know that these drugs alter the normal regulation of mucosal electrolyte and water transport, increasing colonic fluid content, leading to a shorter transit time and increased defecation. Only bisacodyl has been shown to actually stimulate colonic motility.

The past several years have not been without therapeutic breakthroughs. Domperidone and cisapride represent major therapeutic advances in the treatment of gastric emptying and intestinal dysmotility. These drugs are thoroughly discussed by Thomas Dorsey in the first part of this book. For the diarrhea disorders, somatostatin and its analogue, sandostatin, are major advances in the treatment of carcinoid and pancreatic islet cell tumors. They clearly have profound effects on intestinal motility, and only time and clinical experience will reveal their final clinical applications.

Although these drugs help in the management of motility disorders, the clinician is still faced with a significant challenge in the patient who complains of a chronic alteration in gastrointestinal motility such as diarrhea or constipation. These complaints can be the *forme fruste* of multiple diseases, and such patients can be among the most difficult diagnostic and therapeutic problems in clinical gastroenterology. At the minimum, these patients deserve a careful history and physical examination with basic laboratory studies. Stool hemoccult and proctoscopy should also be performed. If the constipation is recent in onset, a barium enema is indicated. An important part of the history is the drug and dietary history. Many patients unintentionally or intentionally omit nonprescription drugs or food items that could explain their symptoms. The over-the-counter availability of many motility drugs has led to the misconception that they are free of adverse effects. The easy access to laxatives has led to their frequent abuse and the paradoxical worsening of the constipated state. Fordtran has also shown us the frequency with which cathartics are used to get attention by the mentally ill.

Two of the physician's primary duties to these patients are to educate them about their bowel habits and to explain how different medications may either aid or exacerbate their symptoms. I hope this part will help the physician in those tasks.

Michael S. Gurney

References

1. Burks TF. Actions of drugs on gastrointestinal motility. In LR Johnson (ed), *Physiology of the Gastrointestinal Tract*. New York: Raven Press, 1981.

    A thorough summary of drug effects on gastrointestinal motility. An excellent review.

2. Cannon AE. The mechanical factors of digestion (1911). Science History Publications, Walton Publishing, 1986.

    A reprint of the classic monograph on gastrointestinal motility.

3. Farrar JT. The effects of drugs on intestinal motility. Clin Gastro 1982; 11:673.

    Another good review of drug effects on intestinal motility.

4. Huizinga JD. Electrophysiology of human colonic motility in health and disease. Clin Gastro 1986; 15:879.

    A well-written summary of a difficult topic.

Antidiarrheal Agents

Michael S. Gurney

Kaolin and Pectin

Absorbents and gels have been used for decades to manage the symptoms of diarrhea. The most common preparation now in use is Kaopectate, a combination of kaolin, a hydrated aluminum silicate clay, and pectin, a purified carbohydrate gel derived from apples and citrus fruits.

The Chinese have used kaolin as an antidiarrheal compound for centuries. In the 1920s, both Walker and Braafladt reported that it absorbed bacterial toxins, protected intestinal mucosa, and reduced mortality from cholera. However, in vitro and in vivo studies since then have cast doubt on its clinical efficacy.

Pectin became popular in the 1930s for the symptomatic relief of diarrhea, at a time when apple-pulp and apple-powder diets were popular. Clinical studies in the 1940s, however, cast doubt on its effectiveness, and it has generally been abandoned as a single-agent therapy for diarrhea.

PHARMACOLOGY

Kaopectate is not absorbed and remains in the gut lumen after oral administration. It is a nonspecific adsorbent; nutrients, medications, enzymes, salt, and water are all adsorbed in the lumen. Numerous commercial combinations of kaolin and pectin are marketed, varying in content of the two ingredients, the viscosity, and the flavor. Aluminum hydroxide is occasionally included to increase the adsorptive capacity. Neomycin may also be added as an antibacterial agent.

INDICATIONS

Kaopectate is used for the symptomatic relief of diarrhea. However, the efficacy of the preparation is doubtful. Portnoy showed that Kaopectate given to children with acute infectious diarrhea did not decrease either stool frequency or stool water content when compared with either compound alone or with placebo. The only improvement was a tendency for the stools to be more formed. McClung showed that stool losses of water, sodium, and potassium were actually increased with Kaopectate in an experimental model.

Thus, Kaopectate is only of subjective benefit in diarrhea. Since the cornerstone of diarrhea therapy is replacement of stool and electrolyte losses, McClung's work showed that Kaopectate may actually do more harm than good. Its routine use for acute diarrhea is not recommended.

CONTRAINDICATIONS AND SIDE EFFECTS

Kaopectate should not be used in patients with suspected obstructive lesions of the bowel, or in children younger than 3 years of age. It may adsorb concomitant medications, reducing their bioavailability. Kaolin can cause a pneumoconiosis in kaolin-factory workers (it is also commonly used in plastics, paint, and adhesives), but this is not a problem with the medication.

DOSAGE

The dosage is 15 to 30 milliliters, administered 3 or more times daily, as indicated.

PEARLS AND PITFALLS

1. Kaopectate adsorbs other drugs. Concomitant medications should be given 1 hour before or 3 hours after Kaopectate.
2. Sodium and, in particular, potassium losses may be increased by Kaopectate. Electrolytes may need to be followed closely in severe diarrhea or with prolonged therapy.
3. Pectin alone is a form of dietary fiber. Improvements in postprandial insulin and glucose concentrations have been shown in diabetics given supplemental pectin.

Loperamide

Loperamide is a synthetic antidiarrheal agent for oral use in the treatment of both acute and chronic diarrheal conditions. It is unique among antidiarrheal agents in that loperamide appears to have antisecretory effects in addition to prolonging gut transit time.

PHARMACODYNAMICS AND PHARMACOKINETICS

Loperamide is a member of the phenylpiperidine analgesic class, like meperidine and diphenoxylate, but without significant nervous system effects.

After oral ingestion, serum concentrations of loperamide peak at 4 hours, with an elimination half-life of 7 to 14 hours. The drug is incompletely absorbed after oral ingestion, with delays due to inhibition of gastrointestinal motility. The drug is poorly soluble in water. Large oral doses do not cause euphoria and inhibit withdrawal symptoms only modestly. The abuse potential of loperamide is low.

MECHANISM OF ACTION

Loperamide slows intestinal transit time. Basilisco demonstrated delays in breath hydrogen excretion with loperamide during lactulose hydrogen breath-testing, a delay antagonized by concurrent naloxone administration.

Loperamide exerts its effect by virtue of its opiate agonist activity on gut-associated opiate receptors. It inhibits the action of calmodulin. This effect is greatest in the jejunum and is associated with higher frequency and lower duration of irregular motor activity (phase II). Loperamide accentuates segmenting motor activity in the proximal colon.

Besides effects on motor activity, loperamide appears to affect intestinal secretory activity as well. Turnberg showed that loperamide inhibits mucosal secretion by a variety of known intestinal secretagogues. From research in children, Sandhu found a prompt and impressive decrease in secretory diarrhea during steady-state perfusion studies of the jejunum.

Loperamide does not increase the rate of absorption of water or electrolytes from the intestine. During steady-state total gut perfusion of normal volunteers, Schiller found identical volumes of rectal effluent with or without loperamide. However, loperamide did increase the intraluminal volume of the total gut (985 ml without loperamide, compared to 1764 ml with loperamide).

Loperamide appears to exert its effect by local tissue action. Topical application of the drug to the mucosa of the descending and sigmoid colon of volunteers decreases spike activity (the myoelectric equivalent of propulsive movements). No decrease in plasma prostaglandin F alpha, motilin, or amylase activity is demonstrable. Basal gastric acid output and bile salt production are unchanged by loperamide.

INDICATIONS

Loperamide is approved by the Food and Drug Administration for the treatment of chronic diarrhea associated with inflammatory bowel disease, acute nonspecific diarrhea, and high-volume ileostomy output.

Bergman studied the action of loperamide in 29 patients with chronic diarrhea after intestinal resection for Crohn's disease. In comparison to diphenoxylate, 19 of the 29 patients preferred the decrease in stool frequency and increase in stool consistency associated with loperamide. Only five preferred diphenoxylate, while five had no benefit from either agent. Wille-Jorgensen found no patient preference for loperamide over diphenoxylate in a study of 27 patients with iatrogenic short gut (jejunoileal bypass for morbid obesity).

Loperamide serves as a useful adjunct in the treatment of acute nondysenteric diarrhea in children. Karrar in Saudi Arabia, Gasbarrini in Italy, Singh in India, and Vesikar in Scandinavia all found decreases in stool volume and frequency and more rapid weight gain with the use of loperamide (0.8 mg/kg/24 hrs) in conjunction with an oral rehydration regimen. Vesikar did find that cholestyramine, 2 grams daily, was nearly 3 times more effective than loperamide in decreasing stool frequency and inducing weight gain.

Loperamide is also useful in the treatment of postvagotomy diarrhea, although the daily doses required (12–24 mg) were higher than those used in other conditions.

Loperamide may have a useful role in that subgroup of patients with irritable bowel syndrome troubled predominantly by diarrhea. Lavo and Cann both found amelioration of stool frequency, urgency, and pain in separate studies of irritable bowel syndrome patients. Self-titration of dose and nighttime dosing were both safe and effective.

Although the welfare of adult patients with acute infectious diarrhea is not known to be improved by loperamide (Bergstrom et al.), Johnson found loperamide to be more efficacious than bismuth subsalicylate in the treatment (not prevention) of acute traveler's diarrhea, with decreased diarrhea within the first 4 hours of therapy.

ADMINISTRATION

The usual dose is one to two 2-milligram capsules with each liquid bowel movement, not to exceed eight capsules a day. The typical daily dosage ranges from 4 to 8 milligrams.

SIDE EFFECTS

Constipation can occur with loperamide use and is documented to occur in about 10 percent of patients receiving the drug for both acute and chronic diarrheal disorders. Constipation is most likely to occur in the patient receiving loperamide for treatment of irritable bowel syndrome.

Other gastrointestinal side effects include abdominal pain, abdominal distension, bloating, nausea, and vomiting. In higher daily doses (>8 mg/day), central nervous system depression with drowsiness, dizziness, and fatigue can occur.

CONTRAINDICATIONS

The use of agents that inhibit gastrointestinal motility is clearly associated with the development of toxic megacolon in patients suffering from pseudomembranous enterocolitis and acute ulcerative colitis.

The presence of fever and grossly bloody diarrhea (dysentery) precludes the safe use of loperamide.

PEARLS AND PITFALLS

1. The use of naloxone is indicated for the treatment of central nervous system depression and respiratory depression in acute loperamide overdose.
2. Loperamide is contraindicated in the treatment of pseudomembranous enterocolitis, acute ulcerative colitis, and acute dysentery, as it is associated with the development of toxic megacolon.
3. The use of loperamide in irritable bowel syndrome should be restricted to that subgroup plagued with severe urgency, diarrhea, and pain.

References

KAOLIN AND PECTIN

1. Allen MD, et al. Effect of magnesium-aluminum hydroxide and kaolin-pectin on absorption of digoxin from tablets and capsules. J Clin Pharm 1981; 21:26.
   Kaopectate reduced absorption of digoxin tablets.
2. Jenkins DJA, et al. Decrease in postprandial insulin and glucose concentrations by guar and pectin. Ann Intern Med 1977; 86:20.
   Pectin improved the postprandial insulin and glucose profiles in diabetics.
3. Juhl RP. Comparison of kaolin-pectin and activated charcoal for inhibition of aspirin absorption. Am J Hosp Pharm 1979; 36:1097.
   Kaopectate reduced aspirin absorption but not as much as did activated charcoal.
4. McClung HJ, Beck RD, Powers P. The effect of a kaolin-pectin absorbent on stool losses of sodium, potassium, and fat during a lactose-intolerance diarrhea in rats. J Pediat 1980; 96:769.
   Kaopectate increased stool losses of sodium, potassium, and water in this experimental model.
5. Portnoy BL, et al. Antidiarrheal agents in the treatment of acute diarrhea in children. JAMA 1976; 236:844.
   Kaopectate did not decrease stool water loss or stool frequency when compared with placebo in this clinical trial. It did improve stool consistency slightly.

LOPERAMIDE

1. Altaparmakov I, Wienbeck M. Local inhibition of myoelectric activity of human colon by loperamide. Dig Dis Sci 1984; 29:232–238.
   Loperamide reduced the occurrence of groups of spike activity stimulated by neostigmine to 3.8 from 10.3 per hour in the proximal colon after topical application.
2. Basilisco G, et al. Effect of loperamide and naloxone on mouth-to-cecum transit time evaluated by lactulose hydrogen breath test. Gut 1985; 26:700–703.
   Mouth-to-cecum transit time was significantly longer after loperamide treatment. This prolongation was antagonized by the concomitant administration of naloxone.
3. Bergman L, Djarv L. A comparative study of loperamide and diphenoxylate in the treatment of chronic diarrhea caused by intestinal resection. Ann Clin Res 1981; 13:402–405.
   Loperamide was statistically superior to diphenoxylate at reducing the number of stools and improving fecal consistency in 29 patients who had intestinal resection for Crohn's disease.
4. Bergstrom T, et al. Symptomatic treatment of acute infectious diarrhea: Loperamide versus placebo in a double-blind trial. J Infect 1986; 12:35–38.

Neither the duration of pathogen excretion nor the frequency or consistency of diarrheal stools was significantly altered by loperamide in this study of acute infectious diarrhea in adults.

5. Cann PA, et al. Role of loperamide and placebo in management of irritable bowel syndrome (IBS). Dig Dis Sci 1984; 29:239–247.

   Eighteen of 28 patients with IBS received symptomatic benefit from loperamide therapy, with significant improvement in diarrhea, urgency, and borborygmi.

6. Gasbarrini G, et al. A multicenter, double-blind, controlled trial comparing lidamidine HCl and loperamide in the symptomatic treatment of acute diarrhea. Arzneimittel-Forschung 1986; 36:1843–1845.

   Lidamidine and loperamide had comparable effects in the treatment of acute nonspecific diarrhea.

7. Hamdi I, Dodge JA. Toddler diarrhea: Observations on the effects of aspirin and loperamide. J Ped Gastro Nutri 1985; 4:362–365.

   Although aspirin reduced plasma concentrations of prostaglandin F alpha and controlled diarrhea symptoms, loperamide consistently controlled toddler diarrhea but had no effect on plasma prostaglandin F alpha.

8. Johnson PC, et al. Comparison of loperamide with bismuth subsalicylate for the treatment of acute traveler's diarrhea. JAMA 1986; 255:757–760.

   People receiving loperamide passed fewer unformed stools during the first 4 hours of therapy, the first 24 hours of therapy, and the first 48 hours of therapy.

9. Kachel G, et al. Human intestinal motor activity and transport: Effects of a synthetic opiate. Gastroenterology 1986; 90:85–93.

   Loperamide increases the transit time in the jejunum but not in the ileum or the colon. Transport rates of water and electrolytes and transmural electrical potential differences were not significantly affected by the drug.

10. Karrar ZA, et al. Loperamide in acute diarrhea in childhood: Results of a double-blind, placebo-controlled clinical trial. Ann Trop Paediat 1987; 7:122–127.

    Loperamide, 0.8 mg/kg/day, plus standard oral rehydration therapy was compared with placebo plus standard oral rehydration therapy. The use of loperamide was associated with faster recovery and quicker weight gain in the majority of children.

11. Kassem AS, et al. Loperamide in acute childhood diarrhea: A double-blind, controlled trial. J Diarrhoeal Dis Res 1983; 1:10–16.

    The authors believe that the proximal gut is the main site of action of loperamide, with accentuation of segmenting motor activity.

12. Lavo B, Stenstam M, Nielsen AL. Loperamide in treatment of irritable bowel syndrome—A double-blind, placebo-controlled study. Scand J Gastro 1987; 130 (suppl):77–80.

    Significant advantages of loperamide were found to be improvements in stool consistency, pain relief, and diminished urgency.

13. Mellstrand T. Loperamide—Opiate receptor agonist with gastrointestinal motility effects. Scand J Gastro 1987; 130 (suppl):65–66.

    Loperamide is an opiate agonist that inhibits the action of calmodulin.

14. O'Brian JD, et al. Effect of codeine and loperamide on upper intestinal transit and absorption in normal subjects and patients with postvagotomy diarrhea. Gut 1988; 29:312–318.

    Loperamide delayed transit and improved symptoms, but the doses required for this effect (12–24 mg) were higher than usually considered necessary in secretory diarrhea.

15. Rees WD, et al. The effects of an opiate agonist and antagonist on the human upper gastrointestinal tract. Eur J Clin Invest 1983; 13:221–225.

    Plasma motilin was not altered by naloxone, nor did the drug have any effect on basal gastric acid output or bile salt production.

16. Remington M, et al. Abnormalities in gastrointestinal motor activity in patients with short bowels: Effect of a synthetic opiate. Gastroenterology 1983; 85:629–636.

    Loperamide increases feeding activity (phase-II motor activity), thus prolonging intestinal transit time.

17. Sandhu BK, et al. Loperamide in severe protracted diarrhea. Arch Dis Child 1983; 58:39–43.

    Loperamide resulted in a prompt and impressive improvement in the condition of each of six children with life-threatening, protracted secretory diarrhea.

18. Schiller LR, et al. Mechanism of the antidiarrheal effect of loperamide. Gastroenterology 1984; 86:1475–1480.

    While loperamide did not alter the rate of absorption by intestinal mucosal cells, it did substantially increase the intraluminal volume of the total gut.

19. Sninsky CA, et al. Effect of lidamidine hydrochloride and loperamide on gastric emptying and transit of the small intestine. Gastroenterology 1986; 90:68–73.

    Loperamide significantly slowed transit when compared with placebo or lidamidine.

20. Turnberg LA. Antisecretory activity of opiates in vitro and in vivo in man. Scand J Gastro 1983; 84 (suppl):79–83.

    Loperamide inhibits secretion induced by a variety of different secretagogues. Experimentally induced secretion in the human jejunum is reduced by loperamide.

21. Vesikari T, Isolaur E. A comparative trial of cholestyramine and loperamide for acute diarrhea in infants treated as outpatients. Acta Pediat Scand 1985; 74:650–654.

    The duration of watery diarrhea in a group of children with acute diarrhea (rotavirus, 66%) from the beginning of treatment was 0.9 days in the cholestyramine group, 2.5 days in the loperamide group, and 3.3 days in the placebo group.

22. Wille-Jorgensen P, et al. Diarrhea following jejunoileostomy for morbid obesity: A randomized trial of loperamide and diphenoxylate. Acta Chir Scand 1982; 148:157–158.

    Both loperamide and diphenoxylate had a significant effect on diarrhea when compared with no treatment, but no significant difference was found between the two drugs.

Bile Salt Binders

Michael S. Gurney

It has been known for centuries that bile is an excellent laxative, hence the use of animal bile for the relief of chronic constipation. However, only in the last several decades have the bile acids been identified as the compounds responsible for this effect. The inappropriate passage of bile acids into the colon is responsible for the clinical entity of bile acid diarrhea, a chronic, watery secretory diarrhea. Such patients typically have frequent bowel movements after meals but not at night. The stool weight is only mildly increased, and significant steatorrhea is rarely present. The diarrhea is usually more bothersome than debilitating; dehydration and electrolyte abnormalities are uncommon. We now know that the dehydroxy bile acids cause this syndrome by stimulation of colonic cyclic AMP, with secondary secretion of water and electrolytes. The bile salt binding agents, cholestyramine and colestipol, have been employed with great success in such patients, and their use has earned physicians many grateful patients for the relief they provide. The two resins are very similar and are discussed together.

PHARMACOLOGY AND MECHANISM OF ACTION

The resins are high-molecular-weight anion-exchange resins. Cholestyramine has quarternary ammonium groups on the resin, whereas colestipol contains secondary and tertiary amines. Both are protonated with chloride.

Following oral administration, both resins release their chloride ions and absorb bile acids in the small intestine. An insoluble, nonabsorbable complex is formed and excreted unchanged in the feces. In vitro, each gram of cholestyramine binds about 1100 micromoles of taurocholate and 913 micromoles of glycocholate. Colestipol binds 938 micromoles of taurocholate and 825 micromoles of glycocholate. Since both drugs are nonspecific anion-exchange resins, other compounds and drugs, especially those with an acid pH, are bound.

INDICATIONS

Bile acid diarrhea is divided on the basis of etiology into three groups. Type I is probably the most common form and is caused by ileal disease, resection, or bypass. The bile acids, which only have receptors in the terminal ileum, are unable to be reabsorbed and pass into the colon, causing secretory diarrhea. Type II is less common and seems to be due to a selective ileal transport defect of bile acids. Type III occurs after surgical truncal vagotomy, or more commonly, postcholecystectomy. The exact mechanism is unknown. Cholestyramine and colestipol are indicated in the treatment of all three types and are extremely effective. However, it must be remembered that patients with more than 100 centimeters of ileum resected do not actually have bile acid diarrhea. Their diarrhea is caused by a reduced bile salt pool from significant chronic intestinal loss. The lack of bile salts causes poor fat micelle formation in the small intestine and subsequent malabsorption and steatorrhea. Bile acid binders actually worsen the diarrhea in such patients.

Both colestipol and cholestyramine have been shown to bind the toxin of *Clostridia difficile*. In vitro, colestipol binds 4 times the amount of toxin that cholestyramine does. However, the two have not been tested against each other in a clinical study. Thus, mild *C. difficile*–induced pseudomembranous colitis responds to treatment with either resin. Moderate to severe disease, however, does not improve significantly with resin therapy and is better treated with antibiotics.

Chronic cholestatic liver disease, such as primary biliary cirrhosis and sclerosing cholangitis, is often complicated by chronic pruritis. The pruritis is thought to be due to elevated serum levels of bile acids and other pruritogens. This very bothersome complaint is usually improved with bile salt binders.

SIDE EFFECTS

There are no absolute contraindications to the use of either colestipol or cholestyramine. In patients with intestinal strictures, however, the drugs must be used carefully, in reduced amounts, since there are reports of obstruction caused by the resins.

The most common side effects are gastrointestinal, especially with high doses and in patients older than 60 years of age. Constipation is the most frequent complaint in patients taking the drugs for lipid disorders; this is, of course, less of a problem when treating diarrhea illnesses. Bloating, abdominal pain, belching, flatulence, nausea, and vomiting are other less common intestinal side effects.

Of more practical concern is the resin binding of concomitant medications. Table 33–1 is a list of medications ab-

Table 33–1. Medications absorbed by cholestyramine or colestipol

Digitoxin
Thyroid hormone
Warfarin (coumadin)
Iron
Phenylbutazone
Thiazide diuretics
Phenobarbital
Tetracycline
Penicillin

sorbed by colestipol and cholestyramine. All drugs, and especially those on the list, should be given either 1 hour before or 4 hours after the resins are taken. Occasionally, a rebound effect, such as prolonged anticoagulation with coumadin, is noted when resin therapy is stopped abruptly.

Cholestyramine and colestipol occasionally interfere with the absorption of fat. Deficiency of the fat-soluble vitamins (A, D, E, and K) may occur with long-term therapy and thus supplementation may be needed. Folate deficiency has also been reported with chronic therapy, and folate supplements should be given, especially in children.

DOSAGE

Colestipol is usually the preferred medication of the two resins, since cholestyramine has an unpleasant taste. The starting dose for colestipol is one 5-gram packet 3 times daily, just before meals. The dose may be increased up to 30 grams/day if needed. The starting dose for cholestyramine is one 4-gram packet 3 times daily, just before meals. It may be increased to 24 grams/day if needed. Both resins should be mixed with at least 120 milliliters of a liquid. After the mixture is ingested, the glass should be rinsed with additional liquid and drunk to ensure that the entire dose has been taken. The resins should not be taken in the dry form, since this is associated with esophageal irritation or obstruction. Alternatively, either resin may be mixed with a soup or a pulpy fruit with a high moisture content, such as crushed pineapple or applesauce.

For pseudomembranous colitis, the resins should be given 4 times a day initially, and the dose may later be reduced if needed. When given to patients with pruritus, improvement is usually noted in 1 to 3 weeks.

Once the desired clinical response has been achieved, the dose can be reduced. When reducing the dose, it should be remembered that the most important dose is the morning dose, since the gallbladder is then filled with bile from the overnight fast. Often, only a breakfast dose is ultimately needed for the control of symptoms.

PEARLS AND PITFALLS

1. In ileal dysfunction from Crohn's disease, one morning dose is often enough to relieve the bile salt diarrhea.
2. Some patients with idiopathic diarrhea have a bile salt transport defect and secondary bile salt diarrhea. Since this condition is difficult to diagnose, an empiric trial of colestipol can be rewarding in these challenging patients.
3. The binding resins should not be used in patients with partial small intestinal obstruction, since they can precipitate total obstruction.
4. Other medications should be given either 1 hour before or 4 hours after resins. If the evening dose of cholestyramine or colestipol is stopped as the dose is reduced, this is a convenient time to give other medications.

5. Fat-soluble vitamin and folate supplementation may be needed for patients on long-term resin therapy. This is especially important for patients receiving resins for cholestatic liver disease such as primary biliary cirrhosis.
6. Patients taking both coumadin and a binding resin may have a significant increase in their prothrombin time if the binding resin is stopped.

References

1. Aldini R, et al. Bile acid malabsorption and bile acid diarrhea in intestinal resection. Dig Dis Sci 1982; 27:495.

    Aldini studied patients with large and small ileal resections and colectomy versus normal controls, and found that stool pH and free fatty acids were as important as bile salts in causing diarrhea. This may explain why patients with large ileal resections usually respond well to low-fat diets.
2. Balistreri WF, Partin JC, Schubert WK. Bile acid malabsorption: A consequence of terminal ileal dysfunction in protracted diarrhea of infancy. J Pediat 1977; 89:21.

    Two infants with the enigmatic condition of protracted diarrhea of infancy were shown to have bile acid diarrhea due to ileal dysfunction.
3. Chang TW, Onderdonk AB, Bartlett JG. Anion-exchange resins in antibiotic-associated colitis. *Lancet* 1978; 2:258–259.

    Both colestipol and cholestyramine were mixed in vitro with *C. difficile* toxin. Both resins bound the toxin, but colestipol was 4 times more effective on a weight basis.
4. Fromm H, Malavolti M. Bile acid–induced diarrhea. Clin Gastro 1986; 15:567.

    An excellent discussion of bile acid diarrhea and its pathophysiology.
5. Garbutt JT, Kenney TJ. Effect of cholestyramine on bile acid metabolism in normal man. J Clin Invest 1972; 51:2781.

    An exhaustive study of the effect of resin-binding therapy on bile acid metabolism.
6. Hofmann AF, Poley JR. Cholestyramine treatment of diarrhea associated with ileal resection. NEJM 1969; 281:397.

    Hofmann and Poley are the first to make the distinction between large and small ileal resections with respect to postoperative diarrhea. A well-written classic.
7. Hutcheon DF, Bayless TM, Gadacz TR. Postcholecystectomy diarrhea. JAMA 1979; 241:823.

    Postcholecystectomy diarrhea was shown to be associated with bile acid malabsorption and it responded well to cholestyramine resin. Truncal vagotomy with cholecystectomy is particularly associated with postoperative diarrhea.
8. Merrick MV, Eastwood MA, Ford MJ. Is bile acid malabsorption underdiagnosed? An evaluation of accuracy of diagnosis by measurement of SeHCAT retention. BMJ 1985; 280:665.

    The investigators used a radio-labeled synthetic bile acid to study ileal function. They found that 5 of 42 patients with diarrhea and the irritable bowel syndrome actually had bile

acid malabsorption. Cholestyramine relieved their symptoms.
9. Thaysen EH. Idiopathic bile acid diarrhea reconsidered. Scand J Gastro 1985; 20:452.

Thaysen reports several more cases of idiopathic bile acid diarrhea and proposes that in the proper clinical setting—chronic, watery diarrhea without any other demonstrable abnormality—an empiric trial of resin is worthwhile.

34

Anticonstipation Agents

Michael Carboni and Michael S. Gurney

Bulk-Forming Agents

The average American gets only 15 to 20 grams of dietary fiber a day, when 20 to 50 grams are needed for normal bowel function. In order to normalize bowel function, bulk-forming agents are used as dietary fiber supplements. This chapter discusses and compares the more commonly used bulking agents: Citrucel, Fiberall, Metamucil, and Perdiem.

DIETARY FIBER

Dietary fiber is that portion of the plant cell wall that escapes digestion and is composed of lignins and polysaccharides (i.e., cellulose, hemicellulose, pectin, gums, and mucilage). These components exercise a variety of important mechanistic and metabolic functions and influence bacterial flora in the large intestine. Different sources of dietary fiber (i.e., brans, grains, fruits, and vegetables) vary in their fiber content and composition, as do the different bulk-forming agents. The differences in composition account for the differences in the water-holding capacity and mechanism of action of bulking agents.

COMPOSITION AND FORMULATION

Bulk-forming agents are more refined and concentrated than the usual dietary sources of fiber and are generally more effective. Most bulk-forming agents are composed of one of three major components of dietary fiber—psyllium, semisynthetic cellulose, or synthetic polycarbophil—in varying proportions.

1. Psyllium hydrophilic colloid (Metamucil, Fiberall, Perdiem). The refined colloid obtained from psyllium seeds is rich in mucilage. This mucilloid preparation forms a gelatinous mass when mixed with water. Metamucil does contain dextrose as a dispersing agent, but sugar-free preparations are available. Various flavors can also be found. Powders are the usual form of psyllium preparations, but Perdiem is formulated as psyllium granules. The sodium content varies with each individual preparation.
2. Carboxymethylcellulose and methylcellulose (Citrucel). The indigestible and nonabsorbable semisynthetic derivatives of cellulose form a bulky, hydrophilic colloid when mixed with water. The carboxymethyl preparation contains high amounts of sodium, which may lead to fluid retention and should be avoided in patients on sodium restrictions. Citrucel is available as a powder in regular

and orange flavors. Forms of other preparations include liquids, capsules, and tablets.
3. Polycarbophil and calcium polycarbophil (Mitrolan). The polycarbophils are synthetic polyacrylic resins that are nonabsorbable, indigestible, and metabolically inert. They have more water-binding activity than the other two types of agent, absorbing 60 to 100 times their weight in water. The sodium content is lower, but free calcium is released in the intestine and so they should be avoided in patients on calcium restriction or using tetracyclines. Tablets are the most common form used.

MECHANISM OF ACTION

The hydrophilic properties of dietary fiber in bulk-forming agents add weight and provide bulk to the stool through the absorption of water. This increase in water content normalizes transit time through the intestine, prevents overabsorption of water by the colon, and keeps the feces soft and bulky. In addition, dietary fiber components are digested by and stimulate the growth of colonic bacteria, thus adding to fecal mass. Movement of soft stools through the colon requires less pressure, thereby decreasing the colonic intraluminal pressures important in the treatment of diverticular disease. Bulk-forming agents usually take effect within 12 to 24 hours and with repeated administration a maximal effect can be reached in a few days.

In addition, bulk-forming agents have been shown to possess certain important metabolic properties. For example, water-soluble fibers (i.e., mucilages and pectins) are known to delay gastric emptying, to slow the absorption of glucose from the intestine, and to substantially reduce postprandial hyperglycemia. These properties are important in the management of diabetes and other conditions associated with the rapid breakdown of carbohydrates.

Cholesterol metabolism is also affected by soluble fibers, which bind bile acids and increase bile acid excretion in the feces. Decreased bile acid reuptake causes an increase in bile acid synthesis from cholesterol precursors, thus decreasing the plasma cholesterol concentration of low-density lipoproteins (LDLs). Water-insoluble fibers such as cellulose are not associated with the lowering of cholesterol levels.

INDICATIONS

1. Constipation. One of the most widely accepted therapeutic uses of bulk-forming agents is for the management of constipation. Constipation results from excessive absorption of water from fecal material due to slow passage through the colon. Bulk-forming agents absorb water, increase fecal bulk, alter stool consistency, and activate propulsive motility, preventing constipation.

Bulk-forming agents are used for the treatment and prevention of constipation in the elderly, pre- and postpartum women, chronically bedridden or immobilized pa-

tients, postoperative patients, patients receiving narcotics, and in fiber-deficient patients.
2. Diverticular disease. Constipation is the number 1 cause of increased pressure in the colon. By preventing constipation, one of the most common causes of diverticular disease can be avoided. Preexisting diverticulae cannot be eliminated, but further diverticula formation and symptoms of diverticulosis can be prevented through the use of bulk-forming agents. The addition of dietary fiber decreases intestinal transit time, increases fecal weight, and decreases intracolonic pressures, which are all important factors in the treatment of diverticular disease.
3. Irritable bowel syndrome. Dietary fiber supplements can normalize bowel transit times and ameliorate the symptoms of diarrhea or constipation associated with irritable bowel syndrome (IBS). Because each IBS patient has different symptoms, the dose of bulk-forming agents should be prescribed to meet individual needs. With prolonged treatment and dose adjustment, the IBS patient's symptoms should be well controlled.
4. Hemorrhoids, anal fissures, and anal surgical patients. Because bulk-forming agents act as stool softeners, patients who need to resist straining or to soften their stools are recommended to use bulking agents.
5. Diarrhea. Bulk-forming agents, especially methylcellulose and polycarbophil, are useful in the symptomatic relief of acute and chronic watery diarrhea by increasing bulk and consistency of the stool. They are also helpful in reducing the number of evacuations in the patient with an ileostomy or colostomy. However, bulk agents can increase losses of sodium, potassium, and water in these patients.
6. Diabetes. Since the water-soluble fiber components slow gastric emptying and the absorption of glucose, bulk-forming agents add an attractive dimension to the treatment of diabetics. Postprandial blood sugars have been lowered in patients on dietary fiber supplements, reducing their need for insulin. Although the exact mechanisms remain a mystery, the advantages of increased soluble fiber in the diabetic patient have been well documented.

DOSAGE AND ADMINISTRATION

The dosages and general information for some of the more common bulk-forming agents are presented in Table 34–1. The grams of dietary fiber in each dose are compared, as well as sodium content, sugar content, and calories.

In Table 34–2, the average cost of the bulk-forming agents per gram of dietary fiber and per dose are presented.

It is important to remember that each oral dose of any bulk-forming agent must be taken concurrently with one or more glasses of water or juice to ensure that an obstruction does not develop from an improperly hydrated bolus.

Doses are usually taken in the morning—and evening, when taking two doses a day. The number of doses per day

Table 34–1. Common bulk-forming agents

Product	Preparation	Oral dose (grams)	Dietary fiber (gm/dose)	Sodium (mg/dose)	Carbohydrate (gm/dose)	Calories (dose)
Citrucel	Regular	19 (1 Tbsp)	2	3	15	60
	Orange	19 (1 Tbsp)	2	3	15	60
Fiberall	Sugar-free	5 (1 tsp)	3.4	10		6
Metamucil	Regular	7 (1 tsp)	3.4	1	3.5	14
	Orange	11 (1 Tbsp)	3.4	1	7.1	30
	Sugar-free Regular	3.7 (1 tsp)	3.4	1	0.3	1
	Sugar-free Orange	4.3 (1 tsp)	3.4	1	0.6	2
	Instant Mix	1 pkt (.19 oz)	3.4	2		1
Perdiem Fiber		6 (1 tsp)	4.03	1.8		4
Perdiem		6 (1 tsp)	3.25	1.8		4

Table 34–2. Average cost of bulking agents

Product	Preparation	Product weight (gm)	Dietary fiber (gm/dose)	Cost/gm dietary fiber	Cost/dose	Dose/day
Citrucel	Regular	283	2	$.23	$.47	1–3
	Orange	852	2	$.11	$.22	1–3
Fiberall	Sugar-free	284	3.4	$.03	$.11	1–3
Metamucil	Regular	907	3.4	$.03	$.10	1–3
	Orange	907	3.4	$.05	$.16	1–3
	Sugar-free Regular	558	3.4	$.03	$.09	1–3
	Sugar-free Orange	527	3.4	$.03	$.11	1–3
	Instant Mix	30/.19-oz pkt	3.4	$.06	$.21	1–3
Perdiem Fiber		250	4.03	$.05	$.20	1–4
Perdiem		250	3.25	$.06	$.21	1–4

is determined by the patient's needs and titrated during therapy to meet those needs.

CONTRAINDICATIONS AND SIDE EFFECTS

Since no systemic side effects occur with the use of bulk-forming agents, prolonged therapy is not a risk. Also, unlike other laxatives and cathartics, no dependence can develop, allowing for long-term therapy with bulking agents. In addition, children's doses are available when indicated, with no major risks.

A caution should be given to phenylketonurics, as Sugar-Free Metamucil contains phenylalanine.

Contraindications for the administration of bulk-forming agents include any suspicion of bowel obstruction or impaction, an undiagnosed change in bowel habits, or an acute abdomen.

Fecal impaction or intestinal obstruction can occur in any condition that stops the progression of the bulk-forming agent through the intestine, including stenoses, ulceration with fibrosis, or obstructing adhesions of the alimentary canal. Water is reabsorbed from the bulking agent and the bolus can become inspissated within the bowel lumen. Thus, any narrowing of the intestinal lumen represents a risk. Obstruction can also occur within the esophagus and intestine if too little water is taken with the bulk-forming agent.

Allergic reactions (urticaria, rhinitis, dermatitis, and bronchial asthma) to bulk-forming agents are rare but possible. Workers involved in the production of psyllium powder can become sensitized from chronic exposure and may experience asthmatic symptoms on inhalation of the powder. The sugar added to some preparations can be hazardous if used by diabetics.

Cellulose can bind cardiac glycosides, salicylates, and nitrofurantoin and decreases their intestinal absorption. These interactions are not usually clinically significant. However, psyllium preparations may bind coumarin derivatives, with adverse clinical effect. Information on this interaction is sparse, but the potential effects are serious enough that close monitoring of prothrombin times in the care of patients taking coumarin is important.

Carboxymethylcellulose and some psyllium colloids may contain significant quantities of sodium and should not be used when sodium and water retention present a problem.

PEARLS AND PITFALLS

1. Citrucel and Regular Metamucil may be more palatable when mixed with juice.
2. Sugar-Free Metamucil has fewer calories and comes in assorted flavors.
3. Perdiem requires large amounts of water to prevent the formation of bezoars.

Contact Laxatives

Contact (stimulant) laxatives are nonprescription preparations that usually promote a bowel movement within 6 to 12 hours. This rapid response is appealing to many in the general population, who are in search of an easy, inexpensive "quick fix" to the problem of constipation. The availability, low cost, rapid onset of action, and constant promotion of these products have led to their status as one of the most frequently used, misused, and least understood of all the classes of drugs in our therapeutic armamentarium. These laxatives are generally thought of as stimulants, under the common misconception that they cause propulsive peristaltic activity either through local irritation of the mucosa or a selective stimulation of colonic intramucosal nerve plexus. Actually, most contact laxatives have no such peristaltic actions. In addition, there is a lack of awareness among the population of the potential complications of these medications.

The contact laxatives can be divided into several classes, based on their structure and mechanism of action. The classes include the anthraquinones, the diphenylmethanes, ricinoleic acid (castor oil), and docusate.

INDICATIONS

Contact laxatives are not indicated for chronic use, and their use in children at all should be discouraged. Failure to heed these warnings can result in laxative-dependent constipation. Situations for which their use is indicated are:

1. To ease the pain of defecation in patients with painful episiotomies, thrombosed hemorrhoids, anal fissures, or perianal abscesses.
2. To decrease the need to administer Valsalva to patients with abdominal-wall or diaphragmatic hernias, anal stenosis, and aneurysms or other diseases of the cerebral or coronary arteries.
3. To relieve constipation during puerperium.
4. In geriatric patients with poor abdominal and perineal tone.
5. For the temporary alteration of bowel motility due to other drugs.
6. To prepare the colon for radiologic or endoscopic examination.
7. To provide a fresh stool for ova and parasite analysis.
8. For the relief of temporary constipation in a healthy patient.

Anthraquinones

Anthraquinones are among the most used and abused of the contact laxatives. Most produce a soft or formed stool within 6 to 12 hours. The preparations range from the mildest (senna) to those that are too strong and often cause colic (aloe, aloin, or rhubarb).

Aloe is the dried latex of the leaves of various species of the *Aloe* plant, found in Africa and the West Indies. The drug has a bitter taste and a disagreeable odor. Aloin is a microcrystalline powder consisting of a mixture of active ingredients extracted from aloe. Cascara sagrada is the dried bark of the buckthorn tree. The active ingredients are four anthraquinone glycosides (cascarasides A through D). Senna is the dried leaflet of the *Cassia* plant, and the active ingredients are sennosides A and B, another two anthraquinone glycosides.

The anthraquinones are poorly absorbed from the small intestine and hydrolyzed by colonic bacteria to the pharmacologically active free anthraquinones. Any absorbed anthraquinones are metabolized by the liver and then secreted into the bile or urine. Low levels may be excreted in breast milk.

MECHANISM OF ACTION

The anthraquinones' actions are restricted to the distal ileum and colon. The compounds stimulate fluid and electrolyte secretion and impair sodium absorption. These actions may be mediated by cyclic AMP, which is increased in colonic mucosal cells after anthraquinone administration. Contrary to popular belief, there is no good evidence for any action on the colonic nerve plexus or colonic motility.

CONTRAINDICATIONS AND SIDE EFFECTS

All laxatives are contraindicated in patients with acute or undiagnosed abdominal pain, nausea, or vomiting. Stimulant cathartics are contraindicated in intestinal obstruction.

Anthraquinone derivatives used chronically (more than 4 months) may cause melanosis coli, an accumulation of dark pigment in the mucosa of the cecum and rectum. There does not appear to be a problem with the accumulation of the pigment alone. The condition resolves in 3 to 6 months after discontinuation of the drug.

Other consequences of chronic use of stimulant laxatives include "cathartic colon" and metabolic alkalosis or acidosis. Cathartic colon occurs after many years of use and is defined as colonic dilatation and poor motor function. Such patients require colon stimulants for defecation or a prolonged colon retraining program.

All stimulant cathartics can result in severe cramping and diarrhea after ingestion.

DOSAGE

Table 34–3 shows the usual dose of the various drugs. The dose should be reduced by half in geriatric and obstetric patients, and in children weighing over 27 kilograms.

Table 34-3. Contact laxatives*

Agent	Brand names	Adult dosage
Anthraquinones		
Cascara	Generic: 325-mg tablets fluid extract aromatic fluid extract	200–400 mg 0.5–1.5 ml 5 ml
Senna	Senokot tablets granules	2–4 tablets/day 1–2 tsp bid
Bisacodyl	Dulcolax tablets (5-mg) suppositories (10-mg) Fleet Bisacodyl tablets (5-mg) suppositories (10-mg)	5–15 mg orally or 10 mg rectally
Castor oil	Generic liquid Emulsoil Neoloid Purge Concentrate	15–60 ml
Docusate	Sodium: Colace, 50 & 100 mg Regutol, 100 mg Modane Soft, 100 mg Kasof, 240 mg Potassium: Dialose, 100 mg Calcium: Surfak, 240 mg	50–400 mg daily
Phenolphthalein	Ex-Lax, 90-mg tablets Feen-A-Mint Gum, 97-mg chewable tablets Modane, Mild, 60-mg tablets Prulet, 60-mg tablets Yellolax	30–270 mg daily

*Combination preparations are not listed.

Diphenylmethane Derivatives

This family of contact laxatives consists of the bisacodyl preparations (Dulcolax, Fleet's Bisacodyl) and the phenolphthaleins (Modane, Phillips' Laxcaps, Prulet, Correctol, Doxidan, Ex-Lax, Feen-A-Mint, Yellolax). Both types of preparation produce a bowel movement within 6 to 8 hours after ingestion.

Bisacodyl is only minimally absorbed after oral administration, but 15 percent of oral phenolphthalein is absorbed and enters the enterohepatic circulation. Small amounts are excreted in the urine and breast milk.

Both the diphenylmethanes and the phenolphthaleins stimulate colonic fluid and electrolyte secretion, similar to the anthraquinones. Bisacodyl also causes stimulation of the submucosal neural plexus, increasing peristalsis. Phenolphthalein may interfere with fluid and electrolyte conservation in the small intestine.

CONTRAINDICATIONS AND SIDE EFFECTS

The contraindications and side effects mentioned under the heading Anthraquinones also apply to use of the diphenylmethanes.

Phenolphthalein can cause dermatologic reactions in sensitive patients. Fixed drug eruptions, pruritis, burning, and pigmentation have all been reported. It also imparts a pink color to alkaline urine or feces, and patients should be forewarned. Because of a prolonged enterohepatic circulation, phenolphthalein's action may last for several days after only a single dose in sensitive patients.

Although bisacodyl usually produces soft stools with little or no colic, an enteric coating is required to minimize gastric irritation. The suppository preparation may cause stinging, tenesmus, and mild proctitis in a few patients. If the oral form is chewed and the enteric coating disrupted, oral and gastric irritation may result.

DOSAGE

See Table 34–3 for adult dosages. Children 6 years and older may receive either bisacodyl (5 mg orally or 10 mg by suppository) or phenolphthalein (30–60 mg orally).

Ricinoleic Acid

Castor oil is hydrolyzed in the small intestine to ricinoleic acid, a long-chain fatty acid. Castor oil produces one or more copious, watery evacuations 2 to 6 hours after ingestion. The colon is emptied so completely that passage of normal stool afterward may be delayed for 2 days or more. Because of its strong action, castor oil is principally used to prepare patients for radiologic examination. It should not be used to treat common constipation.

MECHANISM OF ACTION

Ricinoleic acid stimulates anion secretion in the small intestine and causes net accumulation of fluid and electrolytes. Some studies have shown that it may erode villous tips, disorganize the microvillous surface, and increase mucosal permeability to molecules with molecular weights as large as 16,000.

CONTRAINDICATIONS AND SIDE EFFECTS

Castor oil has the same general contraindications and side effects as other contact cathartics. In addition, because of its strong action, it is more likely to cause cramping, dehydration, and electrolyte disturbances.

DOSAGE

Table 34–3 states the usual dosage for castor oil. Palatability is improved by administering chilled castor oil along with fruit juice, or with a carbonated beverage afterwards. Neoloid is a flavored emulsion of castor oil and is more palatable.

Docusate (Dioctyl Sulfosuccinate)

The docusate salts—calcium (Surfak), potassium (Dialose, Kasof), and sodium (Colase Regutol, Modane Soft) are anionic surfactants promoted as stool-softening agents. It is now known that, in addition to their emollient properties, these drugs are also mild contact laxatives. They appear to be absorbed to some extent in the duodenum and jejunum and subsequently excreted in the bile. These drugs produce a softer bowel movement within 3 to 5 days of administration.

CONTRAINDICATIONS AND SIDE EFFECTS

The docusate salts are so mild that many of the side effects of other contact laxatives are not a problem. However, docusate does increase intestinal permeability, and other laxatives or mineral oil should not be given concomitantly. Increased toxicity, including hepatotoxicity, has been reported in such cases. Diarrhea and morphologic intestinal mucosal changes have also been reported.

DOSAGE

See Table 34–3 for dosage. It is recommended that 240 to 340 milliliters of water be taken with each dose.

PEARLS AND PITFALLS

1. An enema or suppository 20 minutes after breakfast or dinner, followed by 30 minutes on the toilet can psychologically and physiologically (via the gastrocolic reflex) help a constipated patient return to normal bowel habits.
2. Contact laxatives should be avoided in children; too frequent use can result in dependence. The key task is to educate their parents about the normal variability in bowel habits.
3. Laxatives confer no benefit for weight loss, contrary to popular belief.

4. Exercise, a high-fiber diet, generous fluid intake, abdominal strengthening exercises, and education by physicians are of more benefit for chronic constipation than are contact laxatives.
5. A patient who is taking laxatives chronically should have the drugs discontinued gradually. Stopping the laxatives abruptly results in a flare of the constipation and possible impaction.
6. Some elderly patients have difficulty with defecation because of weak abdominal muscles. Elevating the feet on a stepstool while sitting on the toilet increases the pelvic tilt and eases defecation.
7. Surreptitious abuse of phenolphthalein laxatives can be detected by alkalinizing the stool. The proper method is to add one drop of 1N sodium hydroxide to 3 milliliters of stool supernatant or urine. If a pink or red color develops, check for absorption in a spectrophotometer at 550 to 555 micrometers to confirm phenolphthalein. Also, further alkalinization with 10N sodium hydroxide should cause the color to disappear at higher pH levels.

Lubricants

The general population is preoccupied by the idea of constipation. An important cause of this preoccupation is the misconception that lack of a regular, daily bowel movement is associated with the accumulation of toxins and leads to various disquieting somatic complaints. The public frequently turns to over-the-counter preparations in an effort to avoid this dreaded condition. A time-honored, simple, and seemingly innocuous drug used quite often is the lubricant laxative—primarily mineral oil. In 1982, use of mineral oil accounted for 15 percent of all over-the-counter laxatives, at a total cost of over 55 million dollars.

Mineral oil is a complex mixture of saturated hydrocarbons derived from crude petroleum. It is a colorless, transparent, oily liquid with a specific gravity of 0.818 to 0.880 and is insoluble in water or alcohol. The palatability, and possibly the effectiveness, is improved when it is emulsified with acacia. It is also often combined with milk of magnesia, bulk agents, or contact laxatives.

PHARMACOLOGY

Absorption of mineral oil is negligible after rectal administration, but as much as 30 percent may be absorbed after an oral dose. Absorbed mineral oil is distributed to the intestinal mucosa, mesenteric lymph nodes, liver, and spleen.

Mineral oil coats the feces in the colonic lumen, decreasing water reabsorption. The increased water content adds to the bulk of the stool and softens it significantly. Emulsified mineral oil reportedly has better wetting properties than does nonemulsified mineral oil, and penetration of the feces may thus be enhanced. Enemas of mineral oil exert their effect by lubrication of the stool, penetration and softening of the stool, and simple physical distention of the rectum.

INDICATIONS

Mineral oil is indicated for softening of the stool and easing defecation. It should generally be used for only short periods of time, preferably no longer than a week. Ideal patients are postoperative or postpartum patients, or those for whom straining at stool should be avoided, such as post–myocardial infarction patients. Oral or rectal mineral oil is also the laxative of choice for fecal impaction.

Mineral oil has also been shown by Sondheimer to be effective in the management of chronic functional constipation in children. At the other end of the spectrum, Mulinos showed that an emulsion of equal parts of mineral oil and milk of magnesia was effective in chronic constipation of the elderly. However, there is some concern about the toxicity of chronic use, so other laxatives, such as fiber supplements or lactulose, should be used for these long-term indications if possible.

CONTRAINDICATIONS AND SIDE EFFECTS

Pulmonary aspiration of mineral oil causes a lipoid pneumonia that can be severe or even fatal. Thus, it is contraindicated in debilitated patients who are at risk for aspiration, in patients with poor esophageal emptying (such as Zenker's diverticulum), and in those with gastroesophageal reflux disease.

Chronic mineral oil ingestion leads to lipogranulomas in the mesenteric lymph nodes, liver, and spleen. The clinical importance of these granulomas is uncertain, but several cases of organ failure, possibly caused by mineral oil, have been reported.

A common complaint of patients taking mineral oil is anal leakage and secondary pruritis. This usually improves with a decrease in dosage and reportedly is less common with emulsion preparations. Chronic mineral oil use can also cause malabsorption of the fat-soluble vitamins.

DOSAGE

The adult dose is 15 to 45 milliliters of mineral oil orally, or 60 to 150 milliliters rectally. Children over 6 years may take 10 to 15 milliliters orally, or 60 milliliters per rectum. The onset of action is usually within 6 to 8 hours following an oral dose.

For fecal impaction, give 30 milliliters of mineral oil orally every hour while awake, until it begins to seep from the anus (usually within 24–48 hours). Mineral oil retention enemas can also be given, to soften the mass. At this point, digital disimpaction with 5 percent lidocaine jelly is safer, more comfortable, and more successful. Saline enemas and oral cathartics can then expel the remainder. Careful attention to good hydration is important. The risk of mineral oil aspiration can be minimized by keeping the patient upright and avoiding doses within 2 hours of sleep.

PEARLS AND PITFALLS

1. Stool softeners such as calcium or sodium docusate should not be given with mineral oil. The stool softeners enhance mineral oil absorption, increasing its toxicity.
2. Since mineral oil primarily acts by increasing the stool water content, good oral hydration is important and increases the efficacy of therapy.
3. To reduce the risk of mineral oil aspiration, it should not be given within 2 hours of bedtime.
4. Mineral oil should not be given chronically to pregnant patients. Administration for prolonged periods during gestation has been associated with vitamin K malabsorption and subsequent hypoprothrombinemia and hemorrhagic disease of the newborn.

References

BULK-FORMING AGENTS

1. Almy TP. Dietary fiber: Current role in therapy and preventive medicine. Drug Therapy 1984; 14:51–59.

    A comprehensive review of dietary fiber's role in therapy and preventive medicine.

2. Almy TP, Howell DA. Medical progress: Diverticular disease of the colon. NEJM 1980; 302:324–331.

    An in-depth look at diverticular disease, its etiology, and its treatment.

3. Anderson JW. Dietary fiber and diabetics. In GV Vanhouny, D Kritchevsky (eds), *Dietary Fiber in Health and Disease*. New York: Plenum Press, 1982. Pp. 151–165.

    An excellent chapter on dietary fiber's effect on diabetes.

4. Anderson JW, Lin Chen WJ. Plant fiber, carbohydrate, and lipid metabolism. Am J Clin Nut 1979; 2:346–363.

    An article reviewing the evidence that plant-fiber diets greatly influence the absorption and metabolism of carbohydrates and fats.

5. Anderson JW, Seiling B. High-fiber diets for diabetics: Unconventional but effective. Geriatrics 1981; 5:64–72.

    An in-depth discussion of the effects of a high-fiber diet on diabetics.

6. Anderson JW, Ward KW. High-carbohydrate, high-fiber diets for insulin-treated men with diabetes mellitus. Am J Clin Nut 1979; 11:2312–2321.

    A study determining the effects of high-carbohydrate, high-plant-fiber diets on glucose and lipid metabolism in 20 male diabetics receiving insulin therapy.

7. Brodribb AM. Treatment of symptomatic diverticular disease with a high-fiber diet. *Lancet* 1977; 1:664.

    A double-blind, controlled trial of 18 patients over 3 months assessing the therapeutic value of increased daily dietary fiber intake.

8. Brunton LL. Laxatives. In AG Gilman, LS Goodman (eds), *Goodman and Gilman's The Pharmacological Basis of Therapeutics* 7th ed. New York: Macmillan, 1985. Pp. 994–997.

    An in-depth discussion of laxatives—their effects on the colon, their uses, and their classifications.

9. Burkitt DP. Dietary fiber: Is it really helpful? Geriatrics 1982; 1:119–126.

    A discussion on how fiber-rich diets can protect against large-bowel cancer, diabetes, and other diseases.

10. Burkitt DP. Fiber as protection against gastrointestinal diseases. Am J Gastro 1984; 79:249–252.

    A discussion of the importance of fiber in the prevention of gastrointestinal disease.

11. Burkitt DP, Meisner P. How to manage constipation with high-fiber diet. Geriatrics 1979; 2:33–40.

    Valuable information on the treatment of constipation with high-fiber diets.

12. Kallman H. Constipation in the elderly. Am Fam Phys 1983; 27:178–184.

    An article discussing the etiology and treatment of constipation.

13. Kirby RW, et al. Oat-bran intake selectively lowers serum LDL cholesterol concentrations of hypercholesterolemic men. Am J Clin Nut 1981; 5:824–829.

    Eight men with hypercholesterolemia were fed one of two different diets, one with 100 gm of oat bran, the other without. Fecal bile acids, serum cholesterol (LDLs and HDLs), triglycerides, insulin, and glucose were all measured.

14. Mendeloff AI. Dietary fiber and human health. NEJM 1977; 297:811.

    An early look at the effects of dietary fiber on human health.

15. Painter NS, Burkitt DP. Diverticular disease of the colon, a 20th-century problem. Clin Gastro 1975; 39:320.

    A short discussion of diverticular disease and its treatment.

16. Stephen AM, Cummings JH. Mechanism of action of dietary fiber in the human colon. Nature 1980; 284:283–284.

    An excellent explanation of the effects of dietary fiber on the colon.

17. Tedesco FJ, et al. Laxative use in constipation. Am J Gastro 1985; 80:303–309.

    A paper by the American College of Gastroenterology's Committee on FDA-related Matters reviewing laxatives and their use in the treatment of constipation.

18. Tedesco FJ, et al. Laxatives and cathartics. In *AMA Drug Evaluations* 6th ed. Chicago: American Medical Association, 1986. Pp. 977–981.

    A comprehensive discussion of laxatives, individually and as a group, and their uses.

CONTACT LAXATIVES

1. Donowitz M, Binder HJ. Effect of dioctyl sodium sulfosuccinate on colonic fluid and electrolyte movement. Gastroenterology 1975; 69:941.

This study demonstrated that so-called stool softeners were actually mild contact laxatives, with fluid and electrolyte secretion mediated by cyclic AMP.

2. Gullikson GW, et al. Effects of anionic surfactants on hamster small intestinal membrane structure and function: Relationship to surface activity. Gastroenterology 1977; 73: 501.

   Docusate and ricinoleic acid were shown to cause structural damage to small intestinal membrane cells and to increase permeability.

3. Kallman H. Constipation in the elderly. Am Fam Phys 1983; 1:179.

   A well-written guide to the management of this common problem in the elderly.

4. Klein H. Constipation and fecal impaction. Med Clin N Am 1982; 5:1135.

   An excellent commentary on the management of fecal impaction.

5. Meisel JL, et al. Human rectal mucosa: Proctoscopic and morphological changes caused by laxatives. Gastroenterology 1977; 72:1274.

   Fleet's enemas or bisacodyl enemas and suppositories altered the endoscopic and histologic findings in normal patients, giving the misleading appearance of proctitis.

6. Smith B. Pathologic changes in the colon produced by anthraquinone purgatives. Dis Col Rect 1972; 16:455.

   A classic article by the first author to detail the histologic changes from chronic laxative abuse.

7. Tedesco FJ. Laxative use in constipation. Am J Gastro 1985; 80:303.

   A position paper from the American College of Gastroenterology on laxatives and their use. This paper is also a good reference on the different classes of laxatives and their commercial preparations.

LUBRICANTS

1. Blewitt RW, et al. Hepatic damage associated with mineral oil deposits. Gut 1977; 18:476.

   Hepatic inflammation and fibrosis were associated with mineral oil deposits in the liver in this case report.

2. Klein H. Constipation and fecal impaction. Med Clin N Am 1982; 66:1135.

   An excellent guide to the management of fecal impaction.

3. Mulinos MG, Maloney AJ. Treatment of constipation in the aged. J Med Soc NJ 1969; 66:619.

   An emulsion of milk of magnesia and mineral oil was shown to be effective over a 5-month course of treatment for chronic constipation. Side effects were minimal, but lipoid pneumonia was not specifically looked for.

4. Nochomovitz LE, et al. Massive deposition of mineral oil after prolonged ingestion. SA Med J 1975; 49:2187.

   Chronic mineral oil ingestion was associated with debilitation, malnutrition, and death. At autopsy, massive deposition of mineral oil in the liver and spleen were found.

5. Sondheimer JM, Gervaise EP. Lubricant versus laxative in the treatment of chronic functional constipation of children: A comparative study. J Pediat Gastro Nut 1982; 1:223.

   Mineral oil was superior to Senokot in the treatment of chronic functional constipation in children. Toxicity other than fecal soiling was not addressed.

6. Tedesco FJ. Laxative use in constipation. Am J Gastro 1985; 80:303.

   An excellent guide to the indications, complications, and uses of laxatives.

7. Wanless IR, Geddie WR. Mineral oil lipogranulomata in liver and spleen. Arch Pathol Lab Med 1985; 109:283.

   Wanless reviewed 465 consecutive autopsies at the University of Toronto and found lipogranulomata in 48% of the livers and 46% of the spleens. Wanless believed that the lipid depositions were due to chronic mineral oil ingestion, which is often used in the food industry.

Smooth-Muscle Relaxants

William F. Siebert, Jr.

Smooth-muscle relaxants are used with increasing frequency in the treatment of diseases of the upper and lower gastrointestinal tract.

Many diseases of the gastrointestinal tract cause pain. For example, 30 percent of patients undergoing cardiac catheterization for evaluation of chest pain have no demonstrable cardiac defect, but instead have an esophageal disorder such as diffuse esophageal spasm, achalasia, vigorous achalasia, or nutcracker esophagus. Other painful gastrointestinal disorders include duodenal ulcer disease, irritable bowel syndrome, and biliary dyskinesia. In these disease states, smooth-muscle relaxants such as nitroglycerin, calcium channel-blockers, dicyclomine hydrochloride, and other antimuscarinic agents may have useful therapeutic actions and applications.

Nitroglycerin

Nitroglycerin, first compounded in 1846, has been used sublingually for angina pectoris therapy for many years. Since the mid-1970s, Nitroglycerin has provided symptomatic improvement for patients with esophageal motility disorders.

MECHANISM OF ACTION

Nitroglycerin and other nitrate-containing compounds activate guanylate cyclase, increasing the synthesis of cyclic GMP (Guanosine 3', 5' monophosphate) in smooth muscle. The protein kinase produced by the interaction of guanylate cyclase with nitric acid alters the phosphorylation process in smooth muscle, resulting in dephosphorylation of the light chain of myosin and inhibition of the normal contractile process of smooth muscle.

INDICATIONS

Current use of nitrates in gastrointestinal disease includes treatment of patients with esophageal motility disorders, biliary tract dyskinesia (including spasm of the sphincter of Oddi), and relief of elevated biliary pressure in patients with T tubes. Gelfond found that treatment of achalasia patients leads to a maximum fall in the lower esophageal sphincter (LES) pressure of as much as 63.5 percent. This reduction in LES pressure led to improved esophageal emptying and decreased food retention within the middle and distal esophagus (documented by radionuclide cine studies). The most notable finding of this study was symptomatic relief of dysphagia in 86 percent (13 out of 15) of the patients.

In patients with diffuse esophageal spasm and nutcracker esophagus, nitrates primarily improve chest pain; they may also improve the symptoms of dysphagia. Nitrates are often successful even when the chest pain is unresponsive to anticholinergics such as propantheline bromide.

A trial of nitrates should be strongly considered in the treatment of sphincter of Oddi dysfunction. Bar-Meir et al. demonstrated that medical therapy for papillary dysfunction may be an alternative to endoscopic sphincterotomy. They studied a patient with an elevated basal sphincter pressure of 43 mm Hg and a phasic sphincter pressure of 158 mm Hg (normal range 18 ± 6 mm Hg and 101 ± 50 mm Hg, respectively). Following administration of 0.65 milligrams of Nitroglycerin sublingually, the basal and phasic sphincter pressures dropped to zero within 90 seconds. Long-term treatment with long-acting nitrates led to resolution of the patient's symptoms and persistent reduction of the basal and phasic sphincter pressures to the normal range.

DOSAGE AND ADMINISTRATION

Isosorbide dinitrate (Isordil) is dispensed in sublingual and tablet formulations. Sublingual therapy yields maximum plasma concentration in 6 minutes but has a rapid fall-off. Isordil provides prolonged therapeutic effect, most likely due to isosorbide-2-mononitrate and isosorbide-5-mononitrate, because these compounds have longer half-lives (2–5 hours). Isordil is prescribed as 10 to 30 milligrams orally 30 minutes before meals. Equivalent dosages of erythrityl tetranitrate (Cardilate) are 10 to 15 milligrams 30 minutes before meals. Should the sublingual route be chosen, the dosage is 0.4 milligrams after meals and as needed. Sphincter of Oddi dysfunction due to a hyperdynamic sphincter can be treated with either sublingual or long-acting oral therapy.

SIDE EFFECTS

The primary dose-limiting side effect of nitrates is headache, which may be severe. However, headache may improve with continued treatment. Unfortunately, decreasing the nitrate dosage in order to alleviate headache frequently leads to recurrence of symptoms. Other, less common side effects include dizziness, weakness, and flushing. Orthostatic hypotension occurs and is accentuated by alcohol usage.

PEARLS AND PITFALLS

1. Long-term use of nitrates is not often seen because (a) as many as two-thirds of patients discontinue nitrates due to side effects; (b) symptoms often recur even without dosage reduction; and (c) the sporadic nature of symptoms makes the 3-to-4 times a day regimen difficult to follow.

2. Achalasia patients should be given sublingual therapy because of possible prolonged esophageal transit and the resultant delayed gastric absorption.
3. If a patient who you believe to have sphincter of Oddi dysfunction fails to respond to sublingual nitrates, consider that the etiology is sphincter stenosis rather than a hyperdynamic sphincter.

Calcium Channel-Blocking Agents

Calcium channel-blocking agents have been shown in numerous clinical trials to be effective in the treatment of disorders of gastrointestinal motility. These drugs effect a decrease in the contractility of smooth muscle, leading to (1) decreased amplitude of peristalsis; (2) decreased lower esophageal pressure; and (3) a significant reduction in the amplitude of esophageal contractions.

MECHANISM OF ACTIONS

Normal smooth-muscle contraction is dependent on calcium binding to calmodulin. This complex then activates myosin light-chain kinase, which results in phosphorylation of light-chain myosin. Phosphorylation promotes actin-myosin interaction, leading to smooth muscle contraction. The blockade of calcium-ion influx during membrane depolarization by these agents leads to smooth-muscle relaxation.

INDICATIONS

Calcium channel blockers have been studied in many of the esophageal motility disorders. Diffuse esophageal spasm responds well to nifedipine, the usual effective dose range being 10 to 30 milligrams sublingually as needed. Blackwell et al., using nifedipine 20 milligrams orally, reported a significant fall in lower esophageal sphincter pressure and amplitude of esophageal body contractions in a small group of patients. Similarly, Weiner et al. documented a significant reduction in lower esophageal pressure in both control and achalasia patients. The reduction in pressure occurred approximately 30 to 40 minutes after the nifedipine, and the duration of dysphagia relief was as long as several hours.

The symptoms of nutcracker esophagus respond to diltiazem. In an uncontrolled trial involving nine patients, diltiazem provided significant improvement in the incidence and severity of recurrent chest pain while exhibiting no effect on the lower esophageal pressure. On the other hand, nifedipine decreases the lower esophageal pressure, the maximum amplitude of the distal esophageal contractions, and the duration of esophageal contractions. The reduction in contraction amplitude was as high as 86 percent (average reduction, 54%) after one 30-milligram oral dose. The maximum effect occurred in 15 to 30 minutes. The duration of amplitude reduction was prolonged with larger doses, up to 75 minutes after 30 milligrams of nifedipine. Richter et al.

studied nifedipine in 10 patients with nutcracker esophagus and five normal controls; mean distal esophageal contraction amplitude and duration in both nifedipine-treated groups significantly improved. Most important, the response to nifedipine was significantly greater than that to placebo. As Traube and McCallum note, the mode of administration (oral versus sublingual) may be important; achalasia patients often have delayed esophageal transit time, resulting in variable peak nifedipine concentrations. There have been reports of wide variability in plasma levels of calcium blockers, and Richter has raised the possibility of slow and rapid absorption rate as the etiology for this occurrence. Gelfond et al. reported good results in their study of 15 achalasia patients treated with nifedipine, 20 milligrams sublingually 30 minutes prior to food ingestion. Fifty-three percent reported improvement in dysphagia and chest-pain symptoms.

Verapamil causes reduction in the amplitude of esophageal contractions, as well as lower esophageal pressure, in animal models, but human studies have yet to duplicate these results.

Calcium channel blockers may have a role to play in the treatment of the irritable bowel syndrome (IBS). Blume et al. found that nifedipine, 20 milligrams orally, significantly diminishes the abnormal colonic motor response to distention seen in patients with irritable bowel syndrome.

Animal studies by Potter et al. regarding the use of this class of agents in sphincter of Oddi dyskinesia have shown minimal effect on the canine biliary sphincter. Nifedipine bolus and verapamil infusion caused a barely significant reduction in the peak canine sphincter of Oddi pressure. Verapamil and diltiazem bolus therapy caused no statistically significant decrease in sphincter of Oddi pressure.

DOSAGE AND ADMINISTRATION

Nifedipine is supplied as 10-milligram capsules. It may be given orally or sublingually; the sublingual route is preferred for achalasia patients. Therapy should begin with 10 milligrams 3 times a day for several days, with dose titration to relief of symptoms versus tolerance of side effects. Diltiazem is supplied in 30- and 60-milligram tablets; initial therapy is 30 milligrams 4 times a day, again increased as necessary for symptom relief and as side effects allow. Maximum suggested daily diltiazem intake is 240 milligrams.

SIDE EFFECTS

The dose-limiting side effect of nifedipine results from vasodilation. Ten percent of patients develop peripheral edema, dizziness, flushing, paresthesias, nausea, vomiting, and sedation. Orthostatic hypotension (5%), headache (8%), palpitations (2%), and syncope (1%) may also occur. Contraindications to nifedipine include aortic stenosis (due to the potential for coronary steal syndrome secondary to vasodilation), hypotension, and known hypersensitivity to the drug.

Diltiazem has no effect on the peripheral vasculature, but significant atrioventricular conduction defects are possible. It is contraindicated in patients with sick sinus syndrome, second- or third-degree heart block, digitalis toxicity, and known diltiazem hypersensitivity.

PEARLS AND PITFALLS

1. The overall response rate for diltiazem and nifedipine in the treatment of diffuse esophageal spasm, achalasia, and nutcracker esophagus is approximately 40 to 50 percent.
2. Nifedipine is more effective for esophageal pain and dysphagia associated with achalasia. Diltiazem is more effective for the pain of esophageal spasm.
3. Hypertensive lower esophageal sphincter syndrome, in combination with nutcracker esophagus, responds very well to nifedipine. Nifedipine (10 to 30 mg sublingually 30 minutes before eating) used with an anticholinergic such as propantheline (15 mg 30 minutes after meals and again at bedtime) for the treatment of diffuse esophageal spasm leads to an additive reduction in esophageal contraction amplitude and an almost additive reduction in the lower esophageal sphincter pressure.
4. The side effect profiles of diltiazem and nifedipine are very different. McCallum advocates combination drug therapy to avoid side effects that might occur with higher doses of either drug alone.

Dicyclomine Hydrochloride

Dicyclomine hydrochloride (Bentyl), the prototypical anticholinergic agent, has been used for the treatment of irritable bowel syndrome for many years.

MECHANISM OF ACTION

Bentyl is a nonspecific smooth-muscle relaxant. It reduces gastrointestinal tract smooth-muscle spasm by decreasing spontaneous smooth muscle activity. Page and Dirnberger have demonstrated Bentyl's antagonism for the stimulant effect of agonists that act directly on smooth muscle, such as bradykinin.

INDICATIONS

Bentyl is indicated for the symptomatic treatment of irritable bowel syndrome. In one controlled, double-blind, randomized trial involving 71 patients, Page and Dirnberger demonstrated that 84 percent of Bentyl-treated (and 54% of placebo-treated) patients reported a noticeable reduction in abdominal tenderness and pain, along with improved bowel habits. Six percent of the patients taking Bentyl, compared to 35 percent of the placebo-treated, complained of an exacerbation of abdominal pain by the second week of the trial.

The response of the esophageal motility disorders to anticholinergic therapy has been disappointing; however, some authors still recommend a trial of antispasmodics as the initial pharmacological intervention for esophageal motility disorders.

The abdominal pain and cramping of Crohn's disease may respond to low-dose anticholinergic therapy. Confusion may arise should a bowel obstruction occur during anticholinergic therapy. Therefore, careful counseling is necessary if anticholinergic agents are used for symptomatic treatment of Crohn's disease.

DOSAGE AND ADMINISTRATION

Bentyl is available as 10- and 20-milligram tablets, as a syrup concentrate, and in an injectable form. Treatment should begin with 10 to 20 milligrams 4 times a day. The clinician should remember that the oral-dosage form is most efficacious in the alleviation of irritable bowel symptoms if given 30 to 60 minutes before meals and at bedtime on a daily basis and at relatively high doses (i.e., 40 mg 4 times a day). Ideally, therapy begins with 20 milligrams 4 times a day for 7 days; the dosage may then be increased to 40 milligrams 4 times a day unless side effects occur. Intramuscular Bentyl is indicated only for short-term management of NPO patients. Given the increased bioavailability of the injectable form of Bentyl, injectable dosages should be half the usual oral dosage.

SIDE EFFECTS

The most common side effects are dry mouth, blurred vision, and dizziness. These are seen in as many as one-third of patients prescribed this drug. Less frequently seen are decreased gastric secretions, urinary retention, and glaucoma exacerbation. Forty-four percent of the patients in one study were able to tolerate the side effects without decreasing the dosage; between 10 and 15 percent of patients discontinue therapy due to side effects. Contraindications to dicyclomine therapy include obstructive uropathy, mechanical or nonmechanical bowel obstruction, hemodynamic instability, severe flares of ulcerative colitis with or without toxic megacolon, glaucoma, or myasthenia gravis.

Belladonna and Similar Antimuscarinics

Belladonna and its related compounds (Atropine, Bellergal, etc.) are agents that inhibit the effects of acetylcholine on autonomic effectors innervated by the postganglionic nerves and on smooth muscle that lacks cholinergic innervation. They antagonize the muscarinic effects of acetylcholine. Antimuscarinics are useful adjuncts in the treatment of peptic ulcer disease and as antispasmodics in hypermotility syndromes. They may play a role in the treatment of biliary dyskinesia in the near future.

The specific effects of the antimuscarinics vary, depending on the organ system discussed. Small doses decrease sweating, salivation, and bronchial secretions; modest doses cause pupillary dilation and heart rate increase. Larger doses block parasympathetic control of the urinary, bladder, and gastrointestinal tract, leading to inhibition of micturition and decreased tone and motility of the gut. Still larger doses are required to inhibit gastric secretions and motility. Reduction in tone, amplitude, and frequency of peristaltic contractions in the stomach, duodenum, jejunum, ileum, and colon occur when therapeutic doses of antimuscarinics are used. However, multiple side effects common to lower doses are often too severe to permit long-term usage, due to poor patient compliance.

INDICATIONS

When used alone, antimuscarinics (i.e., Atropine 0.4–0.6 mg before meals sublingually) inhibit gastric acid secretion 15 to 25 percent; when used with H_2 blockers, these agents greatly enhance the effectiveness of the H_2 blocker chosen. Unfortunately, at the necessary dosages, adverse side effects such as pupillary dilation, tachycardia, gastric retention, urinary retention, and aggravation of glaucoma preclude their widespread application. Conversely, pepsin secretion is blocked at relatively small doses. The agents in this class are also used as adjunctive therapy in the medical treatment of gastrinoma patients when gastric acid hypersecretion is not controlled by H_2-receptor antagonists alone.

Schuster prefers to use anticholinergics with more antisecretory activity than spasmolytic activity when treating dyspepsia symptoms in his irritable bowel syndrome patients. Tincture of Belladonna, beginning with 10 drops 4 times a day and increasing as symptoms and side effects warrant and permit, may be used. Probanthine, 15 milligrams 3 times a day, and 15 to 30 milligrams at bedtime is another alternative.

Garrigues et al. compared the effects of Atropine, 0.5 milligram intravenously, and pirenzepine 10 milligrams intravenously (a new antimuscarinic), on sphincter of Oddi (SO) motility. Atropine failed to modify the basal SO pressure; the amplitude of the phasic contractions decreased very slightly; and the frequency of phasic contractions decreased significantly during the first and second minutes after drug administration. Pirenzepine significantly decreased the basal SO pressure and the amplitude and frequency of the phasic contractions from the second minute after drug injection. The effect of Pirenzepine was maintained for 3 minutes with respect to the basal pressure decrease, for 4 minutes regarding suppression of the phasic contractions, and for more than 6 minutes regarding the reduced frequency of phasic contractions.

At the present time, no study has supported the use of an antimuscarinic as the sole agent in the treatment of duodenal ulcer disease.

DOSAGE AND ADMINISTRATION

In addition to Belladonna, there are many similar agents, some combining several drugs to provide anticholinergic and antispasmodic effects. Donnatal, a combination of Phenobarbital, Atropine, and Scopolamine, is dispensed in capsule (1–2 capsules 3–4 times a day) and elixir (1–2 tsp 3–4 times a day) forms. It is used extensively in the treatment of motor symptoms associated with irritable bowel syndrome. Bellergal-S, a sustained-release agent containing Phenobarbital, Ergotamine, and Alkaloids of Belladonna, is prescribed as one tablet twice a day. There are several other agents in this class; it is best to become familiar with a few agents and their particular dosage regimens.

SIDE EFFECTS

Major side effects include xerostomia, cycloplegia, mydriasis, constipation, urinary retention, palpitations, tachycardia, bloating, and dysphagia. The first four side effects are dose-dependent, whereas the remaining side effects are not—they may occur at any dosage. Contraindications to the use of antimuscarinics include glaucoma, obstructive uropathy, achalasia, pyloric stenosis, gastric outlet obstruction, ileus, severe ulcerative colitis with or without toxic megacolon, and myasthenia gravis.

PEARLS AND PITFALLS

1. The majority of disorders discussed under the Belladonna heading, with the exception of irritable bowel syndrome, are best approached using other, more proven and effective medications. The antimuscarinics are best used as adjuncts, when necessary, considering the fairly high percentage of unpleasant side effects patients may need to tolerate when prescribed one of these drugs.

References

1. Bar-Meir S, et al. Nitrate therapy in a patient with papillary dysfunction. Am J Gastro 1983; 78:94.

    The authors advocate a trial of nitrates to distinguish functional vs. organic sphincter of Oddi pathology. They advocate nitrate therapy trial for papillary dysfunction first, then sphincterectomy only if nitrates do not provide the desired response.

2. Benjamin SB, et al. High amplitude, peristaltic esophageal contractions associated with chest pain and/or dysphagia. Gastroenterology 1979; 77:478–483. Report on seven patients with high-pressure esophageal peristaltic waves and chest pain.

    The authors define "nutcracker esophagus" as a mean peristaltic amplitude of 111 torr for patients presenting with esophageal pain and/or dysphagia.

3. Blackwell JN, et al. Effect of nifedipine on esophageal motility and gastric emptying. Digestion 1981; 21:50–56.

    Nifedipine (10, 20, 30 mg) decreased mean esophageal contractile pressure 17%, 38%, and 49% in both normal patients and patients with nutcracker esophagus.

    Nifedipine, 30 mg, had no significant effect on gastric emptying of either solids or liquids.

4. Blume M, et al. Effect of nifedipine on colonic motility in the irritable bowel syndrome (abs). Gastroenterology 1983; 84:1109.

5. Castell DO. Chest pain of esophageal origin. Drug Therapy 1983; November: 129.

    The medical and surgical options for treatment of esophageal disorders.

6. Castell DO. Diagnosing and treating noncardiac chest pain. Prac Gastro 1984; May–June: 22.

    Review of various esophageal etiologies of chest pain and drug therapies available.

7. Castell DO. Calcium channel-blocking agents for gastrointestinal disorders. Am J Cardio 1985; 55:210B.

    A discussion of the pharmacological effects of verapamil, diltiazem, and nifedipine on animal and human subjects.

8. Garrigues V, et al. Effects of atropine and pirenzepine on sphincter of Oddi motility. J Hepatol 1986; 3:247.

    This double-blind, randomized trial with ten patients demonstrated a significant reduction in sphincter of Oddi basal pressure and phasic contractions due to pirenzepine. Atropine did not alter the basal pressure significantly.

9. Geenan JE, Venu RP. Sphincter of Oddi dysfunction in diseases of the liver. In L Schiff and E Schiff (eds) *Diseases of the Liver* 6th ed. Philadelphia: Lippincott, 1987. Pp. 1427–1433.

    The pathophysiology and manometric abnormalities seen in patients with sphincter of Oddi disease.

10. Gelfond M, et al. Isosorbide dinitrate and nifedipine treatment of achalasia: A clinical, manometric, and radionuclide evaluation. Gastroenterology 1982; 83:963.

    The study involved 15 patients and correlated clinical response to radionuclide-documented esophageal emptying time. The authors favor the radionuclide test meal as the most objective way to evaluate drug therapy in achalasia patients.

11. Kahn AA, Castell DO. Managing esophageal chest pain once a cardiac cause is ruled out. J Crit Ill 1987; July: 61.

    The criteria for diagnosis and management of esophageal dysmotility syndromes.

12. Lebovics E, et al. Sphincter of Oddi motility: Developments

in physiology and clinical application. Am J Gastro 1986; 81:736.

A review of sphincter of Oddi motility, the effects of various GI hormones and drugs on sphincter of Oddi function, and clinical use of the manometric data obtained.

13. McCallum RW. The management of esophageal motility disorders. Hosp Prac 1988; February 15:131.

    An extremely thorough and informative review of esophageal motility disorders.

14. Needleman P, et al. Drugs for the treatment of angina. In A Goodman (ed) *Goodman and Gilman's The Pharmacologic Basis for Therapeutics* 7th ed. New York: Macmillan, 1985.

    A review of the mechanisms of action of nitrates and calcium channel blockers.

15. Page JG, Dirnberger GM. Treatment of irritable bowel syndrome with Bentyl. J Clin Gastro 1981; 3:153.

    A 2-week, double-blind trial to compare Bentyl and placebo. Bentyl, 40 mg qid, was superior to placebo; however, 60% of patients taking Bentyl (160 mg/day) reported adverse effects.

16. Potter T, et al. Effects of calcium channel-blocking agents in canine sphincter of Oddi (abs from AGA, NYC May 12–15, 1985). Gastroenterology 1985; 88:1543.

17. Richter JE, et al. Verapamil: A potent inhibitor of esophageal contractions in the baboon. Gastroenterology 1982; 82:882.

    A study showing significant reduction in both esophageal contraction amplitude (in smooth muscle) and LES with verapamil infusion.

18. Richter JE, et al. Nifedipine: A potent inhibitor of contractions in the body of the human esophagus. Gastroenterology 1985; 89:549.

    A comparison of nifedipine and placebo effects on LES and amplitude of esophageal contractions in normal patients as well as those with nutcracker esophagus.

19. Schuster MM. Irritable bowel syndrome. In Bayless T (ed) *Current Therapy in Gastroenterology and Liver Disease*. St. Louis, Mo.: Mosby, 1986. P. 342.

    A full review of the treatment modalities available to patients with irritable bowel syndrome.

20. Sunshine A, Cohen S. Diffuse esophageal spasm and related disorders. In Bayless T (ed) *Current Therapy in Gastroenterology and Liver Disease*. St. Louis, Mo.: Mosby, 1986. P. 34.

    A concise review of algorithms used in the diagnosis of chest pain syndromes.

21. Traube M, McCallum RW. Calcium channel blockers and the gastrointestinal tract. Am J Gastro 1984; 79:892.

    An excellent review of various GI disorders when calcium channel-blocker therapy may be attempted.

22. Weiner N. Atropine, scolpolamine, and related antimuscarinic drugs. In A. Goodman (ed) *Goodman and Gilman's The Pharmacologic Basis of Therapeutics* 7th ed. New York: Macmillan, 1985.

Prokinetic Agents

Thomas Dorsey

Domperidone

Domperidone (Motilium-Janssen) is a benzamidazole derivative related to the butyrophenones and was developed in 1974. It is a specific dopamine antagonist with upper tract prokinetic and antiemetic properties similar to metoclopramide but without the central side effects.

PHARMACOLOGY

Good plasma levels are achieved after oral, rectal, or intramuscular administration. Peak plasma levels are seen 15 to 30 minutes after oral or intramuscular administration and 1 to 2 hours after rectal administration. The bioavailability varies with route, achieving 90 percent after intramuscular administration, but only 13 to 17 percent after oral administration due to significant first-pass hepatic and gut-wall metabolism. Animal studies show levels 2 to 8 times that of plasma in most tissues, but minimal levels in brain, placenta, and breast milk. Domperidone circulates in plasma more than 90 percent protein bound. Metabolism is primarily hepatic via oxidative N-dealkylation and glucoronide conjugation. After oral administration, 7 percent is excreted unchanged in the stool and more than 60 percent appears in the stool as metabolites excreted in bile. About one-third of the dose is excreted as metabolites in the urine. Only 1.4 percent of the dose is excreted as unchanged drug in the urine. Its half-life is 7.5 hours.

MECHANISM OF ACTION

Domperidone has a high affinity for gut tissue, especially the esophagus, stomach, and small bowel. It acts on gastrointestinal smooth muscle by antagonizing the effects of dopamine.

In the esophagus, parenteral domperidone increases the lower esophageal sphincter pressure in healthy volunteers by 15 to 20 mm Hg. The effects of oral domperidone in normals and reflux patients are less clear, and higher doses may be required for effect.

In the stomach, there is no effect on serum gastrin or volume and pH of gastric secretions. It decreases adaptive relaxation in the fundus and increases the amplitude and duration of antral contractions. Pyloric dilatation has been noted endoscopically. Both antroduodenal coordination and the amplitude, frequency, and duration of duodenal contractions are improved. The net effect is increased solid- and liquid-phase gastric emptying.

There is no appreciable colonic effect.

Antiemetic activity is mediated by two mechanisms. First

and most important, domperidone provides a central effect, as evidenced by its antagonism of apomorphine-induced emesis at the level of the chemoreceptor trigger zone. Peripherally, enhancement of gastric emptying plays a role in its antiemetic activity.

INDICATIONS

Delayed Gastric Emptying

Domperidone has been reported to decrease symptoms of delayed gastric emptying in a number of settings, including scleroderma, pancreatitis, reflux esophagitis, anorexia nervosa, and postsurgical states (e.g., postvagotomy).

Diabetic gastroparesis is a common clinical problem, and domperidone has been effective in decreasing symptoms and increasing gastric emptying in the majority of patients. Although when taken chronically there may be a loss of benefit with solid food emptying, symptoms seldom return.

In idiopathic gastric stasis or idiopathic postprandial dyspepsia, domperidone is effective in improving gastric emptying and relieving symptoms such as belching, distention, fullness, burning, nausea, and vomiting.

Nausea and Vomiting

Domperidone has shown activity superior to placebo in nausea and vomiting associated with pancreatitis, radiotherapy, hemodialysis, dysmenorrhea, and head trauma. It decreases nausea and other symptoms associated with the use of levo dopa, bromocriptine and nonsteroidal anti-inflammatory drugs. In migraine headache it appears to abort attacks as well as relieve the nausea associated with acute attacks. Although ineffective prophylactically against postoperative nausea and vomiting, it decreases frequency after the first episode.

Perhaps its most important role will be in the therapy of nausea and vomiting due to antineoplastic chemotherapy. Multiple studies have shown it at least as effective as metoclopramide in both adults and children, but with a much lower incidence of side effects.

Gastroesophageal Reflux Disease

Results of current trials are conflicting, with some series reporting symptomatic, endoscopic, and histological improvement and others failing to show benefit on some or all of these parameters. It appears possibly useful but larger, well-controlled trials are necessary.

Miscellaneous Indications

Domperidone has been shown to decrease variceal blood flow without the hyperaldosteronism seen with metoclopramide. The clinical benefits of this action have not been demonstrated. There are reports of efficacy in healing of peptic ulcer disease. Domperidone has also been used as a premedication for endoscopy, to decrease postprocedure nausea.

SIDE EFFECTS

Acute and chronic use are well tolerated in the majority of patients, with side effects seen in only 7 percent (versus 20% with metoclopramide). As it does not cross the blood–brain barrier, the incidence of neurologic side effects such as tardive dyskinesia, acute dystonic reactions, and sedation, which can occur in 10 percent of patients treated with metoclopramide, are rare. Occasionally, headache and nervousness are reported.

Transient, minor problems include dry mouth, thirst, skin rash, pruritis, and diarrhea.

Elevation of serum prolactin is common but usually clinically silent, although gynecomastia, mastalgia, galactorrhea, and amenorrhea can be seen. Women are affected more often than men. Domperidone antagonizes the dopamine-induced suppression of prolactin release. It does not appear to further exacerbate the high levels seen with acromegaly or prolactinomas.

There have been no changes in hematologic or biochemical parameters, including growth hormone and the renin–angiotensin–aldosterone system with acute or chronic use.

Initial studies have shown no effect on heart rate, blood pressure or electrocardiogram, but several reports of sudden death after high doses (60–200 mg) of intravenous domperidone for chemotherapy-induced emesis prompted further investigation. High-dose parenteral therapy causes prolongation of the QT interval, which can be complicated by *torsade des pointes,* ventricular tachycardia, and ventricular fibrillation.

To date, drug interactions are limited to decreased bioavailability when used with cimetidine, and bicarbonate or other antacids.

Animal studies have shown low concentrations in the fetus and no tetratogenic or carcinogenic potential. Human studies have shown low concentrations in breast milk.

There is no accumulation in mild to moderate renal insufficiency. There are few data on use in liver disease.

DOSAGE AND ADMINISTRATION

Domperidone is available as a 10-milligram tablet and a 1% solution (0.3 mg/ml). It is available in suppository form in Europe. Parenteral forms were discontinued in 1984. It should be given on an empty stomach 15 to 30 minutes before meals. Concurrent H_2 blockers or antacids should be avoided. An oral dose in adults is 10 to 30 milligrams orally twice or 4 times a day; and in children, 0.3 to 0.6 milligrams/kilogram twice or 4 times a day. In adults a 60-milligram suppository twice or 4 times a day is recommended.

Cisapride

Cisapride (R 51619-Janssen) is a benzamide derivative with a mechanism of action different from the antidopaminergic agents, thus avoiding their side effects. In addition, it is the first prokinetic drug to show activity in the colon.

PHARMACOLOGY

The drug is well absorbed after parenteral, oral, or rectal administration. The bioavailability after an oral dose is 35 to 40 percent, indicating significant first-pass metabolism. Peak plasma levels occur at 1.5 to 2 hours. Cisapride circulates 90 percent protein bound. It is extensively metabolized by the liver via N-dealkylation, aromatic hydroxylation, and glucoronide conjugation. Fifty percent of a dose is excreted as metabolites into the feces via bile, and the remaining 50 percent is excreted in the urine as metabolites. Its half-life is 14.9 hours. Animal studies show specific gut uptake but low levels in the brain and placenta. In animal studies the drug is secreted in breast milk.

MECHANISM OF ACTION

Cisapride has no antidopaminergic effects (unlike domperidone and metoclopramide). Its primary action is facilitation of acetylcholine release via an indirect cholinergic mechanism mediated by an unknown receptor on postganglionic nerve endings at the myenteric plexus. It does not activate muscarinic cholinergic receptors. In addition, it displays activity as a serotonin antagonist in guinea pig intestinal mucosa.

In the esophagus, it increases both the amplitude of contractions and the lower esophageal sphincter pressure in normals and reflux patients. In the stomach, it stimulates digestive and interdigestive antroduodenal motility and coordination. It decreases adaptive relaxation of the fundus. As with domperidone, the increase in gastric emptying is accomplished without effects on gastric secretion. In the small bowel, both jejunal and ileal activity are increased in amplitude and frequency. A unique action is induction of propulsive activity in the colon, with increased slow-wave activity and increased duration of spike activity. Clinically one sees increased solid and liquid gastric emptying, decreased mouth-to-cecum transit time, and decreased colonic transit time.

As cisapride lacks antidopaminergic activity, its antiemetic activity is less than domperidone's and results solely from increased gastric emptying.

INDICATIONS

Gastroesophageal Reflux Disease

Cucchiara showed cisapride superior to placebo in a randomized, double-blind trial in 20 children with reflux esophagitis. Improvement was documented by pH monitoring, endoscopy, and histology. In adults, doses of 20 milligrams orally increase lower esophageal sphincter pressure without affecting other parameters of esophageal function.

Chronic Dyspepsia

Deruytte demonstrated symptomatic improvement in 75 percent of patients with chronic functional dyspepsia in a randomized, double-blind, crossover trial of cisapride, 4 to 8 milligrams orally twice a day. Rosch showed significant improvement in a group of 118 patients with nonulcer dyspepsia on cisapride, 10 milligrams orally twice a day, in a randomized, double-blind trial. Finally, Urbain studied patients with dyspepsia and abnormal gastric emptying. Cisapride, 10 milligrams orally 4 times a day, increased emptying and decreased symptoms.

Gastroparesis

Horowitz treated 20 diabetics with gastroparesis with cisapride, 10 milligrams orally 4 times a day, and demonstrated symptomatic improvement and increased emptying. Reports have also demonstrated effectiveness in delayed gastric emptying associated with idiopathic gastroparesis, anorexia nervosa, scleroderma, cystic fibrosis, and the postvagotomy state. Cisapride may also be effective in bile reflux gastritis.

Postoperative Ileus

Verlinden studied 118 postoperative patients in a placebo-controlled trial of intravenous cisapride at doses of 2 to 8 milligrams. The 8-milligram dose repeated at 1 hour showed a significant increase in motility as documented by passage of flatus. Boghaert studied 53 postoperative patients in a double-blind, placebo-controlled trial of cisapride, 4 milligrams intravenously. When two 4-milligram doses were given 1 hour apart, 50 percent of patients developed bowel sounds and 43 percent passed flatus within the next hour.

Chronic Constipation

Muller-Lissner, in a randomized, double-blind, placebo-controlled trial of 126 patients with chronic constipation, showed that cisapride, 20 milligrams orally twice a day, significantly increased spontaneous bowel movements and decreased laxative use, compared to placebo.

Chronic Intestinal Pseudo-Obstruction

Camilleri showed increased pyloris-to-cecum transit in eight patients treated with cisapride, 40 milligrams/day, and Cohen reported a case of pseudo-obstruction in a child that responded to cisapride but had been unresponsive to all other therapy.

Miscellaneous Indications

Several authors have indicated cisapride may be of use in therapy of the irritable bowel syndrome, and it has also been suggested that it may be of benefit in the carcinoid syndrome. Trials are needed to study these indications.

SIDE EFFECTS

Initial studies in over 1600 patients, including geriatric and pediatric populations, have shown a low incidence of side effects. The most common adverse effects, occurring in 4 percent of patients, are abdominal cramping, diarrhea, and increased flatus. No genitourinary symptoms have been noted.

Major neurological side effects such as tardive dyskinesia and acute dystonic reactions have not been noted, and neurologic side effects are limited to headache and mild fatigue. There have been no changes in psychomotor function.

On chronic therapy (mean > 2 months), 200 patients manifested no hematologic or biochemical abnormalities. No changes were noted in gastrin, insulin, or prolactin levels. Acute therapy stimulates the release of pancreatic polypeptide and CCK via atropine-sensitive mechanisms, while chronic use causes diminished CCK release by an unknown mechanism.

Although no electrocardiographic changes have been seen, slight but significant elevations of systolic blood pressure and heart rate are noted.

Drug interactions are few. Cimetidine, but not antacids, decreases its bioavailability. No changes in digoxin, propranolol, or tolbutamide bioavailability or action have been discovered.

Animal studies indicate low placental levels but human data are lacking. Although animal studies suggest that cisapride is secreted in breast milk, human studies show only very low levels.

DOSAGE AND ADMINISTRATION

In Europe, cisapride is available as 5- and 10-milligram tablets and a 1-milligram/milliliter suspension. Oral dosages of 10 to 20 milligrams orally twice or 4 times a day before meals have been utilized. A suppository form is available in Europe.

PEARLS AND PITFALLS

1. Domperidone and cisapride are new prokinetic agents awaiting approval in the United States.
2. Domperidone, like metoclopramide, acts via dopamine antagonism in the upper digestive tract and chemoreceptor trigger zone, but does not cross the blood–brain barrier and has a much lower incidence of side effects. Cisapride has a novel mechanism of action in its facilitation of acetylcholine release in the myenteric plexus. Unlike domperidone and metoclopramide, cisapride enhances colonic motility.
3. Major indications for domperidone will be in the therapy of gastric emptying disorders, most notably diabetic and idiopathic gastroparesis, and as an emetic in the setting of cancer chemotherapy. Cisapride has less antiemetic ac-

tivity but appears to be as effective in gastric emptying disorders. In addition, it shows promise in the therapy of postoperative ileus, chronic intestinal pseudo-obstruction, and constipation.
4. Both are well tolerated acutely and chronically. Neither demonstrates the extrapyramidal effects associated with metoclopramide. Domperidone causes elevation of prolactin levels, especially in women, and this may cause clinical symptoms. Cisapride has no effect on prolactin levels. Its major side effects are abdominal cramping and diarrhea.
5. Domperidone should be given on an empty stomach; concomitant use of cimetidine and antacid decreases bioavailability. Cisapride bioavailability is not decreased with antacids but is decreased with cimetidine. Both show first-pass metabolism.
6. Use during pregnancy and in nursing mothers has yet to be fully explored. Caution in these settings is appropriate.
7. As with any new drug, well-designed trials and long-term use in large numbers of patients are needed to fully appreciate appropriate indications and potential side effects of drug interaction.

References

1. Boghaert A, et al. Placebo-controlled trial of cisapride in postoperative ileus. Acta Anaesthesiol Belg 1987; 38:195–199.
   Cisapride increases bowel sounds and the passage of flatus.
2. Brogden RN, et al. Domperidone. Drugs 1982; 24:360–400.
   A comprehensive review of its pharmacology and clinical use.
3. Camilleri M, Brown MD, Malagelada JR. Impaired transit of chyme in chronic intestinal pseudo-obstruction. Gastroenterology 1986; 91:619–626.
   Cisapride increases pylorus-to-cecum transit in adult patients with chronic intestinal pseudo-obstruction.
4. Champion MC, Hartnett M, Yen M. Domperidone, a new dopamine antagonist. Canad Med Assoc J 1986; 135:457–461.
   A recent review of the clinical indications for domperidone.
5. Cohen NP, et al. Successful management of idiopathic intestinal pseudo-obstruction with cisapride. J Pediat Surg 1988; 23:229–230.
   A case report of cisapride's effectiveness in a pediatric patient.
6. Cucchiara S, et al. Cisapride for gastroesophageal reflux and peptic esophagitis. Arch Dis Child 1987; 62:454–457.
   Cisapride showed benefit in children according to pH monitoring, endoscopy, and histology.
7. Deruyttere M, et al. Cisapride in the management of chronic functional dyspepsia. Clin Ther 1987; 10:44–51.

A randomized, double-blind trial showing symptomatic improvement in 75% of subjects.
8. D'Souza DP, Reyntjens A, Thornes RD. Domperidone in the prevention of nausea and vomiting induced by antineoplastic agents. Curr Ther Res 1980; 27:384–390.
   Domperidone is as effective as metoclopramide in this setting, without major side effects.
9. First International Cisapride Investigators' Meeting. Digestion 1986; 34:137–160.
   A collection of abstracts covering pharmacology and clinical uses.
10. Horowitz M, et al. Acute and chronic effects of domperidone on gastric emptying in diabetic autonomic neuropathy. Dig Dis Sci 1988; 30:1–9.
    A study of domperidone in diabetic gastroparesis.
11. Horowitz M, et al. Effect of cisapride on gastric and esophageal emptying in insulin-dependent diabetes mellitus. Gastroenterology 1987; 92:1899–1907.
    Chronic cisapride therapy is effective in diabetic gastroparesis.
12. McCallum RW. Review of the current status of prokinetic agents in gastroenterology. Am J Gastro 1985; 80:1008–1016.
    An excellent overview of a variety of prokinetics.
13. Muller-Lissner SA. Treatment of chronic constipation with cisapride and placebo. Gut 1987; 28:1033–1038.
    A study showing decreased laxative use and increases in spontaneous bowel movements with cisapride.
14. Rosch W. Cisapride in nonulcer dyspepsia. Scand J Gastro 1987; 22:161–164.
    Cisapride decreases symptoms in nonulcer dyspepsia.
15. Urbain JL, et al. Effect of cisapride on gastric emptying in dyspeptic patients. Dig Dis Sci 1988; 33:779–783.
    A study showing symptomatic and imaging evidence of improvement.
16. Verlinden M, et al. Treatment of postoperative gastrointestinal agony. Br J Surg 1987; 74:614–617.
    Intravenous cisapride decreases postoperative ileus.

VI
Gastroenterology Procedure–Related Drugs

Gastrointestinal endoscopy as a discipline is barely 2 decades old. Fiberoptics, the technology that led to endoscopy, was born when Curtiss discovered that by coating a glass fiber with glass of a lower refractile index he could achieve nearly total internal reflection. The transmission of an image then became possible. The first modern endoscopes were subsequently developed in the late 1960s. From that beginning, endoscopy has rapidly flourished; over 1 million endoscopic procedures were performed in the United States in 1982. Today, the endoscopist can utilize laser, thermal coagulation, endoscopic ultrasound, and a variety of other new technologies. Even fiberoptics are now becoming obsolete as video endoscopy and its new capabilities take over the market.

Amid this abundance of technology, it is easy to forget that an endoscopic procedure is basically just an interaction between patient and physician. And, as every experienced endoscopist knows, the key to a successful procedure is a relaxed, cooperative patient. This is accomplished by a thorough, understandable explanation of the procedure, a confident, reassuring manner and technique, and effective use of adjunctive medications.

The application of drugs for endoscopic procedures is an art learned very much like endoscopy itself: by first observing their use by an experienced endoscopist, then by a gradual accumulation of one's own experience. Unfortunately for the trainee, it is difficult to find a thorough discussion of gastrointestinal procedure–related drugs, even in textbooks of gastroenterology or endoscopy. This part is intended to help the trainee bridge the gap between naivete and experience; the pharmacology, indications, contraindications, side effects, and dosage are discussed for each drug used during endoscopic procedures. Even the experienced endoscopist can find some unknown facts or pearls that may contribute to effective daily practice.

Michael S. Gurney

Bacteremia Prophylaxis Agents

Eugene Killeavy

With the introduction and refinement of multiple diagnostic and interventional gastrointestinal procedures, there has been increasing interest in the role of antimicrobial prophylaxis to prevent endocarditis in potentially susceptible individuals. While it is well accepted that susceptible individuals should receive chemoprophylaxis before procedures likely to cause significant bacteremia, there are no clinical trials showing the efficacy of antimicrobial prophylaxis for endocarditis, and it is unlikely that clinical trials will ever be performed because of the numbers of patients needed to prove the efficacy of these regimens.

Furthermore, as Kaye has pointed out, most cases of endocarditis are not prevented by antimicrobial prophylaxis, since about one-half of patients have unrecognized, predisposing cardiac lesions for which prophylaxis would be considered; and only about 40 percent of patients with endocarditis caused by *Enterococci* (10% of cases) and less than 25 percent of patients with endocarditis caused by oral *Streptococci* (<50% of cases) develop endocarditis after a procedure for which prophylaxis could be given.

Combining this information with the rarity of well-documented cases of endocarditis after gastrointestinal procedures and the low percentage of patients who develop significant bacteremia after most gastrointestinal procedures makes the issue of prophylaxis of gastrointestinal procedures quite controversial. Furthermore, antibiotic regimens previously recommended by the American Heart Association have not been followed by many gastroenterologists, indicating either difficulty in adhering to them or lack of belief in their necessity or efficacy.

It was with this in mind that the British Society of Antimicrobial Chemotherapy removed all recommendations for antibiotic prophylaxis for gastrointestinal endoscopy in patients with cardiac disease, except for patients with prosthetic heart valves.

However, for the purposes of this review, the guidelines established by the American Heart Association are used as a reference, with a caveat that the recommendations are not based on clinical trials, that they may continue to change as more data accrue on oral prophylaxis in patients not at the highest risk of endocarditis, and that the decision to use prophylaxis should be based on case-by-case risk assessment.

Bacteremia

Bacteremia is reported to occur in a small percentage of patients following upper gastrointestinal endoscopic procedures. In various studies, the incidence ranged from 0 to 10 percent and did not increase with biopsy sampling. Appropriate cleansing of endoscopes and attention to the dental health of these individuals might decrease these percentages. Despite conflicting studies, endoscopic injection sclerotherapy of esophageal varices and esophageal dilatation are apt to produce higher rates of bacteremia, with some studies reporting an incidence of up to 50 percent following these procedures.

Bacteremia following lower gastrointestinal tract procedures, including proctosigmoidoscopy, colonoscopy, and barium enema, varies from 0 to 23 percent. This wide variance is probably based on the small numbers of patients studied, the numbers of blood samples drawn, and the duration of sampling. The incidence of reported bacteremia following colonoscopy is not significantly different than that following barium enema. Also, there does not appear to be a correlation with radiographic or anatomic findings and bacteremia. Likewise, biopsy or fulguration does not seem to increase the risk of bacteremia.

Bacteremia and cholangitis may occur after percutaneous and endoscopic cholangiography. Bacteremia rates between 0 and 14 percent have been reported following ERCP. Overall, the greatest risks to these patients is cholangitis and septicemia, not endocarditis. Bacteremic rates between 3 and 13 percent have been reported following liver biopsy.

A few important points must be considered when evaluating the reported incidence of bacteremia resulting from these procedures. First, most bacteremic episodes after gastrointestinal-tract manipulation are of brief duration and associated with a very low level of bacteremia, as assessed by pour-plate methods. Second, as Durack has pointed out, the majority of organisms isolated are due to anaerobes or commensal gut organisms, which are unlikely to cause endocarditis because of their poor adherence to the endocardium.

INDICATIONS

In December, 1984, the American Heart Association Committee on Rheumatic Fever and Infectious Endocarditis issued a special report outlining their recommendations for the antimicrobial prophylaxis of bacterial endocarditis. Table 37–1 lists the cardiac conditions for which antimicrobial prophylaxis was recommended. These include ventricular septal defects, primum atrial septal defects, patent ductus arteriosis, coarctation of the aorta, Marfan's syndrome, hypertrophic cardiomyopathy, acquired and congenital valvular heart disease, as well as cardiac and systemic-to-pulmonary shunts. Patients with an isolated secundum atrial septal defect or surgically corrected cardiac lesions without prosthetic implants more than 6 months after the operation have a negligible risk of endocarditis and prophylaxis is not warranted. Likewise, patients with coronary artery disease, with or without prior coronary artery revascularization, are not at an increased risk of infective endocarditis and do not warrant prophylaxis.

Gastrointestinal procedures for which endocarditis pro-

Table 37–1. Cardiac conditions for which endocarditis prophylaxis is and is not recommended

Recommended:
  Prosthetic cardiac valves (including biosynthetic valves)
  Most congenital cardiac malformations
  Surgically constructed systemic-pulmonary shunts
  Rheumatic and other acquired valvular dysfunction
  Hypertrophic cardiomyopathy
  Previous history of endocarditis
  Mitral valve prolapse with insufficiency

Not recommended:
  Isolated secundum atrial septal defect
  Secundum atrial septal defect repaired without a patch 6 or more months earlier
  Patent ductus arteriosus ligated and divided 6 or more months earlier
  Postoperative coronary artery bypass graft (CABG) surgery

Table 37–2. Gastrointestinal tract procedures for which endocarditis prophylaxis is recommended in susceptible individuals

Gallbladder surgery

Colonic surgery

Esophageal dilatation

Sclerotherapy of esophageal varices

Colonoscopy

Upper gastrointestinal endoscopy with biopsy

Proctosigmoidoscopy with biopsy

phylaxis was recommended are listed in Table 37–2. The Committee did not recommend routine prophylaxis after procedures that infrequently produced bacteremia, or produced a bacteremia that was felt to be of brief duration and quantitatively negligible. These include percutaneous liver biopsy, upper gastrointestinal endoscopy, proctosigmoidoscopy without biopsy, and barium enema. It is interesting to note that routine prophylaxis was recommended for patients undergoing colonoscopy and upper endoscopy with biopsy, despite the lack of clinical trials demonstrating a higher incidence of bacteremia or endocarditis following these procedures, as compared with barium enema and upper endoscopy without biopsy. The Committee did recommend, however, that patients with prosthetic heart valves (mechanical or bioprosthetic) should be considered for antimicrobial prophylaxis when undergoing these usually low-risk gastrointestinal procedures. This seems reasonable in light of the significant morbidity and mortality occurring in patients with prosthetic heart valves who develop bacterial endocarditis.

The Committee did not address antimicrobial prophylaxis during percutaneous or endoscopic cholangiography. It seems prudent to recommend prophylaxis in patients with prosthetic heart valves or prior endocarditis, and to consider prophylaxis in patients with other cardiac abnormalities who are at higher risk of infection after ERCP because of biliary stasis due to partial or complete obstruction.

DOSAGE AND ADMINISTRATION

Current antimicrobial recommendations for endocarditis prophylaxis of gastrointestinal procedures are listed in Table 37–3. The standard regimen consists of a single dose of injectable Ampicillin and Gentamicin, with an optional follow-up dose 8 hours later if the period of risk is prolonged (which is unlikely). There is also an oral regimen for minor procedures in low-risk patients, though the Committee does not specifically define which patients would qualify for this regimen. Animal studies reveal that single-dose Amoxicillin, given in doses similar to that achieved in humans after a 3-gram oral dose, was highly effective in preventing en-

Table 37–3. Summary of recommended antibiotic regimens for gastrointestinal procedures

Standard regimen	
	Ampicillin, 2 gm IM or IV, plus gentamicin, 1.5 mg/kg IM or IV, given 0.5–1 hour before procedure. One follow-up dose may be given 8 hours later.
Special regimens	
Oral regimen for minor or repetitive procedures in low-risk patients	Amoxycillin, 3 gm orally 1 hour before procedure and 1.5 gm orally 6 hours later
For patients allergic to penicillin	Vancomycin, 1 gm IV given *slowly* over 1 hour, plus gentamicin 1.5 mg/kg IM or IV given 1 hour before procedure. Dose may repeated once 8–12 hours later.
For pediatric patients	Ampicillin, 50 mg/kg/dose; gentamicin, 2 mg/kg dose; amoxycillin, 50 mg/kg/dose; vancomycin, 20 mg/kg/dose. The intervals between doses are the same as those for adults, and the total dose should not exceed adult doses.

terococcal endocarditis. Oral prophylaxis should not be utilized in patients at high risk of infective endocarditis, such as those with prosthetic heart valves or those with a history of previous endocarditis.

PEARLS AND PITFALLS

1. Despite the fact that endocarditis has been reported after dental or surgical procedures in patients with indwelling transvenous cardiac pacemakers, the overall risk of endocarditis is generally quite low. In these cases, antimicrobial prophylaxis for gastrointestinal procedures is unnecessary.
2. Patients with noncardiac prosthetic devices (arterial grafts or orthopedic devices) are unlikely to develop prosthetic infections after gastrointestinal procedures. As Hirschmann has pointed out, except for patients with prosthetic cardiac valves, convincing cases of hematogenous infections of prosthetic devices after dental or surgical procedures are virtually unknown. Instead, almost all reports of infections are secondary to contamination at surgery, spread from contiguous infected areas, or hematogenous-spread from sites of established distal suppurative infections. However, studies in dogs reveal that arterial grafts are susceptible to infection for the first few months following placement. This risk subsequently declines as a pseudointima develops around the graft. Intimal lining is by no means complete at late follow-up in many experimental animals; however, with the rarity of human graft infections of hematogenous origin, it is probably not necessary to prophylax patients with well-healed arterial grafts. Patients with recently placed arterial grafts may theoretically benefit from antimicrobial prophylaxis. Patients with other prosthetic devices (i.e., orthopedic prostheses) should not receive antimicrobial prophylaxis unless the procedure is in association with drainage of a focus of infection such as suppurative cholecystitis.
3. Mitral valve prolapse is now the underlying lesion in 15 to 30 percent of cases of native valve endocarditis. While patients with mitral valve prolapse are 5 to 8 times more likely to develop endocarditis than normals, their overall risk is quite low due to the low prevalence of infectious endocarditis and the estimated 4-percent incidence of mitral valve prolapse in the general population. It is estimated, however, that patients with mitral valve prolapse and a history of a systolic murmur have about a 10-fold increased risk of endocarditis when compared to normals, while the risk of endocarditis in patients with mitral valve prolapse, but without a systolic murmur, has been estimated to be no different than the risk to the general population. Therefore, it is recommended that only patients with mitral valve prolapse and a history of systolic murmur receive endocarditis prophylaxis, which complies with the guidelines established by the American Heart Association.

4. Intramuscular injections are contraindicated in patients receiving anticoagulants because of the risk of an intramuscular hematoma. Oral or parenteral antibiotic regimens should be appropriately substituted.
5. If vancomycin is administered as part of a prophylactic regimen, it must be administered slowly over 1 hour because of the risk of flushing, hypotension, and cardiovascular collapse with a bolus injection.

References

1. Baltch AL, et al. Bacteremia after upper gastrointestinal endoscopy. Arch Intern Med 1977; 5:594.

   Eight percent of 200 upper endoscopies resulted in transient bacteremia. There was no correlation with pathology, bleeding, or endoscopy time. Of the 16 positive cultures, seven were secondary to staphylococcal species and eight secondary to *Streptococci*.

2. Camara DS, et al. Transient bacteremia following endoscopic injection sclerotherapy of esophageal varices. Arch Intern Med 1983; 7:1350.

   Eighteen patients underwent 40 sessions of injection sclerotherapy. There were two cases of transient bacteremia (*Enterobacter cloacae* and *Staphylococcus* species). The authors conclude that the incidence of bacteremia is no higher after sclerotherapy than after routine upper endoscopy.

3. Cohen LB, et al. Bacteremia after endoscopic injection sclerosis. Gastro Endosc 1980; 193:29.

   Fourteen of 28 procedures were associated with transient bacteremia. Seven of the 14 isolates were secondary to alpha-hemolytic *Streptococci*.

4. Durack DT. Current issues in prevention of endocarditis. AJM 1985; 78 (Suppl 6B):149.

   An information paper by the authority on the subject. It classifies high-, intermediate-, and low-risk cardiac abnormalities and makes recommendations for various gastrointestinal procedures based upon underlying cardiac abnormality. The author does not recommend prophylaxis for gastrointestinal procedures in patients with pacemakers. Other recommendations are similar to AHA guidelines.

5. Everett ED, et al. Transient bacteremia and endocarditis prophylaxis: A review. Medicine 1977; 56:61.

   The frequently cited review of the incidence of bacteremia following procedures. The authors recommend prophylaxis after all procedures in patients with prosthetic heart valves.

6. Farber BF. Prophylaxis of endocarditis: Comparison of new regimens. AJM 1987; 3:529.

   A review of the recommendations of the AHA, British Society of Antimicrobial Chemotherapy, and Medical Letter and differences between them.

7. Kaye D. Prophylaxis for infective endocarditis: An update. Ann Intern Med 1986; 3:419.

An excellent review of current issues regarding antibiotic prophylaxis. The author discusses the controversies surrounding prophylaxis for mitral valve prolapse, gastrointestinal procedures in patients without cardiac prosthesis, and the potential role for oral prophylaxis in low-risk patients undergoing gastrointestinal procedures.

8. Le Frock J, et al. Transient bacteremia associated with barium enema. Arch Intern Med 1975; 135:835.

Eleven percent of 135 patients undergoing barium enema studies developed transient bacteremia. The most common organisms identified were *Enterococci, E coli,* and *Klebsiella*. The authors discuss the role the portal venous system may play in clearing bacteria from the circulation, which may decrease the risk of endocarditis.

9. Low DE, et al. Infectious complications of endoscopic retrograde cholangiopancreatography: A prospective assessment. Arch Intern Med 1980; 8:1076.

Ninety-seven patients underwent 101 ERCPs. Blood cultures from all procedures were negative.

10. MacMahon SW, et al. Mitral valve prolapse and endocarditis. Am Heart J 1987; 5:1291.

This article reviews the relative risks of endocarditis in normals and patients with mitral valve prolapse, with and without a history of systolic murmurs. Estimates are that the risk of endocarditis in patients with mitral valve prolapse without a murmur is no different than for the normal population.

11. Mellow MH, et al. Endoscopy-related bacteremia. Arch Intern Med 1976; 6:667.

Three of 100 patients developed transient bacteremia after upper endoscopy. The authors recommend utilizing sterile conditions when dealing with a susceptible host.

12. Shorvon PJ, et al. Gastrointestinal instrumentation, bacteremia, and endocarditis. Gut 1983; 24:1078.

A thorough review of trials determining the incidence of bacteremia after gastrointestinal procedures and the factors predisposing to endocarditis. The authors are not inclined to routinely prophylax patients undergoing gastrointestinal procedures.

13. Shull AJ, et al. Bacteremia with upper gastrointestinal endoscopy. Ann Intern Med 1975; 83:212.

Four of 50 patients had transient, low-grade bacteremia after upper endoscopy. Bacteremia did not correlate with performance of biopsy or type of mucosal abnormality.

14. Shulman ST, et al. Prevention of bacterial endocarditis: A statement for health professionals by the Committee on Rheumatic Fever and Infective Endocarditis of the Council on Cardiovascular Disease in the Young (abs). Circulation 1984; 6:1123.

The consensus policy statement of the AHA on which the guidelines in this chapter are based. The abstract recommends SBE prophylaxis for endoscopy with biopsy, variceal sclerotherapy, colonoscopy, and proctosigmoidoscopy with biopsy. It also recommends prophylaxis for all gastrointestinal procedures in patients with prosthetic heart valves.

15. Welsh JD, et al. Bacteremia associated with esophageal dilatation. J Clin Gastro 1983; 5:109.

    Two of 17 patients undergoing esophageal dilatation grew *Staphylococcus epidermidus* in blood cultures obtained during the procedure. These were felt to be contaminants. The authors do not advise routine prophylaxis for this procedure. They do recommend sterilizing the dilators before use in susceptible patients.

38

Purgatives

Thomas A. Dowgin

Polyethylene Glycol Electrolyte Lavage Solutions

Early endoscopists adopted the standard bowel preparation devised by surgeons and radiologists; i.e., 48 to 72 hours of clear liquids and laxatives, often followed by several enemas preprocedure. Patients complained of the inconvenience, dietary constraints, abdominal cramping, and anal irritation. Significant dehydration was a problem, especially in elderly patients. The preparation was occasionally inadequate, necessitating rescheduling of the study and repeat bowel prep.

In the late 1960s, oral whole-gut irrigation with high volumes (3–4 liters/hour) of isotonic solutions—the oral electrolyte-overload method—was introduced. This technique was very promising; rapid, effective colon cleansing was achieved. However, absorption of 1 to 2 liters of normal saline was common. Because of potential fluid volume and electrolyte changes, oral electrolyte-overload colon cleansing was not recommended for cardiac or renal patients.

In 1980, Davis et al. introduced a polyethylene glycol electrolyte lavage solution (PEG-ELS). This preparation, with sulfate and polyethylene glycol added to create a nonabsorbable isosmotic solution, was capable of improved colonic cleansing in a shorter period of time, better patient tolerance, and virtually no fluid or electrolyte shifts. Whether obtained commercially (e.g., Golytely from Braintree Laboratories or Colyte from Reed and Carnick) or made locally, PEG-ELS has become the preparation method of choice for colonoscopy.

MECHANISM OF ACTION

Active absorption of sodium across the intestinal mucosa occurs when the accompanying anion is chloride. In designing a solution with sodium *sulfate* as the predominate salt, Davis et al. found that sodium absorption was markedly reduced; also, that the sulfate anion is very poorly absorbed. Isonatremic solutions of sodium sulfate, however, are hyposmotic to plasma because plasma anions are monovalent, whereas sulfate is divalent. Therefore, a nonabsorbable solute was added (mannitol, initially) to create an isosmotic solution that, after ingestion, caused no net absorption or secretion of water. Mannitol presented a problem in that it is fermentable by colonic bacteria, with resultant production of hydrogen gas capable of exploding during colonoscopic cauterization. Polyethylene glycol (PEG), essentially nonabsorbable and unable to be metabolized by colonic flora, was chosen to replace mannitol as the nonelectrolyte

Table 38–1. Composition of polyethylene glycol electrolyte lavage solution

Component	Grams/liter
PEG 3350	60
Sodium sulfate	5.68
Sodium bicarbonate	1.68
Sodium chloride	1.46
Potassium chloride	0.745

osmotic additive. Explosions after the use of PEG-ELS have not been reported.

The composition of a standard PEG-ELS is shown in Table 38–1.

DOSAGE AND ADMINISTRATION

PEG-ELS can be given orally or by nasogastric tube. It is usually given the afternoon prior to the examination, after a clear-liquid lunch. Patients should drink approximately 1 liter/hour, to a total of 4 liters. The first bowel movement occurs about 1 hour after beginning lavage. Patients should be reminded to take nothing but clear liquids by mouth once the prep has started and until the study is completed. Alternatively, for patients requiring close supervision or hospitalization, the lavage can be done the morning of the study, allowing at least a 1-hour postlavage waiting period before performing the procedure.

EFFICACY

Multiple clinical trials have shown PEG-ELS to be equal or superior to standard bowel preps in colon cleansing, with no significant changes in patient weight, hematologic, or biochemical parameters. It has been safely used in patients with congestive heart failure, renal failure, diabetes, cirrhosis, and pulmonary disease. All studies show a clear patient preference for the PEG-ELS over standard bowel preps. Specifically, they like the shorter prep, dietary freedom, and avoidance of enemas.

The percentage of outpatient colonoscopies has increased because of the shorter, simpler, safer bowel prep. By producing an almost completely clean colon, PEG-ELS has prompted a trend toward primary colonoscopy, without preliminary barium enema. Colonoscopists, consistently able to examine very clean colons, are more confident that they are not missing small lesions.

Prior to PEG-ELS, early colonoscopy in the evaluation of acute hematochezia was technically limited by a poorly prepared colon. Rapid bowel cleansing by PEG-ELS is well tolerated in acute hematochezia and allows for adequate colonoscopy, with electrocautery if necessary.

Note that with respect to the histology of biopsy specimens, standard bowel preps can flatten the surface epithelial cells and deplete goblet cells, whereas PEG-ELS preserves normal mucosal histology.

It is common to retain 0.5 to 1 liter of lavage fluid in the colon postprep. This residual fluid is easily removed with suction during colonoscopy. There is less retained fluid when PEG-ELS is given the night before. Although not a problem for colonoscopy, this retained fluid interferes with mucosal coating during barium enema. Thus, PEG-ELS alone is not an adequate prep for barium enema, but the addition of bisacodyl (20 mg orally after PEG-ELS) makes oral lavage as good as the standard prep for barium enema. However, it has not been shown to significantly improve either patient tolerance or colonoscopically judged bowel cleanliness when combined with PEG-ELS.

Two small studies using PEG-ELS in children (10 months to 17 years old) showed good tolerance, with excellent bowel cleansing. As with adults, there were no significant changes in hematologic or biochemical parameters. Encopretic children also tolerated it well, with complete colon clean-out, though they required a larger volume of solution over a longer period of time.

SIDE EFFECTS AND CONTRAINDICATIONS

Patients most commonly complain of nausea and abdominal fullness. Brady et al., in two separate prospective studies, found that compared to placebo, neither 10 nor 20 milligrams of metoclopramide improved colonoscopically judged bowel cleanliness. In addition, there was no significant difference in patient symptoms between 10 milligrams of metoclopramide and placebo. Twenty milligrams of metoclopramide resulted in less cramping ($p = 0.02$) but more nausea ($p = 0.03$) than placebo.

Lavage-induced pill malabsorption has been described. An 88-year-old man took his procainamide tablet 1 hour prior to ingesting PEG-ELS. At colonoscopy 4 hours later, the intact tablet was found in the descending colon. Thus, patients should take essential medications more than 1 hour before starting colonic lavage.

PEG-ELS is contraindicated in patients with ileus, bowel perforation, toxic colitis, and gastrointestinal obstruction. Two patients with large rectal carcinomas suffered colonic perforation with oral lavages.

Initial concern over the toxicity and possible carcinogenicity of absorbed PEG has not been borne out by clinical data. PEG 3350 is a mixture of different-sized molecules with a mean molecular weight between 3200 and 3700. The higher molecular weight PEGs (>1000) have little or no gut absorption. Urinary excretion of PEG after oral lavage is minimal, and similar for normal and IBD patients. Likewise, urinary sulfate excretion postlavage is not significantly changed from baseline. Thus, the potential toxicity from absorbed PEG or sulfate during PEG-ELS is very low.

There is a case report of reversible cardiac asystole occurring after a large bowel movement during 1-liter/hour PEG-ELS peroral colonic lavage in an elderly man presenting with massive hematochezia. The arrest was thought to be secondary to the increased vagal tone in a patient with underlying sinoatrial node disease. This episode prompted a study where 22 patients underwent continuous ECG monitoring during a control period, during bowel prep with chilled PEG-ELS, and during colonoscopy. In approximately half of the patients tested, an increase in ventricular ectopy was noted during the colonic lavage period. ECG changes included short runs of ventricular tachycardia (two patients) as well as complex ventricular ectopy without ventricular tachycardia, and significantly increased PVCs (Lown Class IA in four patients; Class II in one patient; and Class IVA in four patients). All patients remained asymptomatic, and all were elderly. No electrolyte abnormalities were noted, and not all had documented heart disease. In patients with or without ischemic heart disease, the significance of this ectopy is unknown.

A Mallory-Weiss tear has been reported as a complication of oral lavage. This complication occurred with the earlier oral electrolyte-overload technique, before PEG-ELS. The patient received 3.5 liters over 40 minutes, about 3 times the recommended PEG-ELS dose rate, precipitating emesis and the resultant Mallory-Weiss tear.

PEARLS AND PITFALLS

1. Supplemental simethicone, as a split oral dose before and after PEG-ELS, significantly reduces the amount of colonic foam noted on subsequent colonoscopy. The amount of residual stool is also reduced. The same results are obtained if the simethicone is added to the PEG-ELS.
2. Patients, particularly the elderly, complain of difficulty ingesting a sufficient amount of PEG-ELS in the required time. This problem can usually be avoided by dividing the dose into one-half the evening prior to and the other half the morning of the study. There is no difference in bowel cleanliness between the single- and split-dose regimens.
3. The salty taste of PEG-ELS may be disagreeable. The solution is made more palatable by chilling it prior to ingestion. Note that a 66-year-old man developed mild hypothermia after drinking 5 liters of chilled PEG-ELS. During cold weather, sufficient care should be taken to minimize this potential complication.

References

1. Brady CE III, DiPalma JA, Pierson WP. Golytely lavage—Is metoclopramide necessary? Am J Gastro 1985; 3:180.
    Neither 10 nor 20 mg of metoclopramide improved colon cleansing or decreased symptoms.
2. Brady CE III, et al. Urinary excretion of PEG 3350 and sulfate after gut lavage with a PEG-ELS. Gastroenterology 1986; 6:1914.

A study showing that there is minimal absorption of these compounds after oral lavage in either normal or IBD patients.
3. Caos A, et al. Colonoscopy after Golytely preparation in acute rectal bleeding. J Clin Gastro 1986; 1:46.
   Urgent colonoscopy in 35 patients with acute hematochezia was well tolerated, with excellent mucosal visualization.
4. Davis GR, et al. Development of a lavage solution associated with minimal water and electrolyte absorption or secretion. Gastroenterology 1980; 78:991.
   The original article describing the development of PEG-ELS.
5. DiPalma JA, Brady CE III, Pierson WP. Golytely colon cleansing—Does bisacodyl improve cleansing? (abs) Clin Res 1984; 5:839A.
   No, in this study it did not.
6. DiPalma JA, et al. Comparison of colon-cleansing methods in preparation for colonoscopy. Gastroenterology 1984; 5:856.
   A randomized trial of 197 patients. Golytely was clearly preferred by patients and colonoscopists.
7. Ernstoff JJ, et al. A randomized, blinded clinical trial of a rapid colonic lavage solution (Golytely), compared with standard preparation for colonoscopy and barium enema. Gastroenterology 1983; 6:1512.
   A well-designed study concluding that Golytely is the prep of choice by both patients and gastroenterologists for colonoscopy, though for barium enema radiologists judged it to be not significantly different from standard preps.
8. Girard CM, et al. Comparison of Golytely lavage with standard diet/cathartic preparation for double-contrast barium enema. AJR 1984; 142:1147.
   This large, well-designed study found that Golytely alone was inadequate as a prep for double-contrast barium enema. However, Golytely plus bisacodyl was as effective as standard preps.
9. Ingebo KB, Heyman MB. Polyethylene glycol electrolyte solution for intestinal clearance in children with refractory encopresis. AJDC 1988; 142:340.
   The best study to date of PEG-ELS use in normal children as well as encopretics.
10. Marsh WH, et al. Ventricular ectopy associated with peroral colonic lavage. Gastro Endosc 1986; 4:259.
    Colonic lavage was associated with significantly increased complex ventricular ectopy. The clinical significance of this finding is unknown.
11. Oral electrolyte solutions for colonic lavage before colonoscopy or barium enema. Med Lett Drugs Ther 1985; 686:39.
    A concise summary of the mechanism of action, dosage, effectiveness, adverse effects, and cost of PEG-ELS.
12. Pockros PJ, Foroozan P. Golytely lavage versus a standard colonoscopy preparation: Effect on normal colonic mucosal histology. Gastroenterology 1985; 2:545.
    The study concludes that standard bowel preps flatten the surface epithelial cells and deplete the goblet cells, whereas PEG-ELS preserves normal mucosal histology.
13. Shaver WA, Storms P, Peterson WL. Improvement of oral

colonic lavage with supplemental simethicone. Dig Dis Sci 1988; 2:185.

The addition of Antifoam C emulsion (Dow Corning Corp.) to Golytely at 15 cc/liter decreased the amount of colonic foam and residual stool.

14. Sogge MR, Butler ML. Mallory-Weiss syndrome induced by the oral electrolyte-overload technique for colonoscopy preparation. Gastro Endosc 1980; 2:51.

    A case report of MW tear induced by rapid (3.5 liters over 40 minutes) consumption of a non-PEG-containing solution.

15. Thomas G, Brozinsky S, Isenberg JI. Patient acceptance and effectiveness of a balanced lavage solution (Golytely) versus the standard preparation for colonoscopy. Gastroenterology 1982; 3:435.

    A 20-patient study supporting better patient tolerance with PEG-ELS.

16. Tolia V, Fleming S, Dubois RS. Use of Golytely in children and adolescents. J Pediat Gastro Nut 1984; 3:468.

    In a prospective study, 12 children (6–18 years old) were treated, with no physiologic disturbances. The only significant side effect was nausea.

39

Tranquilizers

Michael Canty

Benzodiazepines

Proper preparation of the patient for endoscopy is essential for achievement of optimal results. The patient should be relaxed and have minimal spasticity of the buccopharyngeal, esophageal, and gastric musculature but without obliteration of peristaltic movements. This requires full confidence in the endoscopic team, adequate voluntary muscle relaxation, and a relative freedom from discomfort, pain, anxiety, and apprehension. This environment has been achieved by the use of benzodiazepines, primarily diazepam and midazolam, as premedicants for endoscopy. Chlordiazepoxide, the prototype of the benzodiazepines, was first synthesized but inadvertently set aside in 1955. It was rediscovered in 1957 during a laboratory cleaning operation at Hoffman-La Roche, Inc., and found to have sedative, muscle-relaxant, and anticonvulsant properties. Numerous analogs of chlordiazepoxide have been synthesized since that time. Diazepam and midazolam were synthesized in 1959 and 1976, respectively.

Diazepam

Diazepam (Valium) is a colorless, crystalline compound that is relatively lipid soluble and water insoluble. It is one of the most widely used drugs in clinical medicine. Approximately 55 million prescriptions for diazepam were filled at American retail pharmacies in 1972, and the number has progressively increased since.

PHARMACOLOGY

After oral administration, diazepam is rapidly and completely absorbed, reaching peak blood concentrations within 2 hours. Absorption of intramuscular diazepam is slow, erratic, and probably incomplete. This is not surprising since the drug is poorly water soluble at physiologic pH. After intravenous administration, diazepam exhibits the redistribution kinetics typical of highly lipid-soluble agents. Initially it is rapidly distributed centrally (to the brain). Then the concentration in plasma declines rapidly due to redistribution, with an initial distribution half-life of 10 to 15 minutes. However, there is often a return of drowsiness with an increased concentration of diazepam in plasma after 6 to 8 hours. This is probably due to absorption from the gastrointestinal tract after excretion in bile. The injectible form is available as 5 milligrams of diazepam per milliliter of organic solvent. The organic solvent is composed of 40 percent propylene glycol, 10 percent ethyl alcohol, 5 percent sodium benzoate, and 1.5 percent benzyl alcohol. The mixture is a viscous, oily substance with a pH of 6.8. Dilution with water or saline results in transient cloudiness from crystallization of small particles.

Metabolism of diazepam proceeds slowly in the liver, with an elimination half-life of between 20 and 40 hours in most patients. The major metabolic product, desmethyldiazepam, is formed by a removal of the N-1 methyl group. This compound has appreciable sedative and anxiolytic activity, and is biotransformed even more slowly than diazepam. Hydroxylation of desmethyldiazepam at the 3 position yields oxazepam, also an effective sedative, which is rapidly glucuronidated and excreted in the urine as the major urinary metabolite of diazepam. Steady-state concentrations are reached after 5 to 10 days. Diazepam is 99 percent protein bound.

Pharmacokinetic studies have shown that the plasma half-life of Valium increases linearly with age. This is a result of an increase in the initial distribution space and volume of distribution at steady state. Elderly patients appear to have an increased nervous system sensitivity to diazepam, but this is independent of the increased plasma half-life. Patients with liver disease may have a more than twofold increase in plasma half-life as a result of a decrease in plasma clearance. There is no important change in the initial volume of distribution in cirrhosis, but the volume of distribution at steady state increases significantly. This is probably a reflection of decreased diazepam protein binding in cirrhosis.

MECHANISM OF ACTION

Most clinically important effects of benzodiazepines are mediated through the central nervous system. Specific benzodiazepine receptors have been found throughout the mammalian central nervous system, with the highest density of receptors in the cerebral cortex and limbic forebrain. The drugs appear to work by potentiating inhibitory interneurons mediated by gamma-aminobutyric acid that regulate excitatory input from collaterals in many areas of the central nervous system, and by interaction with glycine receptors in the brainstem and spinal cord. Interactions between gamma-aminobutyric acid receptors and benzodiazepine receptors have been shown at the molecular level. The benzodiazepine receptors are membrane proteins located in the immediate vicinity of gamma-aminobutyric acid synapses. They form part of a supramolecular complex of functionally related macromolecules, including the gamma-aminobutyric acid receptor, its associated chloride ionophore, and other proteins. The final result of the activation of benzodiazepine receptors appears to be an increase in the frequency of gamma-aminobutyric acid chloride channel opening, which results in potentiation of gamma-aminobutyric acid release, thus increasing the inhibitory activity of the neuron. The sedative properties of diazepam appear to result from this facilitation of gamma-aminobutyric acid neurotransmission in the cerebral cortex.

The antianxiety action of benzodiazepines has been localized to the limbic system. Electrical discharge from the amygdaloid nuclei and amygdalohippocampal transmission are inhibited by low doses that do not depress the rest of the brain. In essence, they appear to reduce anxiety by means of a pharmacologic amygdalectomy. Benzodiazepines also produce objective muscle relaxation in both healthy patients and patients with neuromuscular diseases. Multiple factors are felt to contribute to muscle relaxation, including facilitation of brainstem inhibitory neurons, influencing of interneuronal activity in the spinal cord and direct depression of motor nerve and muscle function.

It has been proposed that memory consolidation requires neural perseveration in the hippocampus. Benzodiazepines may cause anterograde amnesia by blocking this perseverative activity, which is indispensable to the generation of a memory trace.

INDICATIONS

The most common indication for diazepam is as an anxiolytic agent. Intravenous diazepam is extremely helpful in facilitating endoscopy, colonoscopy, peritoneoscopy, cytoscopy, and bronchoscopy by producing a light anesthesia. This is not a true anesthesia. It is created by sedation and an anterograde amnesia that produce the illusion of anesthesia. The anterograde amnesia is at its peak 2 to 3 minutes after intravenous injection of diazepam. Most patients are also given a parenteral opiate before their procedure. It is unclear whether this significantly enhances sedation or amnesia. It has been shown that 80 to 90 percent of patients given intravenous diazepam and meperidine for gastroscopy have good to excellent relaxation and resolution of apprehension and muscle tension. Administration of diazepam alone is not sufficient for performance of a successful examination, since suppression of the gag reflex is not obtained. This is generally achieved by administering a topical anesthetic or an opiate.

Diazepam has also been shown to be effective in relieving nonspecific muscle spasms in healthy patients as well as the pathological muscle spasticity seen in neuromuscular diseases. Intravenous diazepam is the drug of choice when intractable, repetitive seizure activity mandates parenteral therapy. Diazepam is effective in suppressing the symptoms of alcoholic withdrawal. Its sedative and amnesic effects make it ideal to use as sedation for cardioversion, as a premedicant for surgical procedures, and as an induction agent before general anesthetic administration.

CONTRAINDICATIONS

Injectable diazepam is contraindicated in patients with a known hypersensitivity to the drug, acute narrow-angle glaucoma, and open-angle glaucoma unless patients are receiving appropriate therapy.

SIDE EFFECTS

Dose-related excessive central nervous system depression is the most common side effect of diazepam. Excessive central nervous system depression is more likely to occur in the elderly, in patients with liver disease, in those with low serum albumin, in neonates (because of an inability to biotransform diazepam into inactive metabolites), and in those who are taking other central nervous system depressants. Manifestations of central nervous system depression include drowsiness, somnolence, fatigue, muscle weakness, nystagmus, ataxia, dysarthria, and impairment of memory.

Injection-site complications occur in 3 to 10 percent of patients receiving parenteral diazepam. These range from transient local pain on injection to thrombophlebitis and thrombosis. They may be caused by inherent properties of the diazepam itself, the propylene glycol solvent, or both. Preventive measures that have been employed include using heparin flush, saline flush, use of larger veins, use of a different solvent (cremophor-EL), dilutions, injecting slowly (5 mg/minute), and use of other benzodiazepines.

Diazepam has been shown to cause respiratory and circulatory depression. Overly rapid intravenous administration of Valium may cause apnea, particularly in the setting of concomitant opiate use. Intravenous injection causes a decrease in tidal volume, PaO_2, and pH; and an increase in PCO_2. The decrease in tidal volume appears to be exclusively mediated by a decrease in the abdominal contribution to respiration. Intravenous Valium may also result in a moderate (15–20%) decrease in systemic blood pressure and vascular resistance. Heart rate may show a slight decrease or a moderate increase. These effects are also potentiated by concomitant opiate use. Generally the respiratory and circulatory depression of diazepam is not clinically significant and requires no therapeutic intervention. However, means to administer respiratory and circulatory support should always be readily available when giving intravenous diazepam. Studies have shown that the respiratory changes do not necessarily correlate with the overt sedative effects of diazepam.

There is an increased risk of congenital malformations associated with diazepam use in the first trimester of pregnancy. Diazepam readily crosses the placenta and is associated with fetal sedation and respiratory distress at birth. Diazepam use should be avoided during pregnancy.

Other adverse effects of diazepam include physiologic addiction, sleep disturbances (including hallucinations and nightmares), and paradoxical excitement, hostility, and rage.

DRUG INTERACTIONS

Diazepam produces additive central nervous system depression when administered concomitantly with other central nervous system depressants (opiates, barbiturates, alcohol, etc.). Benzodiazepines have been reported to enhance the activity of digoxin, possibly by decreasing its rate of renal excretion.

DOSAGE AND ADMINISTRATION

The dosage should be titrated to the patient's response. It must be stressed that no specific number of milligrams is important in dosing. Rather, the drug should be titrated to effect by the clinician. The usual recommended dose in adults is between 2 and 20 milligrams intravenously or intramuscularly, depending on the indication. Determinants of the intravenous dose required include age, prior chronic benzodiazepine use, weight, and liver disease. When used for conscious sedation during procedures such as endoscopy, 5 to 15 milligrams intravenously is recommended. Ten milligrams intramuscularly is recommended for use as a preoperative antianxiety agent. The intravenous solution should be injected slowly (5 mg/minute) into a large vein. It should not be mixed or diluted with other drugs in a syringe. Lower (2–5 mg) doses should be used in the elderly, debilitated patients, and patients who have received other premedications.

Midazolam

Midazolam, an imidazobenzodiazepine derivative, is a white to light-yellow crystalline compound whose hydrochloride salt is soluble in water. The unique chemical structure of midazolam confers a number of physicochemical properties that distinguish it from other benzodiazepines in terms of its pharmacologic and pharmacokinetic characteristics.

PHARMACOLOGY

The principal difference between midazolam's structure and that of the older benzodiazepines is a fused imidazole ring. The imidazole ring accounts for the basicity (pK 6.15), stability in aqueous solution, and rapid metabolism. The basicity allows the preparation of salts that are stable in water solution. At a pH of less than 4, part of the drug in solution has an open benzodiazepine ring, imparting water solubility. At physiologic pH the drug is believed to be present in a closed-ring form that results in increased lipid solubility. It is available in an injectible form (intravenous or intramuscular) that is composed of 5 milligrams of midazolam hydrochloride per milliliter of solvent. The solvent is composed of 0.8 percent sodium chloride, 0.01 percent disodium edetate, and 1 percent benzyl alcohol as a preservative. The pH is adjusted to approximately 3. The oral form of midazolam is not available in the U.S.

The effects of midazolam on the central nervous system are dependent on the route of administration, the dose administered, and the presence or absence of other premedications. Sedation after intravenous injection is achieved in 3 to 5 minutes. After intravenous administration of midazolam to healthy young humans, disappearance of midazolam from plasma proceeds in two distinct phases. The initial phase of rapid disappearance is due principally to distribution of the drug, while the final and slower phase of disappearance is attributable mainly to biotransformation. The onset of sedative effects after intramuscular injection are seen in approximately 15 minutes, with peak sedation occurring in 30 to 60 minutes. The mean absolute bioavailability of midazolam after intramuscular injection is greater than 90 percent. Oral midazolam is absorbed very rapidly from the gastrointestinal tract, achieving peak plasma concentrations within 1 hour of ingestion. Only 40 to 50 percent of the drug reaches the systemic circulation in nonmetabolized form because of extensive and rapid first-pass hepatic clearance.

Metabolism of midazolam involves hydroxylation by hepatic microsomal oxidative mechanisms. Microsomal enzymes rapidly hydrolyze the fused imidazole ring. The principal metabolites are 1-hydroxymethylmidazolam (50–70%), 4-hydroxymethylmidazolam (3%), and 1,4-hydroxymethylmidazolam (1%). These metabolites are excreted in the urine in the form of glucuronide conjugates. Very little intact drug is excreted in the urine. The 1- and 4-hydroxymethylmidazolam metabolites have pharmacologic activity, although less than the parent compound. The elimination half-life of midazolam in healthy young humans ranges from 1.5 to 3.5 hours. It is prolonged in obese and elderly patients, liver disease patients, and patients in shock. Midazolam is approximately 96 percent protein bound. The free fraction of the drug is increased in patients with chronic renal failure.

MECHANISM OF ACTION

Midazolam appears to work in a manner similar to diazepam and other benzodiazepines, by facilitating gamma-aminobutyric acid inhibitory neurons and increasing glycine inhibitory neurotransmission. Midazolam's affinity for the benzodiazepine receptor is approximately 2 times that of diazepam.

Midazolam causes anterograde amnesia similar to other benzodiazepines. The incidence and duration of the amnesia is dose-related. The degree of amnesia does not always parallel the drowsiness. The amnesic effect of midazolam may be more intense than that of diazepam.

Midazolam reduces the cerebral metabolic rate for oxygen and cerebral blood flow in a dose-related manner. These findings suggest that midazolam can protect against cerebral hypoxia and be useful for patients who have impaired intracranial compliance or increased intracranial pressure.

The behavioral and central nervous system electrophysiologic effects of midazolam are antagonized by the benzodiazepine agonist RO 15–1788 (Flumazepil). The clinical effects of midazolam may also be nonspecifically reversed by physostigmine and glycopyrrolate in combination.

INDICATIONS

1. Intramuscular midazolam is indicated for preoperative sedation and to impair memory of perioperative events.
2. Intravenous midazolam is indicated for induction of general anesthesia, before administration of other anesthetic agents.
3. Intravenous midazolam is indicated as an agent for conscious sedation prior to short diagnostic or endoscopic procedures, such as gastroscopy, colonoscopy, bronchoscopy, cystoscopy, and cardiac catheterization, either alone or with an opiate. It is titrated to produce sleep, or more commonly, dysarthria. It results in mild sedation and amnesia. The onset of sedation is more rapid than with diazepam.

CONTRAINDICATIONS

As with other benzodiazepines, midazolam is contraindicated in patients with acute narrow-angle glaucoma and should only be used in open-angle glaucoma patients who are on appropriate therapy.

SIDE EFFECTS

Excessive central nervous depression is commonly seen with midazolam. As with other benzodiazepines, this is dose-related. The central nervous system depression is potentiated when used concomitantly with other central nervous system depressants. Paradoxical agitation, anxiety, argumentativeness, and sleep disturbances may also occur.

Midazolam causes a centrally mediated respiratory depression. It reduces the ventilatory and mouth occlusion–pressure response to carbon dioxide (as does diazepam). Intravenous midazolam decreases tidal volume and increases respiratory frequency without a change in minute ventilation. PCO_2 is increased and PaO_2 is decreased. As with diazepam, the fall in tidal volume is mediated by a reduction in the abdominal contribution to respiration. Midazolam causes apnea in a variable percentage of patients (0–77%). The incidence of apnea is related to the total dose and the rate of administration of midazolam. It is more likely to occur in patients who have been premedicated with opiates. Equipotent doses of midazolam and diazepam have approximately the same degree of respiratory depression. Respiratory depression is more marked and prolonged in patients with chronic obstructive pulmonary disease.

The cardiovascular effects of midazolam are more significant than those of diazepam. Intravenous midazolam decreases systolic and diastolic blood pressure by approximately 5 and 10 percent, respectively. Heart rate is increased. Systemic vascular resistance is decreased 15 to 33 percent. Midazolam is felt to decrease myocardial contractility by a direct effect. Other cardiovascular side effects include bigeminy, premature ventricular contractions, vasovagal episodes, and nodal rhythms.

The frequency of local venous complications with midazolam is much lower than with diazepam. However, there is still a low incidence of pain at the injection site (5%), local tenderness (2%), and phlebitis (0.4%). Intramuscular injection can result in local pain (3.7%), induration (0.5%), redness (0.5%), headaches, and muscle stiffness.

Midazolam crosses the placenta. It is not recommended for use during pregnancy. It is not known whether midazolam appears in human breast milk.

Other adverse reactions that have been reported with intravenous midazolam include hiccups, nausea, vomiting, coughing, and headaches.

DRUG INTERACTIONS

The sedative effect of midazolam is accentuated by opiates, barbiturates, and alcohol. Intravenous midazolam may potentiate the antihypertensive effect of beta adrenoceptor–blocking drugs.

DOSAGE AND ADMINISTRATION

The dosage should be titrated to patient response. As a guide, midazolam, 0.05 to 0.07 milligrams/kilogram, is usually given for intravenous conscious sedation. The dose should be lowered in the elderly, debilitated patients, and patients who have received other premedications. Intravenous midazolam for conscious sedation should be administered slowly over 2 to 3 minutes. Rapid injection may cause respiratory depression or apnea. Injectible midazolam is compatible with 5% dextrose in water, 0.9% sodium chloride, and lactated Ringer's solution. It may be mixed in the same syringe with meperidine, morphine sulfate, scopolamine, and atropine. When intravenous midazolam is used, oxygen, resuscitative equipment, and personnel resources for the maintenance of a patent airway should be immediately available.

COMPARISON OF DIAZEPAM AND MIDAZOLAM

Compared with diazepam, midazolam is more potent and faster acting. There are fewer adverse reactions (e.g., pain on injection and thrombophlebitis) with midazolam. Randomized clinical trials have shown similar recovery times using the Trieger test and critical flicker fusion. Endoscopist and patient satisfaction with the agent have also been similar. Patients have generally preferred midazolam, primarily because of its significantly greater amnesic effect. The major differences in the pharmacokinetics of diazepam and midazolam are that the distribution half-life of midazolam is at least one-half that of diazepam, and that the elimination half-life of midazolam is about 10-fold slower. Disadvantages of diazepam include prolonged action, with a second peak effect at 6 to 8 hours, pain on injection, and a high incidence of thrombophlebitis. The primary disadvantage of midazolam is the need to give repeated doses to maintain sedation during prolonged procedures.

PEARLS AND PITFALLS

1. Midazolam is 1.5 to 2 times more potent than diazepam.
2. Benzodiazepines should be avoided during early pregnancy and during labor and delivery.
3. Neither drug has been shown to cause retrograde amnesia.
4. The sedative effects of both drugs are potentiated when other central nervous system depressants are used concomitantly.
5. Low-dose intravenous aminophylline has been shown to decrease recovery time from sedation with diazepam.
6. Apnea is associated with rapid intravenous injection of both drugs. It is dose-related. Patients with underlying lung disease are particularly sensitive to respiratory complications.
7. Injection-site complications with diazepam can be reduced by using larger veins, saline flush, heparin flush, a different solvent, and by injecting slowly.
8. Oxygen, resuscitative equipment, and personnel to maintain a patent airway should be immediately available when either drug is used intravenously.
9. The elimination half-life of midazolam is increased in the elderly, the obese, and patients with liver disease. The half-life of diazepam may be doubled in the setting of liver disease and increases linearly with age.
10. The free fraction of midazolam is increased in patients with renal disease.
11. Both drugs are metabolized to psychopharmacologically active metabolites.
12. The elderly have an increased sensitivity to benzodiazepines that is independent of dose and pharmacokinetics.
13. Specific benzodiazepine agonists, such as RO 15–1788 (Flumazepil), are under development.
14. The dose of midazolam should be titrated to dysarthria, not overt sedation.

References

1. Berggren I, et al. Changes in breathing pattern and chest-wall mechanics after benzodiazepines in combination with meperidine. Acta Anaesth Scand 1987; 31:381–386.

   Benzodiazepines are shown to decrease tidal volume by decreasing the abdominal contribution to respiration.
2. Cole SG, Brozinsky S, Isenberg JI. Midazolam, a new more potent benzodiazepine, compared with diazepam: A ran-

domized, double-blind study of pre-endoscopic sedatives. Gastro Endosc 1983; 3:219–222.

A randomized trial that found midazolam to be significantly more potent, faster acting, and associated with greater amnesia, compared with diazepam.

3. Dalen JE, et al. The hemodynamic and respiratory effects of diazepam. Anesthesiology 1969; 3:259–263.

The hemodynamic and respiratory effects seen in 15 patients given 5–10 mg of diazepam intravenously for cardiac catheterization are discussed.

4. Dundee JW, et al. Midazolam: A review of its pharmacological properties and therapeutic use. Drugs 1984; 28:519–543.

A thorough review of all aspects of midazolam.

5. Foster PN. Low-dose aminophylline accelerates recovery from diazepam premedication for digestive endoscopy. Gastro Endosc 1987; 6:421–424.

A randomized trial of 110 patients given low-dose intravenous aminophylline, versus placebo, after sedation with diazepam. Low-dose aminophylline reduced recovery time.

6. Greenblatt DJ, Shader RI. Benzodiazepines I. NEJM 1974; 19:1011–1015.

The first of a two-part review of benzodiazepines.

7. Greenblatt DJ, Shader RI. Benzodiazepines II. NEJM 1974; 23:1239–1243.

The second of a two-part review of benzodiazepines.

8. Klotz U, et al. The effects of age and liver disease on the disposition and elimination of diazepam in adult man. J Clin Invest 1975; 55:347–359.

An excellent study of the effects of age and liver disease on the pharmacokinetics of diazepam.

9. Magni VC, et al. A randomized comparison of midazolam and diazepam for sedation in upper gastrointestinal endoscopy. Br J Anaesth 1983; 55:1095–1100.

A randomized trial concluding that midazolam produced a greater degree of amnesia and was generally preferred by patients.

10. Mitchell PF. Diazepam-associated thrombophlebitis: A review and discussion of possible prevention. JADA 1980; 101:492–495.

A thorough review of the injection-site complications of diazepam.

11. Reves JG, et al. Midazolam: Pharmacology and uses. Anesthesiology 1985; 62:310–324.

An excellent review of midazolam's pharmacology, pharmacokinetics, and uses.

12. Richter JR. Current theories about the mechanisms of benzodiazepines and neuroleptic drugs. Anesthesiology 1981; 54:66–72.

An excellent discussion of the mechanisms of action of benzodiazepines.

Sclerosing and Hemostatic Agents

David A. Johnson

The initial application of injection therapy to gastrointestinal hemorrhage was for bleeding esophageal varices. Although the bulk of the now voluminous information regarding injection therapy of upper gastrointestinal hemorrhage pertains to variceal bleeding, there has been a more recent blossoming of interest in use of this technique in nonvariceal hemorrhage as well. The advantages of this latter application center around the simplicity, relatively low expense, and efficacy that is comparable to thermal therapy (electrocoagulation, heater probe laser). This method has also been used by several investigators for therapy of nonbleeding angiodysplastic lesions in both the upper and lower digestive tract. This chapter focuses on the agents currently available for injection therapy in the United States: sodium tetradecyl sulfate, sodium morrhuate, absolute alcohol, epinephrine, and vasopressin.

MECHANISM OF ACTION

The acute injury from the injection of sclerosants is characterized by thrombosis of the vessel and ulceration of the overlying tissue. A chronic reaction is also produced and is characterized by an evolution from granulation tissue to mature collagen, with an accompanying chronic inflammatory cellular infiltrate that becomes less prominent with time. Alcohol is a tissue desiccant and causes local dehydration and vasoconstriction. Vascular-wall and endothelial-cell destruction occur, with subsequent thrombogenesis.

Sodium Tetradecyl Sulfate (STS)

This agent is a synthetic anion detergent approved for use in the treatment of small, uncomplicated varicose veins of the lower extremities. However, it is also in widespread use in many medical centers as a sclerotherapy agent for esophageal variceal hemorrhage. It is believed that the surface activity of the fatty acid anions of the soap accounts for the physical properties leading to vessel thrombosis.

DOSAGE AND ADMINISTRATION

STS is available commercially as 1% and 3% solutions. Intravenous injection has been shown to be more effective than perivenous injection in producing vein occlusion. In general, a 1.5% solution of STS is used (mixed with 50% D/W). The work of Jensen has shown that 1.5% STS is comparable to 95-percent ethanol and 5-percent ethanolamine, and slightly better than 5-percent sodium morrhuate. It is recommended by most investigators that no more than 2 milliliters be given per injection, although occasionally larger varices require more. The volume required can be assessed by the degree of distension and blanching of the varix. The total volume of the solution injected during the first procedure is generally less than 25 milliliters with progressively lesser amounts in subsequent procedures.

SIDE EFFECTS

This agent is a sclerosant that causes contact irritation, and care should be taken to protect the patient and endoscopy team from splash contact with the eyes. Allergic reactions are exceedingly rare but anaphylactic reactions have been reported. The effect of long-term esophageal variceal sclerotherapy using this agent has been evaluated, with no serious long- or short-term impairment of lung function with either the 1 or 3% solution.

Sodium Morrhuate

This agent is a mixture of unsaturated fatty acids found in cod liver oil. These fatty acids are capable of injuring endothelial cells and provoking thrombosis as a consequence.

DOSAGE AND ADMINISTRATION

This agent is available as a 5-percent mixture. Restrictions for total and per-injection volume are the same as with sodium tetradecyl sulfate. Efficacy as a sclerosant has been demonstrated in clinical trials, but in animal models Jensen has shown this to be a less effective agent than sodium tetradecyl sulfate or absolute alcohol. The drug is supplied in 5 and 30-milligram ampules, with 50 milligrams/milliliter.

SIDE EFFECTS

The preparation of this agent can be nonuniform, and allergic reactions may be seen. Fever, chest pain, and pleural effusion are more common than with sodium tetradecyl sulfate. Also, since this agent has a higher incidence of deep sclerotherapy-induced ulceration, the complications of esophageal perforation such as bleeding and stricture are also more common. Acute respiratory distress syndrome has been reported in two patients within 24 hours of sclerotherapy with sodium morrhuate. Two of the fatty acids in sodium morrhuate (oleic and linoleic acids) are known to induce experimental pulmonary toxicity. A study of sodium morrhuate delivery to the lung during esophageal sclerotherapy showed that approximately 20 percent of the injected dose reached the pulmonary circulation via the azygos vein. In this study no change in diffusing capacity was noted.

CONTRAINDICATIONS

This drug is contraindicated in patients who have shown a previous hypersensitivity to the drug or the fatty acids of cod liver oil.

Absolute Alcohol

MECHANISM OF ACTION

This agent has been used for intravariceal injection of esophageal varices, but more recently for treatment of nonvariceal bleeding lesions. Alcohol is a tissue desiccant and causes local dehydration and vasoconstriction. Vascular-wall and endothelial-cell destruction then occur, with subsequent thrombogenesis. This thrombogenic effect has particular appeal in the treatment of bleeding nonvariceal lesions. In contrast to vasoconstrictors (e.g., epinephrine), the potential for a more long-lasting hemostasis seems more tenable if a thrombosis is effected, rather than merely inducing a transient vasoconstriction. There are no prospective, controlled studies addressing comparative efficacy, however.

DOSAGE AND ADMINISTRATION

Desiccated alcohol (98%) should be used. Concentrations below 90 percent are not as effective. Most investigators recommend that the total volume injected be less than 1 milliliter. The alcohol is available in 1-cubic centimeter ampules. Approximately 1.5 cubic centimeters are needed to preload a standard sclerotherapy needle. Aliquots of 0.1 to 0.2 milliliters of this agent are then injected circumferentially around a bleeding or visible vessel, with the needle placed 1 to 2 millimeters away from the vessel.

SIDE EFFECTS

The ulcerogenic potential for this agent must be appreciated. Extension of the ulcer may occur, and perforation is reported in about 1 percent of cases.

Epinephrine

The vasoconstrictive effects of epinephrine have great advantage for dealing with ongoing hemorrhage. In particular, local injection of 1:10,000 solution has been helpful in endoscopic therapy of nonvariceal bleeding lesions. Some investigators prefer to use epinephrine in conjunction with another therapy, such as thermal therapy, to allow for a more directed application once active bleeding slows. Leung et al. used endoscopic injection of epinephrine for treatment of bleeding peptic ulcers. These authors injected aliquots of 0.5 milliliter of 1:10,000 epinephrine around and into the bleeding point and the immediately adjacent area until the bleeding stopped. The total volume used ranged from 1.5 to 10 milliliters (mean, 4.1 ml). Local injection of adrenaline has several effects that can impose hemostasis. First, it causes vasoconstriction of the submucosal arterioles of the stomach. Submucosal injection can also cause a local tamponade effect. Furthermore, epinephrine causes platelet aggregation and may promote thrombogenesis.

Other investigators prefer to combine epinephrine with other agents. Hirao et al. have utilized the vasoconstrictive effects of epinephrine and the physiochemical properties of hypertonic sodium chloride as an injection to create the tissue effects of swelling, fibrinoid degeneration of the vascular wall, and consequent thrombosis of the vascular lumen. These authors used a solution of 0.005-percent epinephrine with 3.6% hypertonic saline for injection. In acute nonfibrotic bleeding ulcers, 3 milliliters of the first solution was injected at three to four sites around the base of the exposed vessel. In ulcers with extensive fibrosis (due to previous treatment), 1 milliliter of the second solution was injected in three to four sites around the base of the bleeding vessel. Combining their entire experience (which includes patients treated with only one injection before the "prophylactic" injections were begun), 94 percent of bleeding gastric ulcers and 80 percent of duodenal ulcers achieved permanent hemostasis. Rebleeding occurred in 3.5 percent of gastric ulcers and 13.3 percent of duodenal ulcers, but retreatment was successful in most instances.

Sohendra has used 5 to 10 cubic centimeters of epinephrine 1:10,000, delivered to the submucosa directly around the bleeding vessel, to create hemostasis by compression and vasoconstriction. Following this he injected 5 cubic centimeters of a sclerosant (polidocanol) to provoke thrombosis. Spurting vessels of 16 out of 22 patients were controlled with a single treatment, and retreatment was successful in the remaining six.

SIDE EFFECTS

In that the injection of epinephrine in bleeding lesions is intended to be around and not into a vessel, systemic side effects should not develop. Since epinephrine is a sympathomimetic and acts on both alpha and beta receptors, all actions of the sympathetic nervous system conceivably can develop. Inadvertent venous injection may cause cerebrovascular hemorrhage, resulting from a sharp rise in blood pressure. Fatalities conceivably may also occur, resulting from pulmonary edema due to the peripheral constriction and cardiac stimulation produced. In addition, patients with atherosclerotic vascular disease are at increased risk for infarction secondary to decreased organ perfusion. If intravenous injection is used, immediate follow-up with vasodilators such as nitrates or alpha-blocking agents is recommended, to counteract the vasoconstriction and marked pressor effects of this agent. Also, this product contains sodium bisulfite (an antioxidant) and may cause an allergic-type reaction, including anaphylaxis, in certain susceptible individiuals. Repeated local injections can result in necrosis at the injection sites due to the vascular constriction.

Vasopressin

Vasopressin is a naturally occurring nonapeptide produced by the posterior pituitary gland. Since its discovery, many studies have reported on the use of this agent in acute upper gastrointestinal tract hemorrhage. Trials assessing the efficacy of systemic infusion for nonvariceal hemorrhage have not been successful, although demonstration of the efficacy for selective infusion has had mixed results.

MECHANISM OF ACTION

This agent is a splanchnic vasoconstrictor, and the rationale for its use in variceal hemorrhage is based on the fact that it can reverse (to normal) the increased flow that is known to occur in portal hypertension. Two forms of vasopressin, differing by only one amino acid, are available for clinical use: lysine-vasopressin and arginine-vasopressin. The vasoconstrictive activity of both is similar. In the United States, clinical experience has developed from a mixture of arginine- and lysine-vasopressin (Pitressin). Vasopressin also has a potent antidiuretic effect, ascribed to increasing reabsorption of water by the renal tubules.

INDICATIONS

Although widely used in the treatment of gastrointestinal hemorrhage (in particular, variceal bleeding) Pitressin is only approved for use in the prevention and treatment of postoperative abdominal distension, to dispel interfering gas shadow on abdominal x rays, and for the treatment of diabetes insipidus. Vasopressin has been used for the treatment of other sources of nonvariceal bleeding (i.e., vascular malformation, Mallory-Weis tears, diverticular hemorrhage, and postpolypectomy bleeding), but this treatment usually requires mesenteric intra-arterial infusion and often selective or subselective infusion into the vessel(s) directly supplying the bleeding site. Alcohol- or drug-induced diffuse hemorrhagic gastritis may also respond to vasopressin administration.

DOSAGE AND ADMINISTRATION

Vasopressin can be given intra-arterially as well as intravenously. Since the intra-arterial administration requires special skills and facilities and superimposes complications related to catheterization, continuous intravenous infusion is the route of choice for portal hypertensive bleeding. In addition, continuous intra-arterial infusion has no proven hemodynamic advantage over continuous intravenous infusion at the same rate. Intravenous vasopressin infusion should be started at a dose of 0.3 units/minute for at least 30 minutes and if ineffective, increased at approximately 30- to 60-minute intervals to 0.6, 0.9, 1.2, and 1.5 units/minute. Intra-arterial infusions are begun at 0.1 units/minute for at least 30 minutes and if ineffective, increased at approximately 30- to 60-minute intervals to 0.2, 0.3, 0.4, and 0.5 units/minute. For intravenous use, dosages of up to 1.5 units/minute may be necessary for efficacy, but this significantly increases the toxicity potential. Vasopressin is supplied in ampules containing 0.5 cubic centimeter (10 pressor units). Twenty units of Pitressin mixed in 100 cubic centimeters of 5% D/W provides 0.2 units/cubic centimeter; thus 1 cubic centimeter/minute provides a dose of 0.2 units/minute. Tapering the dose before discontinuation appears to be unnecessary because vasopressin does not prevent rebleeding from varices.

SIDE EFFECTS AND CONTRAINDICATIONS

The list of potential adverse side effects is lengthy. Vasopressin produces increased gut motility, presumably by stimulation of smooth muscle, with attendant abdominal cramps and occasionally diarrhea. The vasoconstrictive effect may result in bowel ischemia with necrosis. An increase in cardiac afterload, baroreceptor-mediated bradycardia, decreased coronary blood flow, and direct impairment of cardiac contractility are factors responsible for the decreased cardiac output and myocardial performance observed with this agent. Severe arrhythmias and myocardial infarction have been reported with the use of vasopressin. Close supervision and cardiac monitoring are therefore advised during infusion. The drug is contraindicated in patients with known, severe coronary artery disease and should be used cautiously in alcoholics, who may have a subclinical cardiomyopathy. Vasopressin has also been associated with respiratory arrest and cerebral hemorrhage. Other dynamic effects include antidiuresis, which may result in hyponatremia. This should be treated with withdrawal of the vasopressin until polyuria occurs. If severe, induction of an osmotic diuresis with mannitol, hypertonic dextrose, or furosemide should be undertaken. Additional side effects include stimulation of endothelial release of plasminogen activator and factor VIII. Administration of vasopressin to nonbleeding patients with cirrhosis, however, has not been associated with chemical evidence of fibrinolysis.

VASOPRESSIN ANALOGUES

An investigational vasopressin analogue, triglycyl-vasopressin, has been studied and compared with vasopressin. Advantages claimed for triglycyl-vasopressin over vasopressin are mesenteric selectivity of action, lack of stimulation of plasminogen, lack of systemic hemodynamic activator release effects, and the ease of intermittent bolus injection over continuous infusion. A comparative study of triglycyl-vasopressin (20 μg/kg) and vasopressin (2.8 mU/kg/minute) in dogs, however, reported equivalent changes in mean arterial pressure and reduction in cardiac output.

NITROGLYCERIN-VASOPRESSIN

Nitrates have been studied in conjunction with vasopressin therapy and may enhance the hemostatic potential and decrease the systemic toxic effects of vasopressin administration alone. As a potent venous and mild arterial dilator, nitroglycerin reverses the cardiotoxic effects of vasopressin. Furthermore, enhancement of portal hypotensive effects is accomplished by reducing the vasopressin-induced increase in portal venous resistance. Results from several clinical trials using this combination are encouraging. It is likely that the combination will become the treatment of choice for pharmacologic management of acutely bleeding varices due to portal hypertension. Nitroglycerin has been administered sublingually, transdermally, and intravenously, although the transdermal route may have an unpredictable absorption. A more rapid titration and control of systolic pressure are possible with intravenous administration, and in most centers this is the route of choice. Dosages used in reported trials range from 40 to 400 micrograms/minute, with a median dose of 250 to 300 micrograms/minute.

CONTRAINDICATIONS

Nitroglycerin (intravenous) is contraindicated in the following situations: hypersensitivity to nitroglycerin, idiosyncratic reactions to nitrates, severe hypotension or uncorrected hypovolemia, increased intracranial pressure (e.g., from head trauma or cerebral hemorrhage), inadequate cerebral circulation, constrictive pericarditis, and pericardial tamponade.

DOSAGE AND ADMINISTRATION

Nitroglycerin must be diluted in a 5% dextrose or 0.9% sodium chloride solution prior to infusion. The fluid requirements of the patient as well as the expected duration of the infusion should be considered in selecting the appropriate dilution. To obtain a concentration of 500 micrograms/milliliter, add 5 milligrams of nitroglycerin to 100 milliliters of dilutent, or 50 milligrams to 1 liter. For a concentration of 100 micrograms/milliliter add 25 milligrams to 250 milliliters, or 100 milligrams to 1 liter. Initial infusion at this concentration should be 5 micrograms/minute (3 ml/hr), with titration of 5 microgram/minute increments every 3 to 5 minutes until some response is noted. If no response is noted at 20 micrograms/minute, then increases can be made with 10- to 20-microgram/minute increments until a pressure effect is noted. The dosage used for sublingual administration in one study was 0.6 milligrams every 30 minutes for 6 hours.

Dosage is titrated to the level of hemodynamic function. Blood pressure, pulse rate, and other physiologic parameters must be monitored continuously to ensure maintainence of adequate systemic blood pressure for critical organ perfusion (target systolic pressure, > 90 mm Hg). Since a fall in pulmonary capillary wedge pressure precedes the onset of arterial hypotension, wedge pressure can serve as a useful guide to safe titration of the drug.

SIDE EFFECTS

Central nervous system complaints of headache are not uncommon. Apprehension, dizziness, restlessness, and muscle twitching have been described. Gastrointestinal side effects are rare but include nausea, vomiting, and abdominal pain. Patients with severely impaired hepatic or renal disease may be more sensitive to this drug and it should be used with great caution in such patients.

DRUG INTERACTIONS

Use with other vasodilators, antihypertensive agents, or alcohol increases the orthostatic hypotensive effect of nitroglycerin. A reduced effect of the following drugs has been noted when they are used concommitantly with nitroglycerin: acetylcholine, norepinephrine, histamine, and sympathomimetics.

PEARLS AND PITFALLS

1. The ulcerogenic potential of all agents used for injection therapy must be appreciated; in particular, even small volumes of ethanol can cause serositis and perforation. The sclerosis achieved is dependent on the balance struck between thrombosis, necrosis, and fibrosis.
2. Sodium morrhuate is thick, viscid, and passed with great difficulty through a 25-gauge sclerotherapy needle.
3. Nitroglycerin is readily absorbed by many plastics. Glass intravenous bottles should be used to dilute and store the drug. Filters that absorb nitroglycerin should be avoided. Common administration sets made of polyvinyl chloride (PVC) can absorb 40 to 80 percent of the total nitroglycerin. Since the loss is neither constant nor self-limited, it cannot be simply calculated or corrected for. Published trials have used PVC tubing and the recommended doses (25 µg/minute or more to start, as is recommended for cardiac patients), but these doses may be too high if administration sets with nonabsorbable materials are used.
4. Paradoxical bradycardia may accompany nitroglycerin-induced hypotension.

References

1. Ayres SJ, Goff JS, Warren GH. Endoscopic sclerotherapy for bleeding esophageal varices: Effects and complications. Ann Intern Med 1983; 98:900–903.

    A paper providing a better understanding of the sclerosing process and the anatomic basis for both the beneficial results and complications.

2. Brooks WS. Variceal sclerosing agents. Am J Gastro 1984; 79:424–428.

    This article discusses agents used in the United States and Europe: sodium morrhuate, tetradecyl sulfate, ethanolamine oleate, and polidocanol.

3. Camara DS. Update in injection sclerotherapy of esophageal varices. J Intens Care Med 1986; 1:171–177.

    Techniques and complications, as well as controlled and uncontrolled studies, are discussed.

4. Connors AF, Bacon BR, Miron SD. Sodium morrhuate delivery to the lung during endoscopic variceal sclerotherapy. Ann Intern Med 1986; 105:532–539.

    This study showed that pulmonary endothelium is exposed to small amounts of sodium morrhuate, and that no change in diffusing capacity is noted.

5. Fleisher D. Endoscopic therapy of upper gastrointestinal bleeding in humans. Gastroenterology 1986; 90:217–234.

    An outstanding overview, with in-depth discussion of the various hemostatic techniques and agents.

6. Groszman RJ. Drug therapy of portal hypertension. Am J Gastro 1987; 82:107–113.

    A review of the vasoconstrictors, vasodilators, and other miscellaneous agents that have shown potential use in the treatment of portal hypertension.

7. Gunson AE, et al. A randomized trial of vasopression plus nitroglycerin in the control of acute variceal hemorrhage. Hepatology 1986; 6:410–413.

    This study demonstrated the efficacy of combination therapy over vasopressin alone (68 versus 44%) in attaining hemostasis after 12 hours.

8. Hirao M, et al. Endoscopic local injection of hypertonic saline–epinephrine solution to arrest hemorrhage from the upper gastrointestinal tract. Gastro Endosc 1985; 31:313–317.

    Hemostasis was attained in 94.7% of bleeding gastric ulcers and 80% of bleeding duodenal ulcers. Retreatment was successful in most cases in which rebleeding occurred.

9. Jensen DM. Sclerosants for injection: Sclerosis of esophageal varices. Gastro Endosc 1983; 29:315–317.

    An article comparing the sclerosant potential of various agents.

10. Leung JWC, Chung SCS. Endoscopic injection of adrenaline in bleeding peptic ulcers. Gastro Endosc 1987; 33:73–75.

    Initial hemostasis was achieved in all patients, with definitive hemostasis in 34 out of 37 (92%).

11. Rector WG. Drug therapy for portal hypertension. Ann Intern Med 1986; 105:96–107.

An in-depth discussion of the pharmacology and rationale for selection of drugs used to treat portal hypertension.

12. Sugawa C, et al. Endoscopic hemostasis of bleeding of the upper gastrointestinal tract by local injection of 98-percent dehydrated ethanol. Surg Gyn Obstet 1986; 162:159–163.

   For bleeding from various lesions, hemostasis was accomplished in 88% of cases.

13. Tsai YT, et al. Controlled trial of vasopressin plus nitroglycerin versus vasopressin alone in the treatment of bleeding esophageal varices. Hepatology 1986; 6:406–409.

   This study demonstrated a strong trend toward efficacy (hemostasis at 24 hours) in favor of the combination therapy using sublingual nitroglycerin (45 versus 21%). Eighty-nine percent of the patients receiving vasopressin alone and 35% receiving the combination had complications.

41

Antimotility Agents

Robert Dolan and Michael S. Gurney

Gastrointestinal endoscopy, long recognized as an excellent diagnostic study, is now gaining wider recognition for its therapeutic potential. Polypectomy has been widely accepted for almost 2 decades. Sclerotherapy of esophageal varices, and now thermal treatment of nonvariceal bleeding, have been shown to be effective. The field of therapeutic biliary endoscopy is currently expanding rapidly.

The ability to suppress the natural motility of the gastrointestinal tract is of immense help in the exacting task of therapeutic endoscopy. Endoscopists have chiefly relied on two medications, atropine and glucagon, to stop peristalsis for these procedures. Their proper use has become part of the art of gastroenterology, yet controlled trials are few and written guidelines for their use are rare.

Atropine

Atropine is the principal alkaloid of the *Atropa belladonna* plant, and is the prototype of the naturally occurring anticholinergic agents. It has been used for centuries for its various potent anticholinergic properties, but has been used recently by endoscopists for its ability to reduce the motility and secretory activity of the gastrointestinal tract.

PHARMACOLOGY

Atropine competitively antagonizes acetylcholine at both M-1 and M-2 muscarinic receptor sites. It does not block transmission at either the neuromuscular junction or autonomic ganglia in clinical doses. This parasympatholytic effect reduces salivary secretion and gastric and intestinal motility.

The antimotility effect is pronounced because the parasympathetic nerves almost exclusively supply the extrinsic nervous motor control of the gut. Atropine has a less potent effect on gastric secretion and the smooth muscle of the bile ducts, gallbladder, ureters, bladder, and myometrium.

Atropine is well absorbed after oral administration and may also be given by the subcutaneous, intramuscular, or intravenous routes. It is also absorbed well when applied locally to any mucosal surface. The half-life is 2.5 hours, and most of the drug is renally excreted within 12 hours.

INDICATIONS

Atropine is rarely used now as a routine adjunct to gastrointestinal procedures. This decline in popularity is due to the high incidence of side effects and the emergence of glucagon as an equally effective but safer drug.

Atropine is very useful in decreasing the sialorrhea associated with esophageal obstruction from malignancy or tumor. It is also used to prevent vasovagal reactions during procedures such as peritoneoscopy, where preprocedure sedation may be minimal.

Anticholinergics may be used as an effective adjunct to histamine 2 antagonists in the treatment of resistant peptic ulcers, but the advent of selective anticholinergics such as pirenzipine has significantly reduced the use of atropine. The irritable bowel syndrome responds to anticholinergic drugs, but the systemic side effects of atropine limit its utility.

CONTRAINDICATIONS AND SIDE EFFECTS

Side effects noted with clinical doses of atropine include dryness of the mouth, anhidrosis, tachycardia, abdominal distension, and acute urinary retention. High doses may cause extreme dryness of the mouth, dysphagia, photophobia, fever, leukocytosis, vomiting, tachycardia, and hypotension or hypertension.

Ileus and toxic megacolon have occurred with atropine use in patients with inflammatory, ischemic, or amebic colitis. Its use in such conditions is generally contraindicated. Physostigmine may counteract these complications.

DOSAGE AND ADMINISTRATION

The usual dose of atropine is 0.3 to 1.0 milligrams every 4 to 6 hours via the oral, subcutaneous, intramuscular, or intravenous routes. Dryness of the mouth, along with the cardiac and cycloplegic effects of atropine, are often seen before gastrointestinal motility is reduced.

Glucagon

Glucagon is now the agent of choice for reducing gastroduodenal motility for upper endoscopy. Compared to anticholinergics, glucagon is superior in effect, causes less patient discomfort, and has fewer contraindications. Because of its prompt and transient antimotility capability, glucagon has become widely used for radiologic examinations as well as endoscopy.

PHARMACOLOGY

Glucagon is a straight-chain polypeptide hormone containing 29 amino acids, normally produced by the alpha cells of the pancreas. Following intravenous administration, glucagon's spasmolytic effect on the gut begins within 30 to 60 seconds and lasts about 7 minutes. Glucagon is extensively degraded in the liver, kidney, and plasma through enzymatic proteolysis. The elimination half-life is 3 to 6 minutes.

Glucagon inhibits gastric, duodenal, and colonic motility as well as gastric and pancreatic secretion. The mechanism by which glucagon includes a spasmolytic effect on the gut remains unexplained. Early studies showed that there was no relation between glucagon's effect on bowel motility and its metabolic effect on glucose and insulin release. It is postulated that glucagon may have a direct effect on smooth muscle, or act indirectly by inducing catecholamine release from the adrenal glands.

Glucagon's metabolic actions are antagonistic to those of insulin. Blood glucose is raised through increased glycogenolysis and gluconeogenesis.

INDICATIONS

Glucagon is indicated for the elective induction of temporary paralysis of the gastrointestinal tract in order to facilitate diagnostic or therapeutic procedures. It is particularly useful as an aid to cannulation of the sphincter of Oddi, for gastric or duodenal polypectomy, and to coagulate difficult bleeding lesions. It is also the most widely used drug for barium studies of the gastrointestinal tract.

DOSAGE

Glucagon should be prepared in a solution with a concentration of 1 milligram/milliliter and given in a dose of 0.1 to 0.5 milligram intravenously. A total dose of 1 milligram can usually be given without problems. Total doses of 1 to 2 milligrams are safe but have an increased incidence of side effects.

CONTRAINDICATIONS AND SIDE EFFECTS

Glucagon is known to stimulate catecholamine and insulin release; therefore, absolute contraindications include pheochromocytoma and insulinoma. In pheochromocytoma, there is a sudden, clinically evident release of catecholamines within minutes, but with insulinoma, the hypoglycemic effects may not be apparent for hours.

The incidence of side effects is markedly lower than with anticholinergic agents. In early studies, in which relatively large doses were used (1–2 mg), nausea, vomiting, and headache were relatively common. These side effects are seen infrequently with the above recommended dose. Interestingly, even with the early, larger doses there was no significant effect on pulse or blood pressure.

PEARLS AND PITFALLS

1. Glucagon is inactivated rapidly after the solution is prepared. It should be reconstituted only immediately prior to administration, or stored in a refrigerator.
2. One milligram of intravenous glucagon can relieve the esophageal spasm associated with meat impaction and allow spontaneous passage of the food bolus.
3. Both atropine and glucagon can cause significant abdominal distension. Endoscopists should be judicious in their

use of air during procedures where these medications are used.
4. Children are much more sensitive than adults to the effects of atropine. Explanation of expected side effects and use of the lowest doses may help avoid some problems.
5. Concomitant use of glucagon and atropine does not provide additional benefit, but does increase the incidence of side effects.
6. Atropine can be very helpful for the reduction of sialorrhea in esophageal obstruction.

References

1. Cattau EL Jr, et al. Efficacy of atropine as an endoscopic premedication. Gastro Endosc 1983; 29:285.

   Atropine, as a routine endoscopic premedication, did not improve the ease of endoscopy or improve patient tolerance. The amount of oral secretions was reduced.

2. Feczko PJ, Haggar AM, Halpert RD. A reappraisal of upper gastrointestinal response to low-dose glucagon. CRC Crit Rev Diag Imag 1986; 23:377.

   A thorough review of the biochemistry, pharmacology, and physiologic actions of glucagon. The article also concisely summarizes the diagnostic and therapeutic uses of glucagon in gastroenterology. An excellent resource.

3. Feczko PJ, et al. Gastroduodenal response to low-dose glucagon. AJR 1983; 140:935.

   A prospective, double-blind clinical study.

4. Gerner T, Myren J, Larsen S. Premedication in upper gastrointestinal endoscopy. Scand J Gastro 1983; 18:925.

   A double-blind, randomized study comparing glucagon and atropine, given in combination with diazepam and prethidine, concluding that glucagon is preferable to atropine.

5. Gilman AG, et al. A concise review of the chemistry and pharmacology of glucagon. In *Goodman and Gilman's The Pharmacologic Basis of Therapeutics* 7th ed. New York: Macmillan, 1985. Pp 1510–1512.

6. Ivey KJ. Are anticholinergics of use in the irritable colon syndrome? Gastroenterology 1975; 68:1300.

   A thorough, critical review on the use of anticholinergics in irritable bowel patients.

Iodinated Contrast Agents

John Mehegan

Iodinated contrast media were introduced in the 1920s to aid in vascular and urographic imaging. They are now among the most widely used diagnostic agents, with over 15 million contrast injections given annually in the United States and Europe. These agents are extremely safe, but with an incidence of anaphylactoid reactions occurring in 1 to 2 percent of cases, there are a significant number of deaths attributable to contrast reactions. For those with a prior history of contrast reactions, a prophylactic treatment to prevent recurrence is of proven benefit.

Standard ionic contrast agents are sodium, meglumine, or mixed salts of a tri-iodinated benzoic acid derivative. These agents are used in concentrations ranging from 24 to 90 percent. For use in endoscopic retrograde cholangiopancreatography (ERCP), a concentration of 30 percent is needed for optimal visualization. At this concentration, contrast media are hyperosmolar, with an osmolarity of 750 milliosmoles/kilogram. These agents have a low molecular weight and are biologically inert. These properties allow them to be freely filtered by the glomerulus, with a half-life for renal clearance of 75 to 128 minutes. Newer contrast media introduced to the U.S. market over the last 5 years are nonionic and have an osmolarity one half that of standard agents. The decreased osmolarity results in significant reduction in toxicity. However, the cost of these agents is 20 times that of standard contrast media and consequently the indications for their general use are still to be defined.

SIDE EFFECTS

Adverse reactions can be separated into chemical effects and hypersensitivity reactions. The chemical effects are the result of the injection of a hyperosmolar ionic solution. This can result in toxicities such as arrhythmias, renal failure, pulmonary edema, and cerebral injury. For the gastroenterologist, these effects are minimized because little contrast agent injected into the pancreatic or biliary systems is absorbed.

Hypersensitivity reactions are immediate and idiosyncratic, resulting in any combination of wheezing, urticaria, angioedema, laryngeal edema, pruritus, hypotension, or vascular collapse. These are not dose-dependent effects and can occur on minimal exposure. No single pathogenic mechanism has been found to explain hypersensitivity to contrast agents. Contrast allergy mimics classic IgE-mediated responses. However, these reactions can occur on first exposure, and circulating antibodies to contrast agents are rarely found. Histamine levels are elevated in some patients after contrast exposure, but do not correlate well with allergic response. Radiocontrast agents can both activate factor XII and inhibit angiotensin-converting enzyme.

These conditions favor the release and potentiation of bradykinin, which is proposed as a major mediator of anaphylactoid reactions. It is likely that several different mechanisms contribute to the allergic response.

Two groups of patients are recognized as being at increased risk for contrast hypersensitivity. Those with a history of clinical allergies are 2 to 3 times as likely to have an acute reaction. The second group consists of those with a prior history of adverse contrast reactions. The likelihood of a subsequent reaction in this group is between 35 and 60 percent. The type of previous reaction does not predict the severity of subsequent response, and at present there are no predictive tests to identify those at high risk for recurrence. The treatment for an anaphylactoid response to contrast is standard, consisting of intravenous fluids, SQ epinephrine (0.3 cc, 1:1000), antihistamines (IV diphenhydramine, 50 mg), steroids (IV hydrocortisone, 200 mg) and observation on a cardiac monitor.

PROPHYLAXIS OF CONTRAST-AGENT ALLERGY

When performing contrast injections in high-risk patients, the physician must ensure that there is an essential indication for the procedure, explain the risks to the patient, attempt to prevent adverse reactions with a pretreatment regimen, and respond with emergency measures as needed. Several different pretreatment regimens have been proposed. There are no randomized, controlled trials demonstrating the benefit of any one regimen for preventing recurrence, but there is convincing evidence, based on historically controlled trials, that pretreatment with steroids does provide protection. A standard regimen would include the following:

1. Fifty milligrams of prednisone given orally 12, 6, and 1 hour prior to the procedure. For emergency procedures, 200 milligrams of hydrocortisone given at least 4 to 6 hours prior to the procedure also appears to provide protection.

2. An antihistamine such as diphenhydramine, 50 milligrams given orally 1 hour before the procedure.

This protocol reduces the incidence of adverse reactions to 5 to 10 percent, and most of these reactions are mild. Some radiologists would include ephedrine sulfate, 25 milligrams orally 1 hour before the procedure. This is reported to decrease the reaction rate to 3 percent. The use of an H_2-antagonist such as cimetidine is controversial. In one trial, the incidence of anaphylactoid reactions increased following the addition of this agent.

Prophylactic treatment regimens greatly reduce the risk of reactions in a patient with previous hypersensitivity. The short-term use of high-dose steroids and antihistamines is extremely safe, and they should be used in patients with any question of previous reaction. Note that there is still concern for a life-threatening reaction despite prophylactic treatment: Three of 15 deaths in a series of 912,000 patients occurred in pretreated patients.

PEARLS AND PITFALLS

1. Radiocontrast agents are extremely safe for general use, with much of their toxicity resulting from their hyperosmolarity. This is not a specific concern in use during ERCP because there is little absorption from the pancreatic or biliary tree.
2. The incidence of anaphylactoid reactions during intravascular procedures is 1 to 2 percent. The incidence during ERCP is significantly less than this. These reactions are idiosyncratic and can occur on exposure to minimal amounts of the agent.
3. In those with prior adverse reactions to contrast, the risk of a repeat reaction on subsequent exposure is as high as 60 percent. Pretreatment regimens that include steroids and diphenhydramine reduce the risk to 5 to 10 percent.
4. Steroids should be administered at least 12 hours prior to elective procedures to derive benefit.

References

1. Abrams HL. The opaque media: Physiologic effects and systemic reactions. In HL Abrams (ed), *Abrams' Angiography*. Boston: Little, Brown, 1983.

    Historic perspective and characterization of the standard contrast media. A review of the adverse effects with emphasis on the chemical toxicities as they pertain to angiography of specific organ systems.

2. Bettmann MA, Morris TW. Recent advances in contrast agents. Rad Clin N Am 1986; 3:347–357.

    Characterization of the newer contrast agents, with emphasis on the biologic properties that provide for lower toxicity. These agents appear safer in human and animal studies; however, the 20-times increase in cost precludes their replacing standard agents for general use.

3. Bilbao MK, et al. Complications of endoscopic retrograde cholangiopancreatography (ERCP): A study of 10,000 cases. Gastroenterology 1976; 70:314–320.

    Fifty-one adverse reactions were attributed to the use of drugs during ERCP. Of these, only three (0.03%) were caused by contrast. This is compared to the 5 to 10% rate for intravascular injections of contrast.

4. Greenberger PA. Contrast media reactions. J Allerg Clin Immunol 1984; 74:600–605.

    A review of the incidence, proposed mechanisms, and efficacy of prophylactic measures in preventing recurrence of hypersensitivity to contrast media.

5. Greenberger PA, Patterson R, Tapio CM. Prophylaxis against repeated radiocontrast media reactions in 857 cases. Arch Intern Med 1985; 145:2197–2200.

    A prospective study comparing different pretreatment regimens in preventing contrast reactions. The best regimen included prednisone, diphenhydramine, and ephedrine, with a 3% reaction rate. The addition of cimetidine appeared to increase the incidence of adverse reactions.

6. Greenberger PA, et al. Emergency administration of radiocontrast media in high-risk patients. J Allérg Clin Immunol 1986; 77:630–634.

    No reactions to contrast occurred in nine patients with a previous history of contrast allergy pretreated with intravenous hydrocortisone, given 2 to 6 hours prior to emergency angiographic procedures.

7. Lasser EC. Adverse reactions to contrast material. In JE Berk (ed), *Bockus Gastroenterology*. Philadelphia: Saunders, 1985.

    A review of contrast allergy and means of prevention.

8. Lasser EC, et al. Pretreatment with corticosteroids to alleviate reactions to intravenous contrast material. NEJM 1987; 317:845–849.

    A randomized, placebo-controlled trial involving 6763 patients that demonstrated the efficacy of a regimen of prednisone given 12 hours prior to contrast exposure in preventing allergic reactions. A regimen of prednisone given 2 hours prior to exposure did not afford any protection. These patients did not have a history of prior contrast allergy.

9. Sable RA, et al. Absorption of contrast medium during ERCP. Dig Dis Sci 1983; 28:801–806.

    Contrast is absorbed during ERCP, as detected by measuring serum levels. The highest level of absorbtion was from pancreatic duct injection.

10. Shehadi WH. Adverse reactions to intravascularly administered contrast media: A comprehensive study based on a prospective survey. Am J Roentgenol 1975; 124:145–152.

    A prospective survey of 112,003 patients undergoing contrast injections. The incidence of reactions ranged from 2 to 5%, depending on the procedure. The incidence of death was 1:10,000.

11. Shehadi WH. Contrast media adverse reactions: Occurrence, recurrence, and distribution patterns. Radiology 1982; 143:11–17.

    An extension of the previous study. A prospective evaluation of contrast reactions in over 300,000 patients, this paper describes the types of reactions that occur in patients with prior adverse reactions. The authors found a general tendency against life-threatening reactions recurring in the same individuals.

43

Naloxone Hydrochloride

Robert Dolan

Naloxone is the agent of choice for narcotic-induced respiratory depression, sedation, and hypotension. It is a "pure" narcotic antagonist, devoid of known agonist activity. Because of naloxone's dramatic ability to rapidly reverse narcotic intoxication with minimal side effects, it has become a popular drug in the emergency ward and the procedure suite.

PHARMACOLOGY

Naloxone is a synthetic N-allyl derivative of oxymorphone. It is usually administered intravenously but may be given subcutaneously, intramuscularly, endotracheally, or intraglossaly. Because of significant first-pass metabolism, an oral dose is only one fiftieth as potent as parenteral administration (Table 43–1). Following parenteral administration, the drug is rapidly distributed throughout the body, with an estimated volume of distribution of about 200 liters. Onset of action is within 1 to 3 minutes following intravenous administration and only slightly longer following intramuscular and subcutaneous administration. Onset of action is related to how rapidly naloxone enters the brain. The brain-to-serum ratio of naloxone is 12 to 15 times higher than that of morphine.

Naloxone is primarily metabolized in the liver, by glucuronide conjugation, and excreted in the urine. The elimination half-life in the adult is 30 to 100 minutes (average, 60 minutes). The duration of action is from 1 to 4 hours, depending on the dose and route of administration.

MECHANISM OF ACTION

Naloxone's mechanism of action is not fully understood, but available evidence suggests that it antagonizes narcotic effects by competing for the same receptor site. Of the known, different opiate receptors, naloxone has no definite agonist effect; i.e., no respiratory depression, pupillary constriction, or psychomimetic effects. It is nonaddicting and not subject to narcotics-control laws.

INDICATIONS

Naloxone is indicated for complete or partial reversal of acute narcotic intoxication and overdose. Signs of acute intoxication include hypothermia, hypotension, stupor, constricted pupils, convulsions, hypoventilation, and irregular pulse.

Untoward or exaggerated reactions to normal doses of narcotics may occur because of underlying illness or concurrent treatment with other drugs. Respiratory depression may be augmented secondary to reduced sensitivity to hy-

Table 43–1. Pharmacological properties of naloxone (intravenous)

Onset of action: 1–3 minutes
Maximum effect: 5–10 minutes
Elimination of half-life: about 1 hour
Duration of effect: 1–4 hours
Doses: 0.1–0.2 mg IV every 1–2 minutes
      up to 0.4–2 mg IV in adults and 0.01 mg/kg in children, neonates
Continuous IV infusion: 2 mg/500 ml for a concentration of 0.004 mg/ml titrated to response (0.4–0.8 mg/hr)

---

percapnia, decreased respiratory reserve, or decreased hepatic metabolism of narcotics, as seen with myxedema, chronic obstructive lung disease, asthma, obesity, severe liver disease, or concurrent cimetidine therapy.

DOSAGE

Naloxone is supplied at a concentration of 0.4 millligrams/milliliter in 1- and 10-milliliter ampules. For known or suspected narcotic overdose, the initial dose should be 0.4 to 2 milligrams intravenously (one to five 1-cc ampules) repeated every 2 to 3 minutes. If there is no clinical response after 10 milligrams (twenty-five 1-cc ampules), acute narcotic intoxication is unlikely.

During diagnostic or therapeutic procedures, naloxone may be given in smaller doses of 0.1 to 0.2 milligrams intravenously every 1 to 2 minutes, titrated to the desired clinical effect. Smaller doses are preferable in patients who have been under the effects of large doses of narcotics for several hours, as they may be acutely physically dependent, and excessive doses of naloxone may precipitate withdrawal. This is clinically apparent as nausea, vomiting, tachypnea, tachycardia, mydriasis, elevated blood pressure, anxiety, and hyperalgesia.

There are no specific dosage adjustments necessary for renal insufficiency. Information is lacking on dosage adjustments for hepatic insufficiency. Investigational uses for naloxone include refractory shock, reversal of alcohol-induced coma, reversal of neurological deficits in the setting of cerebral ischemia, and chronic idiopathic constipation.

SIDE EFFECTS AND CONTRAINDICATIONS

With rare exceptions, the use of naloxone in any dose has been demonstrated to be free of adverse effects. Doses up to 24 milligrams are reported to cause only slight drowsiness. There are several cases of cardiac dysrhythmias and pulmonary edema following naloxone-induced arousal after narcotic anesthesia. However, these cases may have resulted from a sympathetic discharge by the abrupt onset of postoperative pain. The use of naloxone in narcotic addicts may precipitate a withdrawal syndrome, which is not life threatening and is amenable to pharmacologic therapy. There are also case reports of naloxone-induced pulmonary edema.

The only contraindication to naloxone is a previously documented hypersensitivity.

PEARLS AND PITFALLS

1. While waiting for naloxone to reverse narcotic-induced respiratory depression, hypotension, and sedation, remember to always maintain a free airway, provide artificial ventilation, and provide cardiopulmonary resuscitation or intravenous volume, as dictated by the patient's clinical condition.
2. If the patient is hypotensive and without intravenous access, naloxone can be injected into the venous plexus on the inferior surface of the tongue or given endotracheally.
3. During initial narcotic reversal, emesis may occur; therefore, guard against aspiration and have suction available.
4. As naloxone's duration of action is shorter than most narcotics, signs and symptoms of narcotic overdose may recur after 30 to 60 minutes. The requirement for repeat doses (given intravenously at 1- to 2-hour intervals or as a continuous intravenous infusion) is dependent on the amount, type, and route of administration of the narcotic being antagonized.

References

1. Allen T. Narcotic antagonists. In R Rosen (ed), *Emergency Medicine Concepts and Clinical Practice* vol 2. St Louis: Mosby, 1988.

    A thorough and pragmatic approach to narcotic overdose and management.

2. Easom JM, Lovejoy FA. Opiates. In LM Haddal, JF Winchester (eds), *Clinical Management of Poisoning and Drug Overdose*. Philadelphia: Saunders, 1983.

    A comprehensive guide to the diagnosis and management of drug overdoses.

3. Evans LEJ, et al. Treatment of drug overdosage with naloxone, a specific narcotic antagonist. *Lancet* 1973; 1:452.

    This paper details the physiologic changes induced by naloxone in narcotic- and nonnarcotic-induced coma.

4. Handal KA, Schauben JL, Salamone FR. Naloxone. Ann Emerg Med 1983; 12:438.

    A comprehensive review of the biochemistry and clinical use of naloxone.

5. Jaffe J, Martin WR. Opioid analgesics and antagonists. In LS Goodman, A Gilman (eds), *The Pharmacologic Basis of Therapeutics* vol 7. New York: Macmillan, 1985.

    A concise review of opioid antagonists.

6. Martin WR. Naloxone. Ann Intern Med 1976; 85:765.

    A concise review covering the theory and history of narcotic antagonists as well as the approved and unapproved uses of naloxone.
7. McNicholas LF, Martin WR. New experimental and therapeutic roles for naloxone and related opioid antagonists. Drugs 1984., 27:81

    A review of endogenous opioids and their roles in the physiologic regulation of various systems and pathologic processes.
8. Milne B, Jramendas K. Naloxone: New therapeutic roles. Can Anaesth Soc J 1984; 31:3.

    A review of naloxone use for septic shock, spinal cord injury, stroke, and nonopiate—induced respiratory depression.
9. Prough DS, et al. Acute pulmonary edema in healthy teenagers following conservative doses of intravenous naloxone. Anesthesiology 1984; 60:485.

    Two case reports of healthy young males developing acute pulmonary edema after naloxone, without other apparent causes.

VII

Other Agents

44
Somatostatin
Michael S. Gurney

Somatostatin is now at a stage of development similar to that of cimetidine in the late 1970s: It has demonstrated, profound effects on gastrointestinal physiology and diseases, with very few adverse reactions. Initially, it was isolated from the rat hypothalamus and found to inhibit the release of growth hormone. Since then, it has been found to inhibit a long list of regulatory peptides—especially those in the gastrointestinal tract—and has earned the nickname *endocrine cyanide*. It has been applied to hormone-producing tumors of the gastrointestinal tract with remarkable success. Somatostatin's further influence on intestinal functions such as secretion, motility, and absorption has now been realized, and its efficacy for a number of other gastrointestinal problems is being reported as clinical experience grows.

PHARMACOLOGY

Natural somatostatin is a 14-amino-acid peptide with a disulfide bond. Because its half-life is less than 3 minutes and it is not orally absorbed, use is restricted to constant intravenous infusion. To avoid these drawbacks an octapeptide, Sandostatin (SMS 201–995), has been developed and extensively tested. Sandostatin has a half-life of 113 minutes, and plasma levels are detectable up to 12 hours after administration. It retains the activity of the natural hormone and is effective in subcutaneous injections every 6 to 12 hours. Approximately 10 percent of Sandostatin is renally excreted; the remaining 90 percent is systemically metabolized.

Somatostatin and its analogue inhibit release of the following hormones: growth hormone, gastrin, insulin, secretin, cholecystokinin, vasoactive intestinal peptide, gastrin-inhibiting peptide, motilin, and TSH. It does not inhibit prolactin, follicle-stimulating hormone, or leutinizing hormone. Its physiologic properties include inhibition of gastric acid secretion (independent of gastrin inhibition), slowing of gut motility, and inhibition of both carbohydrate absorption and pancreatic enzyme secretion. It also inhibits intestinal secretion in hypersecretory states such as the Zollinger-Ellison syndrome. It is unknown whether these effects are due to its endocrine-modulating properties or an independent effect of the drug.

INDICATIONS

The clearest indication for Sandostatin is in the treatment of hormone-producing islet cell tumors of the gastrointestinal tract. Islet cell tumors are slow growing, and patients can live for many years with metastatic disease. However, because of the release of biologically active peptides, these tumors can produce symptoms out of proportion to their size, and patients may have disabling symptoms or even die as a consequence of the peptide production. Thus, inhibition of these secretagogues is critically important in the management of patients afflicted with these syndromes. For the most part, therapy with other drugs has, to date, been ineffective or associated with significant side effects.

Gastrinoma causes the Zollinger-Ellison syndrome of gastric acid hypersecretioen, peptic ulceration, and diarrhea. It is the one islet cell tumor where therapy is well developed: High-dose H_2 blockers, surgery, and omeprazole have drastically reduced the morbidity and mortality. However, the side effects of high-dose H_2 blockers can be significant, and the issue of carcinoid-tumor patients on long-term omeprazole may limit its use too. Sandostatin may fill a valuable niche in such patients since it is well tolerated and has been shown in several trials to effectively suppress both acid production and gastrin release. Gastrin levels have fallen in 93 percent of treated patients; peptic ulcers, abdominal pain, and diarrhea have been relieved in 70 to 90 percent of patients. The true impact of Sandostatin is unclear, however, since concomitant therapy has not always been clearly stated in reports. One report has shown that chronic Sandostatin therapy reduced basal and maximal acid output, indicating that the medication may be able to reverse the trophic effect of chronically elevated gastrin levels on the stomach. The effectiveness of Sandostatin is dose-related, with starting doses ranging from 50 micrograms twice a day to 150 micrograms 4 times a day. As in other islet cell syndromes, the dose may be increased if greater efficacy is needed. Doses reported for patients receiving chronic therapy have ranged from 50 to 1500 micrograms per day.

VIPoma is also known as the Verner-Morrison syndrome, the WDHA syndrome, or pancreatic cholera. It is characterized by voluminous, watery diarrhea, hypokalemia, hypochlorhydia, and occasionally, hypocalcemia and hypophosphatemia. No clinical trials of Sandostatin use have been reported, but multiple case reports have been published. VIP levels fell during therapy in 16 out of 18 patients, but levels subsequently rose in five. Symptomatic response has been even more impressive, possibly because somatostatin not only inhibits VIP release, but also slows gut motility and combats intestinal secretion at the cellular level. Over 80 percent of patients whose symptoms were resistant to other therapies have had dramatic clinical improvement. Initial treatment doses have ranged from 50 or 100 micrograms twice a day to 150 micrograms 4 times a day. A curious feature is that in some patients the VIP suppression is prolonged, allowing a lengthening of the dosing interval to even an as-needed basis. Sandostatin represents a significant therapeutic advance in the therapy of clinical manifestations in VIPoma.

Glucagonoma, a rare malignancy of the pancreatic alpha cells, is characterized by a unique necrolytic skin rash, anemia, weight loss, glucose intolerance, and occasionally, diarrhea. Twelve patients have been reported to have received

Sandostatin for this disorder. Glucagon levels fell in nine of the 12 but reached normal levels in only one. The rash resolved over several days in eight of the nine patients who had this manifestation of the tumor. Weight loss, anemia, pain, and diarrhea improved in all patients with those symptoms, but the glucose intolerance did not improve. The change in glucagon level did not necessarily correlate with rash improvement. This suggests that the drug may have an independent effect on the skin, which is supported by the fact that Sandostatin is also beneficial in psoriasis. The dose used in the reports ranged from 50 milligrams twice a day to 150 micrograms 4 times a day. Occasionally the rash has recurred despite maintenance Sandostatin; in each case it responded to an increased dose. Sandostatin appears to be an extremely valuable addition to the therapy of glucagonoma.

Insulinoma causes hypoglycemia with associated autonomic symptoms and bizarre behavioral changes. In contrast to the other islet cell tumors, the majority of insulinomas are benign and amenable to surgical removal if identified. Sandostatin has been administered to 20 patients with insulinoma. Although plasma insulin concentrations fell in 12, a reduction in hypoglycemic episodes has been noted only occasionally. In long-term administration, about 50 percent of patients have had improved glucose control. Doses in the long-term cases have ranged from 50 micrograms twice a day to 500 micrograms 4 times a day. Since Sandostatin does not seem to have a dramatic impact on insulinoma, it is fortunate that most patients are either cured by surgery or have symptoms ameliorated by conventional therapy with diazoxide.

The issue of tumor regression with Sandostatin is often discussed. At least 46 patients have had reported islet cell tumor response to Sandostatin. A decrease in the size of metastases was seen in eight, there was no change in 18, and enlarging metastases were noted in 20. This 17-percent response rate may represent an overestimate, since positive results are more apt to be reported. In the study of 22 metastatic islet cell tumors by Kvols, no tumor regression was noted. Nevertheless, the analogue inhibits tumor growth in certain animal models, and considerable interest exists in this aspect of Sandostatin therapy.

The carcinoid syndrome is caused by metastatic gastrointestinal carcinoid tumor or bronchial carcinoid. The tumor's release of serotonin, its precursors, and other peptides into the circulation is associate with flushing, diarrhea, and abdominal pain. The carcinoid syndrome has been well studied with respect to Sandostatin therapy by Kvols. He treated 25 patients with 150 micrograms 4 times a day; flushing and diarrhea were promptly relieved in 22. Three-fourths had a 50-percent or greater reduction in urinary 5HIAA levels. Over 75 percent of the responders had continued symptom relief after a median therapy duration of a year. Vinik treated three such patients with lower doses (50–150 μg bid) and demonstrated relief of symptoms in all, but serotonin levels fell in only one. The effect of the analogue on long-term sequelae, such as right-sided cardiac valve stenosis and mesenteric sclerosis, has not been studied. Sandostatin has also been used successfully to reverse and prevent the "carcinoid crisis" associated with anesthesia induction or surgical manipulation of the tumor. The demonstrated efficacy of Sandostatin in the carcinoid syndrome is far greater than any medical therapy currently available.

Sandostatin may serve as a useful adjunct in the treatment of pancreatic or small intestinal fistulae since it significantly decreases gastrointestinal secretion. Currently, such fistulae are managed by complete bowel rest and total parenteral nutrition; closure occurs slowly, if at all. Two investigators have used natural somatostatin to heal such fistulae. Geerdsen reported closure of four out of four small bowel cutaneous fistulae in an average of 14 days. The average hospital stay for conventional therapy was 95 days, with a mortality rate of 34 percent. He used a constant intravenous infusion of somatostatin, 250 micrograms/hour. Pederzoli treated 45 patients with external pancreatic fistulae with total parenteral nutrition, bowel rest, and either somatostatin, calcitonin, or glucagon. All regimens closed 85 to 100 percent of the fistulae, but only somatostatin significantly reduced the closure time, to 6 days, versus an average of 30 days for all other methods. He gave native somatostatin, 250 micrograms/hour by constant infusion, for the first 3 to 4 days, then decreased the rate to 125 micrograms/hour until fistula closure. Kingsworth reported failure of fistula closure with somatostatin in six patients, but only used the drug for 4 days before stopping.

Somatostatin decreases splanchnic blood flow and suppresses gastric acid secretion, making it an appealing medication for gastrointestinal bleeding. However, clinical trials have shown only mixed results when the drug is given for all bleeding causes. Variceal hemorrhage does seem to benefit from somatostatin. In three prospective trials, somatostatin infusion without sclerotherapy stopped bleeding in nearly 80 percent of patients. No adverse effects were noted. Conventional therapy with vasopressin alone stops bleeding in only 50 percent of cases, with a morbidity rate of 15 to 25 percent from vasopressin itself.

Somatostatin has been shown to improve experimental pancreatitis in animals. However, a trial of somatostatin infusions, 250 micrograms/hour, in moderate to severe pancreatitis did not reduce the rate of complications. The mortality rate was decreased but not significantly so. Perhaps earlier administration of somatostatin or a larger sample size would demonstrate benefit. A trial using prophylactic Sandostatin to prevent ERCP-associated pancreatitis is currently underway.

Because Sandostatin is well tolerated and has a significant effect on gastrointestinal function, it will be given for a wide variety of disorders in the future. Case reports showing efficacy for the following problems already exist: irritable bowel syndrome, diabetic diarrhea, ileostomy diarrhea, idiopathic secretory diarrhea in infancy, and postgastrectomy dumping syndrome. Only imagination, clinical trials, and further clinical experience can tell what the final indications for somatostatin will be.

CONTRAINDICATIONS AND SIDE EFFECTS

There is no absolute contraindication to somatostatin use. Hypersensitivity has not been reported, and the development of a blocking antibody has not occurred in clinical trials. The most common side effect is local irritation at the injection site. This can be minimized by warming the syringe in the palms before injection, and by injecting slowly. Cramping, bloating, or nausea are common complaints during the first week or 2 of therapy but usually disappear with time. If stool fat is analyzed before and during therapy, as many as 60 percent of patients have steatorrhea. This is rarely clinically significant. It is thought to occur from inhibition of gallbladder contraction and pancreatic secretion. The steatorrhea is partially reversible with oral pancreatic enzyme replacement and also improves on its own, with time. Mild glucose intolerance has been noted in some patients, but glucose control in diabetic patients does not change significantly. About 50 percent of patients in clinical trials have had one of the mentioned side effects, but the complaints are usually minor and temporary, and they have never been severe enough to stop the medication. Since gallbladder contraction is decreased by somatostatin, and since cholelithiasis is characteristic of somatostatinomas, there is a theoretic risk of gallstones developing as a consequence of therapy. This complication has not yet been reported.

DOSAGE AND ADMINISTRATION

Natural somatostatin must be given by continuous intravenous infusion. The dose used in clinical trials is 3 to 3.5 micrograms/kilogram/hour.

Sandostatin, the synthetic analogue, is given by subcutaneous injections similar to insulin administration. The starting dose is 50 micrograms 2 or 3 times per day. Clinical benefit is often apparent within days. The dose can be increased without difficulty, if needed, to 150 micrograms 4 times a day. The medication is well tolerated and higher doses can be used, but a favorable response is unlikely if no effect was noted at the lower doses. An oral preparation has shown good absorption and is currently in clinical trials.

PEARLS AND PITFALLS

1. Steatorrhea often develops during somatostatin therapy, but it is usually mild and improves with oral pancreatic enzyme supplements.
2. Preoperative somatostatin treatment can help prevent carcinoid crisis caused by the induction of anesthesia or surgical manipulation of the tumor. Carcinoid crisis is

manifested by an intense flush, profound hypotension, and bronchospasm.
3. Development of a blocking antibody to somatostatin has not been a problem to date. Decreased clinical response in tumor syndromes may be due to increased hormone production or loss of a somatostatin receptor within the tumor.
4. Mild hyperglycemia may develop in nondiabetic patients; this problem often improves after a month of treatment. Paradoxically, diabetics have no decrease (and may have an improvement) in glucose control.
5. VIP can be suppressed for long periods of time with somatostatin, and injections can often be decreased to an as-needed basis.
6. Caution should be used when somatostatin is stopped. There have been several reports of dramatic rebound of tumor hormone secretion when the drug is abruptly discontinued.
7. Warming the syringe prior to injection by rolling it between the palms can reduce local irritation at the injection site. Slower injection rates also decrease pain at the injection site.

References

1. Bauer W, et al. SMS 201–995: A very potent and selective octapeptide analogue of somatostatin with prolonged action. Life Sci 1982; 31:1133.

   An article from the manufacturer about much of the basic pharmacology for their analogue, Sandostatin.

2. Bloom S, Polak J. Somatostatin—Regular review. BMJ 1987; 295:288.

   A short, general review of somatostatin and its analogue.

3. Creutzfeldt W, et al. Effect of somatostatin analogue on pancreatic secretion in humans. AJM 1987; 5b:49.

   An excellent basic-science study of the drug's effect on pancreatic physiology. The data provide an explanation for the common side effect, steatorrhea.

4. Dudl RJ, et al. Treatment of diabetic diarrhea and orthostatic hypotension with somatostatin analogue SMS 201–995. AJM 1987; 83:584.

   A well-documented case report showing good clinical benefit for the unfortunate patient with these complications of severe diabetes.

5. Gordon P, et al. Somatostatin and somatostatin analogue (SMS 201–995) in treatment of hormone-secreting tumors of the pituitary and gastrointestinal tract and non-neoplastic diseases of the gut. AIM 1989; 110:35–50.

   The many uses of somatostatin are reviewed in this comprehensive article. Somatostatin is the drug of choice for non-resectable pituitary thyrotropin-producing tumors, for carcinoid syndrome and carcinoid crisis, and pancreatic islet cell tumors that produce vasoactive intestinal peptide.

6. Jaros W, et al. Successful treatment of idiopathic secretory diarrhea of infancy with the somatostatin analogue SMS 201–995. Gastroenterology 1988; 94:189.

   A case report with a good discussion. Sandostatin safely and effectively reduced stool output from 250 ml/kg/day to 80 ml/kg/day.

7. Jenkins SA, et al. A prospective, controlled clinical trial comparing somatostatin and vasopressin in acute variceal hemorrhage. BMJ 1985; 290:275.

   Somatostatin, in this controlled trial, was superior to vasopressin in both efficacy and side effects.

8. Kvols LK, et al. Rapid reversal of carcinoid crisis with somatostatin analogue. NEJM 1985; 313:1229.

   Sandostatin was used intraoperatively, with dramatic effect, in a carcinoid crisis.

9. Kvols LK, et al. Treatment of the malignant carcinoid syndrome. NEJM 1986; 315:663.

   Sandostatin was used to treat the peripheral effects of metastatic carcinoid tumors. Symptoms were relieved in 22 of 25 patients, and 5HIAA levels fell significantly in 18.

10. Kvols LK, et al. Treatment of metastatic islet cell carcinoma with a somatostatin analogue (SMS 201–995). Ann Int Med 1987; 107:162.

    An excellent study of 22 patients with malignant islet cell carcinoma. These tumors are difficult to manage with conventional therapy, but good results were seen with Sandostatin.

11. Maton PN, Gardner JD, Jensen RT. The use of the long-acting somatostatin analogue SMS 201–995 in patients with pancreatic islet cell tumors. Dig Dis Sci (in press).

    An outstanding review of the published experience with Sandostatin therapy for islet cell tumors of all types.

12. Pederzoli P, et al. Conservative treatment of external pancreatic fistulas with parenteral nutrition alone or in combination with continuous infusion of somatostatin, glucagon, or calcitonin. Surg, Gyn, and Obstet 1986; 162:428.

    Somatostatin decreased the fistula closure time from 31 to 6 days, saving an estimated $2100 per patient.

13. Souquet J, et al. Clinical and hormonal effects of a long-acting somatostatin analogue in pancreatic endocrine tumors and in carcinoid syndrome. Cancer 1987; 59:1654.

    A series of patients treated with Sandostatin is reported. The results were good even though duration of treatment was often short.

14. Talley N, Turner I, Middleton W. Somatostatin and symptomatic relief of irritable bowel syndrome. *Lancet* 1987; 2:1144.

    An intriguing report where somatostatin given for acromegaly completely relieved the symptoms of concomitant, long-standing irritable bowel syndrome.

15. Usadehl K, Uberla K, Leuschner U. Treatment of acute pancreatitis with somatostatin: Results of the multicenter, double-blind trial (abs). Dig Dis Sci 1985; 30:992.

    Despite encouraging experimental results, somatostatin did not improve various clinical parameters in sever pancreatitis. Mortality was decreased with somatostatin but did not reach statistical significance.

16. Vinik A, et al. Somatostatin analogue (SMS 201–995) in the management of gastropancreatic tumors and diarrhea syndromes. AJM 1986; 6b:23.

    A review of a potpourri of conditions treated with Sandostatin.

45

Antiserotonin Agents

Michael S. Gurney

Carcinoid tumors were first described by Lubarsch in 1888, but it was not until 1953 that Waldenstrom and Lundgren associated the peculiar syndrome of flushing, diarrhea, and cardiac valvular disease with elevated levels of serotonin secreted by the tumor. Pharmacotherapy was then directed against serotonin in an effort to ablate the syndrome's debilitating symptoms. Methysergide (Sansert) and various anticholinergics, particularly cyproheptadine (Periactin), were found to have antiserotonin activity and clinical benefit in such patients. The development of somatostatin, which has greater efficacy and fewer side effects, will soon relegate these drugs to lesser roles.

Cyproheptadine (Periactin)

Antihistamines competitively antagonize most of the smooth muscle–stimulating actions of histamine on the H_1-receptors in the gastrointestinal tract. Cyproheptadine also competes with serotonin for receptor-site binding and is felt to be the most effective member of the antihistamine family for the carcinoid syndrome.

PHARMACOLOGY

Cyproheptadine is absorbed rapidly after oral administration. Symptomatic relief begins within 15 to 30 minutes, with full efficacy reached within 1 hour. Less than 5 percent of the drug is excreted unchanged in the stool. Cyproheptadine is metabolized by the liver, and the inactive glucoronide salt is renally excreted. The drug has a longer half-life than many antihistamines and may be given at 6- to 8-hour intervals.

INDICATIONS

In 1960, Brown studied several antiserotonin agents in carcinoid patients and found that cyproheptadine gave the best clinical response with the fewest side effects. Since then, it has gained a reputation as the agent of first choice for relief of the diarrhea and flushing. Severe flushing and diarrhea are unlikely to be completely relieved, but some improvement may be expected. Bronchospasm, on the other hand, is not well managed by this medication.

Antihistamines are notorious for their lack of predictability for both clinical response and side effects in any individual patient. If cyproheptadine is not efficacious or is poorly tolerated, the entire class should not be abandoned. Good alternate choices are prochlorperazine (Compazine) or chlorpromazine (Thorazine).

CONTRAINDICATIONS AND SIDE EFFECTS

Side effects are common with all antihistamines and vary in incidence and severity with both the individual and the drug. However, serious toxicity rarely occurs.

Sedation is a common complaint with all antihistamines. Continued use of the medication or a reduction in dose often results in good tolerance. Dizziness and hypotension are also common side effects and are most common in the elderly.

Antihistamines lower the seizure threshold in patients with convulsive disorders and should be used with caution in such patients. All antihistamines also have anticholinergic activity and should be administered carefully, if at all, to patients with narrow-angle glaucoma, prostatin hypertrophy, or gastric outlet obstruction. Monoamine oxidase inhibitors intensify the anticholinergic side effects of antihistamines and inhibit the breakdown of serotonin. They should not be given to carcinoid patients, particularly those on cyproheptadine.

DOSAGE

The initial dose of cyproheptadine is 4 milligrams 4 times a day, but higher doses are usually needed for relief of carcinoid symptoms; 6 to 8 milligrams 3 times a day are often needed for these patients. Total daily dosage should not exceed 500 micrograms/kilogram of body weight. For acute attacks, 50 to 75 milligrams in 200 milliliters of saline infused intravenously over 1 to 2 hours may be beneficial.

Methysergide (Sansert)

Methysergide is structurally related to methlergonavine maleate. Like cyproheptadine and the ergot alkaloids, it competitively inhibits serotonin binding.

PHARMACOLOGY

Methysergide is rapidly absorbed following oral administration and metabolized by the liver. As a serotonin antagonist, it has not been tested against other compounds, but in animal studies it appears to be as effective as cyproheptadine.

INDICATIONS

Methysergide was shown, in a study at NIH by Brown et al., to reduce steatorrhea and diarrhea in patients with the carcinoid syndrome. Flushing only variably responds, probably because the flush is not due to serotonin alone.

Use of Sansert has been limited because of reports that long-term use is associated with retroperitoneal fibrosis. Less commonly, fibrotic processes involving the aorta, heart, and lungs have occurred. The fibrosis may regress when the drug is withdrawn, but in some patients this regression is only partial. This complication is particularly vexing in carcinoid patients, since fibrosis in the abdomen and cardiac valves can occur late in the carcinoid syndrome and is a serious complication. Use of methysergide, therefore, should be reserved for those patients who are intolerant or unresponsive to other medications and are debilitated by their symptoms.

CONTRAINDICATIONS AND SIDE EFFECTS

Methysergide can cause vascular insufficiency and should not be used in patients with known cardiac or peripheral atherosclerotic vascular disease. It should be given with caution to patients with risk factors for coronary disease, and all patients over 40 should have their cardiac status evaluated prior to therapy.

Renal function must be quantified prior to drug administration and every 4 to 6 months during therapy. If blood urea nitrogen rises, dysuria or flank pain develops, or signs of phlebitis or venous obstruction occur, the medication should be stopped and clinical status evaluated. Patients should also be observed for pleural or cardiac friction rubs, pleural effusions, shortness of breath, and chest pain.

The drug is contraindicated during pregnancy and in patients with severe hepatic or renal disease.

An estimated 30 percent of patients have side effects, and 10 to 20 percent need to discontinue the drug because of them.

DOSAGE

Methysergide is administered orally. The suggested starting dose is 4 to 6 milligrams/day in divided doses, preferably with meals. The dose can be increased to 8 to 12 milligrams/day if tolerated. The drug should be discontinued for several weeks, and the patient reevaluated, after every 6 months of continuous therapy.

PEARLS AND PITFALLS

1. Antihistamines may prevent a positive reaction to skin-testing procedures and should be discontinued several days prior to such testing.
2. Gastrointestinal side effects of the antihistamines such as cyproheptadine include nausea, anorexia, and epigastric distress. Administration of antihistamines with meals or milk usually alleviates these problems.
3. The incidence of peptic ulcer disease is high in the carcinoid syndrome. Not all gastrointestinal complaints should be attributed to the syndrome or the therapy, since ulcer disease may be the culprit.
4. The best study to look for retroperitoneal fibrosis is an intravenous pyelogram. Dilatation or deviation of the ureters are signs of fibrosis with obstruction.
5. Morphine is a serotonin liberator and must be avoided in carcinoid patients.

6. Alpha adrenergic-blocking agents such as aldomet or phenoxybenzamine are often helpful in controlling flushing.
7. The bronchospasm of carcinoid syndrome may respond to low doses of isoproterenol aerosol or corticosteroids. Epinephrine or other adrenergic agonists must never be given to such patients, since they worsen the bronchospasm and may precipitate hypotension and carcinoid crisis.

References

1. Brown RE, et al. Studies on several possible antiserotonin compounds in the functioning carcinoid syndrome. Clin Res 1960; 8:61.

    One of the few studies that compares different medications in symptomatic carcinoid syndrome. Cyproheptadine was the most effective and best tolerated.

2. Melmon KL, et al. Treatment of malabsorption and diarrhea of the carcinoid syndrome with methysergide. Gastroenterology 1965; 48:18.

    A study showing good benefit and tolerance with methysergide in seven patients.

3. Miller R, et al. Anesthesia for the carcinoid syndrome: A report of nine cases. Can Anaesth Soc J 1978; 25:240.

    A fine discussion of the perioperative management of patients with the carcinoid syndrome.

4. Oates JA, Butler C. Pharmacologic and endocrine aspects of the carcinoid syndrome. Adv Pharmacol 1967; 5:109.

    The pathophysiology and treatment of the carcinoid syndrome are well discussed.

5. Roberts LJ, Marney SR, Oates JA. Blockade of the flush associated with metastatic gastric carcinoid by combined H_1- and H_2-receptor antagonists. NEJM 1979; 300:236.

    A patient with metastatic gastric carcinoid had complete relief of flushing only when both histamine receptors were blocked. This therapy is effective only for foregut carcinoids, since they secrete high amounts of histamine, in contrast to midgut and hindgut carcinoids.

6. Warner RRP. Carcinoid tumor. In JE Berk (ed), *Gastroenterology* vol 3. Philadelphia: Saunders, 1985.

    An excellent discussion of the carcinoid syndrome, its pathophysiology, and its therapy.

46

Cyclosporine

Tho D. Le

In the early days of organ transplantation, rejection due to graft-versus-host disease was a major reason for the low success rate of this surgical endeavor. Until recently, azathioprine in combination with steroids was used for immunosuppression after transplantation, with a survival rate of about 30 percent after one year. However, with the discovery of cyclosporine, a cyclic endecapeptide isolated from the soil fungi *Cylindrocarpum lucidum* and *Tolypocladium inflatum,* a great avalanche in human liver transplantations occurred around 1980. One-year survival rates for liver transplants almost doubled overnight with this new form of immunosuppressive therapy. Unlike previous agents, cyclosporine did not cause bone marrow suppression. Consequently, morbidity and mortality due to anemia and infection became much less of a concern. With cyclosporine, the incidence of rejection decreased significantly from past figures. Cyclosporine has significant toxicities but in low doses, in combination with steroids, has been found to be adequate in suppressing rejection, without major adverse effects. Besides liver transplants, cyclosporine is also used for many other solid-organ transplants and is being considered as a possible therapeutic approach for autoimmune diseases such as insulin-dependent diabetes mellitus, primary biliary cirrhosis, and inflammatory bowel disease.

MECHANISM OF ACTION

Cyclosporine prevents host rejection mainly through the inhibition of T-cell proliferation. On exposure to foreign antigens, the immune system responds by activating macrophages to produce interleukin-1 (IL-1). IL-1, in turn, stimulates antigen-primed helper T cells to produce interleukin-2 (IL-2). Cyclosporine inhibits this latter step in the immune response, the production of IL-2. Without IL-2, cytotoxic T cells are unable to complete their growth cycle and proliferate; T-cell-mediated rejection is thus inhibited.

Suppression of the humoral response to antigenic stimulation occurs only for those responses requiring T-cell help. Research has shown that antibody responses to T cell–*independent* antigen is *unimpaired* by cyclosporine, both in vitro and in vivo. Thus, humoral response inhibition probably works through the same mechanism that is responsible for cell-mediated responses. Without IL-2 and subsequent helper T-cell proliferation, those B cell responses that require helper T cells are inhibited.

Cyclosporine has also been shown to induce proliferation of antigen-activated suppressor T cells. With this observation, one could rationalize why immunosuppression sometimes persists in transplanted patients despite removal of cyclosporine therapy. We could postulate that suppressor T cells, once stimulated to divide by cyclosporine, continue to proliferate and mediate immunosuppression even after the removal of the original stimulus. However, neither the maintenance of allografts following discontinuation of cyclosporine nor the emergence of specific suppressor cells has been confirmed in large clinical trials.

ADMINISTRATION AND DOSAGE

Cyclosporine is a hydrophobic compound and must be dissolved in lipids or organic solvents before administration. Cyclosporine can be administered orally, intramuscularly, or intravenously. However, intramuscular administration has been shown to be less effective because of inadequate absorption. Absorption following oral administration is highly variable, with peak levels occurring from 1 to 8 hours after administration. Because of its lipophilicity, cyclosporine accumulates in fat and skin. Therefore, dosage requirements decrease with long-term usage. Cyclosporine is metabolized and excreted mainly by the liver, with about 10 percent excreted by the kidneys. Thus, patients with liver failure have decreased dosage requirements. Pediatric patients require higher doses because of quicker metabolism.

Cyclosporine is usually administered 4 to 10 hours preoperatively and as needed intraoperatively. Postoperatively, patients should be started on intravenous, not oral, cyclosporine because of variable oral absorption. Oral cyclosporine can be added to the regimen as tolerated by the patient, and drug levels should be monitored frequently. When levels indicating oral absorption start to increase, intravenous medication can be tapered and eventually discontinued.

Since cyclosporine has significant toxicities and variable absorption, the monitoring of drug levels takes on great importance. Radioimmunoassay (RIA) and high-pressure liquid chromatography (HPLC) are two methods available for measuring levels. RIA is less specific, since it measures cyclosporine as well as some inactive metabolites. Blood cyclosporine concentration is more reliable than is plasma level because it is not dependent on temperature, hematocrit, or plasma lipoprotein concentration. Levels should be measured before drug administration and every 2 or 3 days thereafter, until a stable clinical condition and drug level are achieved.

A single oral dose of cyclosporine of 15 milligrams/kilogram/day should be administered 4 to 10 hours prior to transplantation. This daily dose is continued postoperatively for 1 to 2 weeks and then tapered by 5 percent per week to a maintenance level of 5 to 10 milligrams/kilogram/day. Patients with variable absorption orally and patients unable to take oral medications can be treated with the intravenous concentrate.

The intravenous dose is approximately one-third of the oral dose. The intravenous concentrate should be diluted, 1 milliliter in 20 to 100 milliliters of 0.9% saline or 5% dextrose, and given in a slow intravenous infusion over approximately 2 to 6 hours.

This regimen should be considered only as a starting

point. Drug therapy should be adjusted based on the blood levels of cyclosporine, the patient's clinical status, biochemical profiles, and immunologic parameters.

SIDE EFFECTS

The most common and clinically important toxic effect of cyclosporine is kidney damage. This effect seems to be reversible with a decrease in dose; only 4 to 17 percent of patients require complete termination of the agent. Nephrotoxicity manifests as a modest increase in serum creatinine that is nonprogressive and usually occurs weeks after the start of therapy. Glomerular filtration rate usually stabilizes at 45 to 60 percent of normal despite continued drug administration. Some patients experience transient oliguria. Hypertension and hyperkalemia, probably secondary to renal damage, are other common side effects. Renal biopsy shows vascular changes that usually do not correspond with the extent of renal failure, thus implicating a functional rather than structural mechanism.

Other, less frequent toxic effects include hepatotoxicity, gingival hyperplasia, hirsutism, and transient tremors. Rises in bilirubin, transaminases, and alkaline phosphatase occur transiently and respond frequently to dose reduction. There have been reported cases of central nervous system toxicity associated with reversible white-matter changes, as well as thrombotic thrombocytopenic purpura after cyclosporine treatment.

The incidence of lymphoma in cyclosporine-treated patients is about 0.7 percent, a figure not significantly different from conventionally treated patients. Furthermore, most patients who developed lymphoma were found to have previous Epstein-Barr virus infection, an infection associated in the past with B cell tumors. Thus, the occurrence of lymphoma could be due to reactivation of the Epstein-Barr virus secondary to immunosuppression, and not due to the cyclosporine itself.

INDICATIONS

Since its discovery in 1980, cyclosporine has become the foremost agent for immunosuppression in solid-organ transplantation, including liver transplants. With the success of cyclosporine treatment, liver transplants have become an acceptable treatment and even the treatment of choice for many liver illnesses. Biliary atresia has been the most common indication for liver transplants overall, with primary biliary cirrhosis and sclerosing cholangitis most common in adults. Survival rates have approached 70 to 75 percent after one year; and higher in the pediatric population than in the adult population. Furthermore, morbidity and mortality now more commonly result from the severity of preexisting disease or technical problems than from rejection or sepsis. In one study, 25 percent of cyclosporine-treated patients had episodes of rejection, compared with 66 percent of those treated conventionally with azathioprine and prednisone. The incidence of severe sepsis has also diminished greatly because cyclosporine is less bone-marrow suppressive than were previous agents.

Besides liver transplants, cyclosporine is indicated after renal transplantation, bone-marrow transplantation, heart and lung transplantation, and pancreas transplantation. Researchers are presently looking into the possibility of small-bowel transplant using cyclosporine for immunosuppression.

Cyclosporine has been tried as medical treatment for many autoimmune disorders, including primary biliary cirrhosis and inflammatory bowel disease. Cases of Crohn's disease refractory to steroid and sulfasalazine that responded to cyclosporine therapy have been reported. Cyclosporine as treatment for ulcerative colitis has also been investigated.

Finally, cyclosporine has made possible a more aggressive approach toward retransplantation. Cases of success after one or two repeated transplants have been reported, with survival rates approaching 50 percent after one year.

PEARLS AND PITFALLS

1. Cyclosporine does not cause bone-marrow suppression in animal models or humans.
2. Oral absorption of cyclosporine is highly variable, with peak levels occurring 1 to 8 hours after administration.
3. Cyclosporine is nephrotoxic and sometimes causes rapid elevation of BUN and creatinine. Since these events are similar to rejection episodes, care must be taken to differentiate between them.
4. Monitoring of renal and liver functions as well as electrolytes is essential because cyclosporine has significant toxicities.
5. Cyclosporine should be used in conjunction with steroids post-transplantation.
6. Cyclosporine is metabolized mainly by the liver, and therefore liver failure necessitates dosage adjustment.
7. Monitoring of blood cyclosporine level by radioimmunoassay can be deceptive because some inactive metabolites are measured in addition to the cyclosporine.

References

1. Cohen DJ, et al. Cyclosporine: A new immunosuppressive agent for organ transplantation. Ann Int Med 1984; 101:667–682.

    A good overall review of cyclosporine emphasizing its role in transplantation.

2. deGroen PC, et al. Central nervous system toxicity after liver transplantation: The role of cyclosporine and cholesterol. NEJM 1987; 14:861–866.

    Thirteen out of 48 patients receiving cyclosporine post–

liver transplantation had symptoms of central nervous system toxicity and radiographic evidence of diffuse white-matter changes.
3. Dzik WH, et al. Cyclosporine-associated thrombotic thrombocytopenic purpura following liver transplantation—Successful treatment with plasma exchange. Transplantation 1987; 4:570–572.

    One reported case of thrombotic thrombocytopenic purpura was treated successfully by plasma exchange.
4. Gordon R, et al. Indications for liver transplantation in the cyclosporine era. Surg Clin N Am 1986; 3:541–556.

    A review of different indications for liver transplantation and their success rates.
5. Grant D, et al. Adverse effects of cyclosporine therapy following liver transplantation. Transpl Proc 1987; 4:3463–3465.

    The side effects of cyclosporine, as observed in 62 orthotopic liver transplants.
6. Iwatsuki S, et al. Nephrotoxicity of cyclosporine in liver transplantation. Transpl Proc 1985; 4(suppl 1):191–193.

    5-year follow-up of the incidence of renal dysfunction with long-term cyclosporine therapy.
7. Parsons H, et al. Effect of cyclosporine A on serum lipid in primary biliary cirrhosis patients. Gastroenterology 1988; 94:A580.

    A report on measurements of plasma lipid, liver function studies, apolipoprotein concentration, and lecithin-cholesterol acyltransferase activity in primary biliary cirrhosis patients treated with cyclosporine.
8. Starzl T, et al. Liver transplantation in the cyclosporine era. Prog Allerg 1986; 38:366–394.

    A general assessment of liver transplantations, including success rate, surgical techniques, tissue matching, and organ procurement.
9. Van Buren, CT, et al. Cyclosporine: Progress, problems, and perspectives. Surg Clin N Am 1986; 3:435–449.

    A good review of cyclosporine.
10. Venkataramanan R, et al. Pharmacokinetics and monitoring of cyclosporine following orthotopic liver transplantation. Sem Liv Dis 1985; 4:357–367.

    An in-depth article on the pharmacokinetics and monitoring of cyclosporine.
11. Wiesner RH, et al. The effects of in vivo cyclosporine on lymphocytes in patients with primary biliary cirrhosis. Gastroenterology 1988; 94:A563.

    The effects of cyclosporine on blood lymphocytes and blastogenesis after one year of treatment are discussed.
12. Williams JW, et al. Survival following hepatic transplantation in the cyclosporine era. Amer Surg 1986; 6:291–293.

    An article on the 6-month follow-up of 50 patients post–liver transplant.
13. Williams JW, et al. Biopsy-directed immunosuppression following hepatic transplantation in man. Transplantation 1985; 6:589–596.

    This paper shows that there is little correlation between

hepatic dysfunction suggesting rejection and the incidence of true rejection diagnosed histologically.

14. Williams R, et al. Long-term use of cyclosporine in liver grafting Quar J Med 1985; 224:897–905.

    Of 29 liver-graft recipients, only three had episodes of rejection, and it was necessary to stop treatment in only five due to cyclosporine toxicity.

15. Wonigeit K, et al. Experiences with a blood level–adjusted cyclosporine regimen in kidney and liver allograft recipients. Transpl Proc 1986; 6(Suppl 5):181–187.

    A study of whole-blood cyclosporine level, measured by radioimmunoassay as an indication of adequate cyclosporine dosage.

Appendix: Drugs and Pregnancy
Michael M. Van Ness

Although drugs probably account for no more than 1 percent of all human congenital anomalies, the thalidomide tragedy of the early 1960s has convinced many of a direct relationship between drug use and congenital defects.

This appendix is a compilation of the drugs in common usage for gastrointestinal disorders. In the final analysis, the practicing clinician must evaluate the relative merits and risks of every drug prescribed for pregnant or lactating patients. To assist in that judgment, the Food and Drug Administration pregnancy categories, the relative risks and benefits of the drug in question, and the breast-feeding categories are presented for the agents discussed in this handbook.

We are indebted to the American College of Gastroenterology's Committee on FDA-Related Matters and James H. Lewis, MD, FACP, FACG, for their inspiration and work in this area.

Drugs and pregnancy

Agent	FDA pregnancy category	Risk vs benefit (by trimester) 1st	2nd	3rd	Breast-feeding category
4-ASA, 5-ASA	B1	B>R	B>R	B>R	II
Acyclovir	C1	R>>B	R>>B	R>>B	IV
Amphotericin	B2	?	?	?	IV
Antacids	B1	?	B>R	B>R	II
Atropine	C2	?	?	?	IV
Azathioprine	D	R>>B	R>>B	R>>B	IV
Belladonna	C1	?	?	?	IIIB
Bismuth	C1	?	?	?	IIIB
Bulk agents	C2	B>R	B>R	B>R	I
Cimetidine	B2	?	B>R	B>R	IV
Cisapride	B1	?	?	?	IV
Colchicine	C1	R>>B	R>>B	R>>B	IV
Corticosteroids	C1	B>R	B>R	B>R	IIIA
Colestipol	C2	?	?	?	IV
Cyclosporin	D	?	?	?	IV
Cyproheptadine	B1	?	?	?	IV
Diazepam	D	R>>B	R>>B	R>>B	IIIB
Dicyclomine	D	?	?	?	

Diltiazem	D	?	?	?	IIIB
Disulfiram	B1	?	?	?	IIIB
Domperidone	B1	?	?	?	IV
Ethanol	D	R>>B?	R>>B?	R>>B?	IIIB
Famotidine	B1	?	?	?	IV
Ganciclovir	C1	R>>B	R>>B	R>>B	IV
Glucagon	C2	?	?	?	IIIB
Hep B Ig	C2	B>R	B>R	B>R	II
Hep B vaccine	C2	B>R	B>R	B>R	I
Immune globulin	C2	?	?	?	II
Iodinated contrast	B1	?	?	?	II
Lactulose	C2	?	?	?	IIIB
Loperamide	C2	?	?	?	IV
Mebendazole	C1	R>>B	R>>B	R>>B	IV
Mercaptopurine	D	R>>B	R>>B	R>>B	IV
Metoclopramide	B1	?	?	?	IV
Metronidazole	C1	R>>B	R>>B	R>>B	IV
Midazolam	D	R>>B	R>>B	R>>B	IV
Misoprostol	C1	R>>B	R>>B	R>>B	IV
Monooctandin	X	R>>B	R>>B	R>>B	IV
Naloxone	B1	B>R	B>R	B>R	IIIB
Neomycin	C1	?	?	?	IIIA
Nifedipine	D	?	?	?	IIIB

Agent	FDA pregnancy category	Risk vs benefit (by trimester) 1st	2nd	3rd	Breast-feeding category
Nitroglycerin	D	?	?	?	IIIB
Nizatidine	B1	?	?	?	IV
Omeprazole	B1	?	?	?	IV
Pancrealipase	C2	?	B>R	B>R	I
Penicillamine	C1	?	?	?	IIIB
Phenobarbitol	D	R>>B?	R>>B?	R>>B?	IIIB
Piperazine	C2	R>>B	R>>B	R>>B	IV
Polyethylene glycol purge	C2	?	?	?	IIIA
Pyrantel	C2	R>>B	R>>B	R>>B	IV
Ranitidine	B1	?	?	?	IV
Sodium tetradecyl sulfate	C2	R>>B?	R>>B?	R>>B?	IIIB
Somatostatin	BI	?	?	?	IIIA
Spiromycin	C1	R>>B	R>>B	R>>B	IV
Sucralfate	B1	B>R	B>R	B>R	IIIA
Sulfasalazine	B1	B>R	B>R	B>R	II
Thiabendazole	C1	R>>B	R>>B	R>>B	IV
Trientine Hcl	C1	?	?	?	IIIB

Vitamin K	B1	?	B>R	II
Zinc	C1	?	B>R	IIIB

FDA pregnancy categories:
A = Well-controlled studies fail to demonstrate risk to the fetus.
B1 = Animal studies fail to demonstrate risk to the fetus but no human studies are available.
B2 = Animal studies show some risk to the fetus but this is not confirmed in human studies.
C1 = Animal studies show risk to the fetus but no human studies are available.
C2 = Animal and human studies are unavailable.
D = Drug associated with birth defects but with potential benefits that may outweigh known risks.
X = Drugs associated with birth defects and with potential risk that clearly outweighs potential benefit.
Risk vs benefit: R>>B = Proven or potential risk outweighs potential benefits.
B>R = Potential benefits outweigh potential risks.
R>>B? = Risks may be outweighed by benefits in some circumstances.
? = Risk-to-benefit ratio is unknown.

Breast-feeding categories:
I = Drug does not enter breast milk.
II = Drug enters breast milk but is not known to be harmful in therapeutic doses.
IIIA = Drug may or may not enter breast milk but no adverse effects are expected.
IIIB = Drug may or may not enter breast milk but drug is systemically absorbed.
IV = Drug enters breast milk and poses a potential risk to the neonate.

Index

Aach, RD, 224
Absolute alcohol, 367
Acetaldehyde syndrome, 262
Acetaminophen
  cimetidine and, 27
  toxicity, ranitidine and, 33
  metabolism, 27
  overdose, 20, 27
Acetylcholine, 2
Achalasia
  calcium channel blockers for, 324
  nitroglycerin for, 320, 322
ACTH, 93
  intravenous administration of, 103–104, 105
Acyclovir, 184–185
  administration of, 186
  indications for, 184–185
  mechanism of action of, 184
  pharmacokinetics of, 184
  side effects of, 185
Aeromonas species, 211
AIDS
  cryptosporidiosis and, 190–191
  hepatitis B vaccine and, 257
  infectious agents and, 157, 159
Albumin, 99
Alcohol
  absolute, 367
  metronidazole and, 130, 194, 196
Alcoholic liver disease, 225
  corticosteroids for, 228
Alcoholism, disulfiram for, 262–264
Alkaline diet, 1
Allopurinol, azathioprine and, 236, 237
Aloe, 310
Aloin, 310
Aluminum hydroxide, 7, 9
Aluminum phosphate, 7
Amebiasis, 193–196
  iodoquinol for, 195–196
  metronidazole for, 128, 193–195
American Heart Association, 341, 345
  Committee on Rheumatic Fever and Infectious Endocarditis, 342–344
Amino acids, in TPN, 149(t)
(4)-aminosalicylate, 115, 116
(5)-aminosalicylate, 115, 116
Aminosalicylic-acid compounds, 94. *See also* 4-ASA; 5-ASA
Ammonia, detoxification of, 266
Amoebic colitis, 158
Amoxicillin
  for prevention of enterococcal endocarditis, 344–345
  for typhoid fever, 162
Amphotericin B, 181–182
  contraindications for, 181
  dosage and administration of, 181–182
  indications for, 181
  notes on, 182
  pharmacokinetics of, 181
  side effects of, 181
Ampicillin, 344
  for shigellosis, 165, 166
  for typhoid fever, 162
Amylopectin sulfate, 59
Anaerobic organisms, metronidazole for, 126, 127–128
Anal fissures, bulk-forming agents and, 305
Ancylostoma duodenale, 200
Anorectal herpes, 184
Antabuse. *See* Disulfiram
Antabuse-ethanol reaction, 262
Antacids, 7–11
  administration of, 10
  cimetidine and, 13, 29
  continuous infusion of, 21
  contraindications for, 10
  dosages of, 7–9, 10
  indications for, 7–10
  intensive program of, 21, 23
  liquid vs. tablets, 7, 8(t)
  notes on, 10–11
  tetracycline and, 10
Antacid therapy, 1
Anthelminthics
  Ascaris lumbricoides, 197–199
  hookworm, 200

Index

Anthelminthics—*Continued*
  Strongyloides stercoralis, 200–201
  treatment of, 198(t)
  Trichuris trichiura, 199
Anthraquinones
  contraindications for, 310
  dosage of, 310
  mechanism of action of, 310
  side effects of, 310
  types of, 309–310
Antibiotics
  for cholera, 167–168
  for diarrhea, 158–159
  for pseudomembranous colitis, 172
Anticholinergics, 326
Anticonstipation agents
  anthraquinones, 309–311
  bulk-forming agents, 303–308
  contact laxatives, 309
  diphenylmethane derivatives, 311–312
  docusate salts, 313–314
  lubricants, 314–316
  ricinoleic acid, 312–313
Anticonvulsants, metronidazole and, 131
Antidiarrheal agents
  kaolin, 291–292
  loperamide, 292–294
  pectin, 291–292
Antihistamines, 397–400
Anti-inflammatory agents, ranitidine and, 32
Antimetabolites
  administration of, 121–123
  contraindications, 121
  indications for, 119–121
  notes on, 123
  pharmacology of, 119
Antimicrobial agents, 4
Antimicrobial prophylaxis, 341
Antimotility agents
  atropine, 375–376, 378
  glucagon, 376–378
Antimuscarinics, 325–327
Antiserotonin agents
  cyproheptadine, 397–398
  methysergide, 398–399
Antiviral drugs, 184–186
Aquamephyton, 255
4-ASA, 94, 96, 115, 116
  for distal proctocolitis, 137–138

5-ASA, 94, 96, 112, 113, 115, 116
  carriers for, 134
  for Crohn's disease, 137
  dosage of, 136
  enemas, 115, 116, 135, 137
  formulation of, 135(t)
  indications for, 135–136
  mechanism of action of, 135
  notes on, 137
  pharmacology of, 134–135
  side effects of, 136–137
Asacol, 134, 136, 137
Ascaris lumbricoides, 197–199
Aspirin-induced mucosal damage, misoprostol and, 65
Atabrine, 188–189, 190
Atropine, 325–327
  contraindications for, 376
  dosage and administration of, 376
  indications for, 375–376
  pharmacology of, 375
  side effects of, 376
Atterbury, CE, 267
Aubaniac, 143
Azathioprine, 119
  administration of, 236
  for chronic autoimmune liver disease, 223, 230, 234, 235
  for chronic hepatitis, 235–236
  for Crohn's disease, 95
  indications for, 234–236
  mechanism of action of, 234
  notes on, 237
  for primary biliary cirrhosis, 234–235
  side effects of, 236–237
Azomysin, 129

Bachrach, WH, 7
Bacillas cereas, 164
Bacitracin, for pseudomembranous colitis, 172
Bacteremia, 341–342
  Salmonella and, 161
Bacteremia prophylaxis agents
  bacteremia and, 341–342
  dosage and administration of, 344–345
  indications for, 342–344
  notes on, 345–346
Bacterial DNA gyrase, 210

Index

Bacterial infections, 161–173
  Campylobacter, 169–171
  Clostridia difficile, 171–173
  metronidazole for, 127–128, 131
  Salmonella, 161–164
  shigellosis, 164–166
  Vibrio cholera, 166–169
Bacteroides fragilis, 127
Bahgat, M, 248–249
Balantidium coli, metronidazole for, 128
Bardham, KD, 31
Bar-Meir, S, 321
Baron, JH, 103
Barreras, RF, 7
Barrett's esophagus, 24
  ranitidine and, 32
Bartlett, JG, 171, 215
Basilisco, G, 292
Beclomethasone dipropionate, 101
Beer, 215
Behar, J, 23
Belladonna
  dosage and administration of, 327
  effects of, 325–326
  indications for, 326–327
  notes on, 327
  side effects of, 327
Bellergal, 325
Bellergal-S, 327
Bentyl, 324–325
Benzodiazepines, 355. *See also* Diazepam; Midazolam
  dosage and administration of, 359
  drug interactions with, 359
  mechanism of action of, 356–357
  notes on, 363
Berenson, MM, 31
Bergman, L, 293
Bernstein, LH, 127
Berstad, A, 7–9, 10
Betamethasone sodium phosphate, topical administration of, 105
1-(B-hydroxyethyl)-2-methyl-5-nitroimidazole, 125
Bile acid diarrhea, 298–301
Bilenzyme, 255
Bile reflux gastritis, sucralfate and, 61

Bile salt binders
  dosage of, 300
  indications for, 298–299
  mechanism of action of, 298
  notes on, 300–301
  pharmacology of, 298
  side effects of, 299–300
Biliary disease, 225
Billroth, 2
Bisacodyl, 311–312
Bismuth, 4, 72–74
  administration of, 73–74
  dosage of, 73–74
  duodenal ulcers and, 74
  gastric ulcers and, 73
  gastritis and, 74
  indications for, 72–73
  mechanism of action of, 72
  notes on, 74
  pharmacokinetics of, 72
  side effects of, 74
Bismuth ion, 72
Bismuth oxide, 72
Bismuth salts, 72
Bismuth subsalicylate, 208
  dosage and administration of, 206
  mechanism of action of, 206
  pharmacology of, 206
  side effects of, 206
Bismuth subsalicylate (Pepto-Bismol), 72, 73, 74
  norfloxacin and, 206–207
  for traveler's diarrhea, 205–206
Bizzozero, 73
Black, M, 27
Blackwell, JN, 322
Blastocystis hominis, metronidazole for, 129
Bleeding, cimetidine and, 20
Bleeding esophageal varices, injection therapy for, 365
Bleeding rates, for stress ulcers, 23(f)
Blichfeldt, P, 126
Blum, AL, 229
Blume, M, 323
B-lymphocytes, 91–92
Bodenheimer, H, 224, 248
Boghaert, A, 334
Borsch, G, 74
Bovera, E, 39–40
Boyer, JL, 249
Boyes, BE, 73, 74

Braafladt, 291
Brady, CE, III, 351
Brand, DL, 65
Breast-feeding, relative risks and benefits of drugs and, 407–411(t)
Bredfeldt, JE, 33
British Society of Antimicrobial Chemotherapy, 341
Brody, M, 7
Brogden, 29
Brooke, BN, 119
Brown, PW, 215
Brown, RE, 397, 398
Buck, GE, 73
Budenoside, 101
Bulk-forming agents
  average cost of, 307(t)
  common, 306(t)
  composition and formulation of, 303–304
  contraindications for, 308
  dietary fiber and, 303
  dosage and administration of, 305–308
  indications for, 304–305
  mechanism of action of, 304
  notes on, 308
  side effects of, 308

Calcium carbonate, 7, 9
Calcium channel-blocking agents
  dosage and administration of, 323
  indications for, 322–323
  mechanism of action of, 322
  notes on, 324
  side effects of, 323–324
Calcium polycarbophil, 304
CALD. See Chronic autoimmune liver disease (CALD)
Calicivirus, 164
Camilleri, M, 334
Campylobacter, 158, 164, 169–171, 203
Campylobacter fetus, 169–170
Campylobacter jejuni, 169, 211
Campylobacter pylori, 4, 19
Candida albicans, 178
Candidiasis, amphotericin B for, 181–182
Cann, PA, 294
Cannon, AE, 287
Capurso, L, 15

Carboxymethylcellulose, 303, 308
Carcinoid tumors
  antiserotonin agents for, 397–400
  somatostatin for, 391–392, 393–394
Cardilate, 321
Carling, L, 61
Cascara sagrada, 310
Castor oil, 312–313
CBG, 99
CDAI, 95
Cefoperazone, for typhoid fever, 163
Ceftriaxone, for typhoid fever, 163
Centers for Disease Control, 193, 195
  Parasitic Disease Division, 196
Central vein feedings, 144
Cerulli, MA, 40
Chappius, CW, 215
Chemotherapy-induced emesis, metoclopramide and, 78
Chenix, 271
Chenodeoxycholic acid, 271
Chenodiol, 280
  dosage of, 274–275
  indications for, 272–273
  pharmacology of, 271–272
  side effects of, 273–274
Chlorambucil, for PBC, 224
Chloramphenicol
  for cholera, 167
  for meningitis, 171
  for typhoid fever, 162
Chloridiazepoxide, 355
Cholangitis, 342
Choledocholithiasis, 225
Cholelithiasis, 225
  chenodiol for, 271–272
  dosage of, 274–275
  indications for, 272–273
  prevalence of, 271
  side effects of, 273–274
Cholera, 166–169
  dehydration from, 167
  immunization for, 168
  rehydration therapy for, 167–169
Cholesterol metabolism, bulk-forming agents and, 304
Cholestyramine
  for bile acid diarrhea, 298–300

medications absorbed by, 299(t)
for pseudomembranous colitis, 172
sulfasalazine and, 115
Chondroitin sulfate, 59
Chronic autoimmune liver disease (CALD), 223–224
azathioprine for, 234, 235
corticosteroids for, 227, 230
Chugai Pharmaceutical Company, 59
Cigarette smoking
cimetidine and, 18
ranitidine and, 30–31
Cimetidine, 2, 3, 4, 9
administration of, 28
adverse reactions to, 25(t)
antacids and, 13
anti-androgenic effects of, 26
cigarette smoking and, 18
continuous infusion of, 20–24, 28
drug interactions with, 26–27
duodenal ulcers and, 15–19
vs. famotidine, 35
gastric ulcers and, 19
gastroesophageal reflux disease and, 23–24
hepatotoxicity and, 24
indications for, 15–24, 17(t)
intravenous use, of 25(t)
mechanism of action of, 13
mental status changes and, 24–25
metronidazole and, 131
notes on, 28–29
pharmacokinetic properties of, 13, 16(t)
potency of, 35
renal disease and, 25
side effects of, 24–28
sinus bradycardia and, 25
stress-related mucosal bleeding and, 20–23
structure and formula of, 14(f)
vs. sucralfate, 61
theophylline level and, 27(t)
transaminase elevation and, 24
for Zollinger-Ellison syndrome, 19–20
Ciprofloxacin, 159, 208
for *Campylobacter,* 170, 171
contraindications for, 212
dosage of, 212
for enteritis, 170
indications for, 211
mechanism of action of, 210
notes on, 212–213
pharmacology of, 210
for typhoid fever, 163
Cirrhosis, colchicine for, 257(t), 248–249. *See also* Primary biliary cirrhosis (PBC)
Cisapride, 77, 288
dosage and administration of, 335
indications for, 333–334
mechanism of action of, 332–333
notes on, 335–336
pharmacology of, 333
side effects of, 335
Cisplatin, 78
Citrucel, 303, 308
Clostridia difficile, 171–173, 299
notes on, 173
treatment for, 172–173
Clostridium difficile–associated colitis, metronidazole for, 128
Clotrimazole, 178–179
contraindications for, 179
dosage and administration of, 179
indications for, 178
pharmacokinetics of, 178
side effects of, 179
Cocco, AE, 20
Cohen, A, 24, 33
Cohen, NP, 334
Cohn, I, 215
Colase Regutol, 313
Colchicine
for cirrhosis, 248–249
contraindications for, 249
indications for, 246–249
mechanism of action of, 246
notes on, 249–250
for PBC, 224
pharmacodynamics, 246
for primary biliary cirrhosis, 246–247
side effects of, 249
Colectomy, 93, 94
Colestipol
for bile acid diarrhea, 298–300
medications absorbed by, 299(t)
for pseudomembranous colitis, 172

Colin-Jones, DG, 30
Colitis
  Clostridia difficile–related, 128
  pseudomembranous, 171–173
  severe, criteria for, 103(t)
  ulcerative, 91, 92–94, 103–104, 113, 126
Collen, MJ, 18, 20, 31, 32, 36–37
Colonoscopy, PEG-ELS for, 349, 350–352
Constipation
  bulk-forming agents and, 304–305
  motility disorder drugs and, 288
Contact laxatives, 311(t)
  anthraquinones, 309–310
  diphenylmethane derivatives, 311–312
  docusate salts, 313–314
  indications for, 309
  notes on, 313–314
  ricinoleic acid, 312–313
Continuous infusion antacids, 21
Continuous infusion cimetidine therapy, 20–24
Corboy, ED, 65–66
Corleto, V, 37
Correctol, 311
Corticosteroids, 92
  administration of, 103–105, 230
  for alcoholic liver disease, 228
  for chronic autoimmune liver disease, 227, 230
  contraindications for, 105–106
  for Crohn's disease, 104–105
  dosages of, 99–101
  enemas, 93
  foams, 93
  indications for, 103–105, 227–230
  intravenous administration of, 103–104
  mechanism of action of, 102, 227
  notes on, 106–108, 230–231
  oral administration of, 93, 103
  parenteral, 93
  pharmacokinetics of, 99–101
  pharmacology of, 99–101
  for primary biliary cirrhosis, 229–230
  rectally-instilled steroids, 93
  retention enemas, 93
  side effects of, 106, 230
  steroid suppositories, 93
  topical administration of, 104
  for ulcerative colitis, 92–94, 103–104
  for viral hepatitis, 228–229
Corticotropin (ACTH), 93, 103–104, 105
Cortisol, 99
Cortisol-binding globulin (CBG), 99
Cosar, 125
Crohn's disease, 91, 94–96
  5-ASA for, 136, 137
  corticosteroids for, 104–105
  cyclosporine and, 404
  dicyclomine hydrochloride for, 325
  6-mercaptopurine for, 119–121
  metronidazole for, 126–127, 131
  nutrition and diet therapy for, 144–146
  prednisolone and, 100–101
  sulfasalazine for, 113
  total parenteral nutrition and, 144–146
Crohn's disease activity index (CDAI), 95
Crowe, J, 234
Cruveilhier, 215
Cryptosporidiosis, 190–191
Cryptosporidium, 190–191
Cucchiara, S, 333
Cuckler, AC, 157
Curtiss, 339
Cyclosporine
  administration and dosage of, 402–403
  indications for, 403–404
  mechanism of action of, 401–402
  notes on, 404
  side effects of, 403
Cyproheptadine
  contraindications for, 398
  dosage of, 398
  indications for, 397
  pharmacology of, 397
Cytoprotection, 3–4
  agents of, 59–66
  misoprostol and, 63–66
  sucralfate and, 59–63
Czaja, AJ, 229

Danilewitz, M, 32
Davies, PS, 126
Davis, GR, 349
Dawson, J, 31
Dazopride, 77
DeLattre, M, 17
Delayed gastric emptying, domperidone for, 331
DeRitis, R, 229
Deruytte, M, 334
Desmethyldiazepam, 356
Dexamethasone, for typhoid fever, 162
Dexamethasone sodium phosphate, topical administration of, 105
Diabetes, bulk-forming agents and, 305
Diabetic gastroparesis
  domperidone for, 331
  metoclopramide and, 78, 79–80
Dialose, 313
Diarrhea. *See also* Traveler's diarrhea
  acute infectious, 157
  bile acids and, 298–301
  bloody, 166
  bulk-forming agents and, 305
  Campylobacter and, 169–171
  ciprofloxacin for, 211, 212
  Clostridia difficile and, 171
  incidence of, 2
  infectious, 157–159
  kaolin for, 291–292
  Kaopectate for, 291–292
  loperamide for, 292–294
  mild, 157–158
  motility disorder drugs and, 288
  pectin for, 291–292
  Salmonella and, 161, 163
  severe, 158
  Shigella and, 164, 166
  Vibrio cholera and, 166–168
Diazepam (Valium)
  contraindications for, 357–358
  dosage and administration of, 359
  drug interactions, 359
  indications for, 357
  mechanism of action of, 356–357
  notes on, 363
  pharmacology of, 355–356
  side effects of, 358

Dickson, ER, 241
Dicyclomine hydrochloride (Bentyl)
  dosage and administration of, 325
  indications for, 324–325
  mechanism of action of, 324
  side effects of, 325
Dietary fiber
  bulk-forming agents and, 303–305
  diverticulitis and, 219
Digepepsin, 255
Diidohydroxyquin, 195–196
Diloxanide furanoate, 195
Diltiazem, 323, 324
Dioctyl Sulfosuccinate, 313–314
Dipentum, 134
Diphenoxylate, 208
Diphenylmethane derivatives, 311–312
  contraindications for, 312
  dosage of, 312
  side effects of, 312
Dirnberger, GM, 324
Disaccharidase deficiency, *Giardia* and, 190
Distal proctocolitis, 4-ASA for, 137–138
Distal sigmoiditis, 93
Di Stefano, R, 31
Disulfiram, 225
  administration of, 252–263
  ethanol and, 263(t)
  indications for, 252–263
  mechanism of action of, 262
  notes on, 263–264
  side effects of, 262
Diverticular disease
  bulk-forming agents and, 305
  perforative, 217(t)
Diverticulitis, acute
  complications of, 216–217
  incidence of, 215
  medical therapy for, 217–218
  notes on, 218–219
  pathogenesis of, 215
  presentation and diagnosis of, 216
Dobbs, JH, 33
Docusate salts (Dioctyl Sulfosuccinate)
  contraindications for, 313
  dosage of, 313
  notes on, 313–314
  side effects of, 313

Doenges, 73
Domperidone, 288
    dosage and administration of, 332
    indications for, 331
    mechanism of action of, 330–331
    notes on, 335–336
    pharmacology of, 330
    side effects of, 332
Donnatal, 327
Dooley, CP, 19, 73
Dorsey, Thomas, 288
Doxidan, 311
Doxycycline
    dosage and administration of, 205
    mechanism of action of, 205
    pharmacology of, 205
    side effects of, 205
    for traveler's diarrhea, 204–205
D-penicillamine, for Wilson's disease, 240, 241–242, 244
Dracuncula medinensis, 129
Dracunculiasis, metronidazole for, 129
Driks, MR, 61
Drug-induced gastritis, sucralfate and, 61
Ducolax, 311
Dudley, FJ, 229
Dudrik, 143
Duodenal ulcer disease
    acute, sucralfate treatment for, 3
    antacid treatment of, 7, 9, 10
    bismuth and, 4, 74
    chronic gastritis and, 19
    cimetidine for, 15–19
    famotidine and, 36
    H2-receptor antagonists for, 2
    misoprostol and, 65
    nizatidine for, 38, 39–40
    omeprazole for, 3, 84–85
    perforated, 18
    ranitidine and, 30, 32
    recurrence of, 18–19
    refractory, 65
    smoking and, 18
    sucralfate and, 61
DuPont, HL, 205
Durack, DT, 342
Dysentery, 157, 164

ECCDS, 96
Electrolyte ranges, for TPN, 147, 148(t)
Emesis, chemotherapy-induced, 78
Endocarditis prophylaxis, 341–345
    indications for 342–343(t)
Endocrine cyanide. *See* Somatostatin
Endogenous prostaglandins, 3
Endoscopic retrograde cholangiopancreatography (ERCP), 379, 381
Endoscopy
    antimotility agents and, 375
    bacteremis prophylaxis agents for, 341–346
    fiberoptics, 159, 339
    iodinated contrast agents and, 379
    tranquilizers for, 355
Enemas, 349
Enprostil, 4
Entamoeba histolytica
    iodoquinol for, 195–196
    metronidazole for, 125, 128, 193–195
Entamoeba polecki,
    metronidazole for, 129
Enteral nutrition, 143, 145, 146
Enteric fever. *See* Typhoid fever
Enteritis, 170–171
    cryptosporidium, 190–191
Enterocutaneous fistulae, 96
Enteropathogenic *Escherichia coli,* 158
Enterotoxigenic *Escherichia coli* (ETEC), 2–3, 158, 164
    bismuth subsalicylate and, 206
    ciprofloxacin for, 211
    TMP/SMX and, 204
    traveler's diarrhea and, 203
Epinephrine, 367–369
Epstein, O, 241
ERCP, 379, 381
Erosive reflux esophagitis, omeprazole for, 84
Erythrityl tetranitrate, 321
Erythromycin
    for *Campylobacter,* 170, 171
    for cholera, 167
    for enteritis, 170
Esophageal diseases, 159

Esophageal motility disorders
  calcium channel blockers for, 324
  dicyclomine hydrochloride for, 325
  smooth-muscle relaxants and, 322–323
ETEC. *See* Enterotoxigenic *Escherichia coli* (ETEC)
Ethanol, disulfiram and, 263(t)
European Cooperative Crohn's Disease Study (ECCDS), 96
Exceed, 158
Ex-Lax, 311
Exogenous prostaglandinlike drugs, 3

Famotidine
  administration of, 38
  continuous infusion of, 38
  dosages of, 36–38
  duodenal ulcer and, 36
  gastric ulcer and, 37
  indications for, 17(t), 36–37
  mechanism of action of, 35, 36
  notes on, 38
  pharmacodynamics of, 35, 36
  pharmacokinetics of, 35, 36
  potency of, 35
  for stress-related mucosal damage, 37
  structure and formula of, 14(f)
  Zollinger-Ellison syndrome and, 36–37
Fass, RJ, 215
FDA. *See* Food and Drug Administration (FDA)
Fecal leukocyte test, 158
Feen-A-Mint, 311
Ferrous sulfate, sulfasalazine and, 115
Fiber. *See* Dietary fiber
Fiberall, 303
Fiberoptic endoscopy, 159, 339
Finklestein, M, 249
Flagyl. *See* Metronidazole
Fleet's Bisacodyl, 311
Fluoroquinolones, 165, 210. *See also* Ciprofloxacin
Food and Drug Administration (FDA), 2, 35, 72, 77, 191, 234, 249, 293
Fordtran, JS, 7, 288
Frager, 215
Frank, WO, 22

Fungal infections, 159
  amphotericin B for, 181–182
  clotrimazole for, 178–179
  ketoconazole for, 179–180
  nystatin for, 178–179
Furazolidone (Furoxone), 208
  for *Campylobacter,* 171
  for cholera, 168
  for enteritis, 171
  for giardiasis, 188, 189–190
Furoxone. *See* Furazolidone

Gallstones
  chenodiol for, 271–275
  deciding to treat, 272–273
  medical dissolution therapy for, 272(t), 273(t)
  monooctanoin for, 276–280
  prevalence of, 271
  recurrence of, 275
  ursodeoxycholic acid for, 275–276
Ganciclovir, 185–186
  administration of, 186
  indications for, 186
  mechanism of action of, 185–186
  pharmacokinetics of, 186
  side effects of, 186
Garrigues, V, 326
Gasbarrini, G, 293
Gastric acid
  antacids and, 7
  neutralization of, 20
  ranitidine and, 32
Gastric pH
  increasing, 20
  ranitidine and, 31–32
Gastric resection, 2
Gastric ulcer disease
  bismuth and, 73
  cimetidine and, 19
  famotidine and, 35, 36
  misoprostol and, 64, 65
  omeprazole for, 84
  ranitidine and, 30–31
Gastrin, 2
Gastritis
  bismuth and, 74
  chronic, duodenal ulcer disease and, 19
Gastroduodenostomy, 2
Gastroenteritis, *Salmonella* and, 161

Gastroesophageal reflux disease
  advances in treatment of, 1
  cimetidine and, 23–24
  domperidone for, 331
  metoclopramide and, 78, 79
  ranitidine and, 31, 35
  sucralfate and, 61
Gastrointestinal disease, acute infectious, 157–160. *See also specific diseases*
Gastrointestinal endoscopy. *See* Endoscopy
Gastrointestinal hemorrhage, injection therapy for, 365
Gastrointestinal motility, 287–288
Gastrointestinal system
  bacterial infections of, 161–174
  protozoal infections of, 188–191
  smooth-muscle relaxants for, 320
  viral infections of, 184–186
Gastrojejunostomy, 2
Gatorade, 158
Geerdsen, 392
Gelfond, M, 320, 323
Gentamicin, 171, 344
Giardia, 164, 203
Giardia lamblia, 188
  metronidazole and, 125, 129
Giardiasis, 188–190
  metronidazole for, 129
Gledhill, T, 15
Glucagon
  contraindications for, 377
  dosage of, 377
  indications for, 377
  notes on, 377–378
  pharmacology of, 376–377
  side effects of, 377
Glucagonoma, Sandostatin for, 390–391
Glucocorticoids, 99–101
Goldenberg, MM, 73
Gonvers, JJ, 65
Gorbach, SL, 178
Gough, KR, 30
Gray, N, 229

H2-receptor antagonists, 1, 2, 9, 13–39
  cimetidine, 13–29
  dosage of, 17(t)
  famotidine, 35–38
  indications for, 17(t)
  nizatidine, 38–40
  pharmacokinetic properties of, 16(t)
  ranitidine, 29–35
Haber, CJ, 121
Halloran, LG, 21
Hamilton, I, 72, 74
Hansky, J, 18
Harris, AI, 229
Hasan, M, 17–18
HDL cholesterol, 26(t)
Heathcote, J, 234
Heavy metal antagonists
  administration of, 243
  indications for, 240–242
  mechanism of action of, 240
  notes on, 242–244
  side effects of, 242–243
  for Wilson's disease, 240–242
Helman, 228
Hemoccult reaction, cimetidine and, 27–28
Hemorrhoids, bulk-forming agents and, 305
Hentschel, E, 19
Hepatitis, chronic, azathioprine for, 235–236
Hepatitis B, 224–225
  immune globulin, 258
Hepatitis B vaccines
  clinical trials for, 258
  contraindications for, 260
  development of, 257–258
  indications for, 258–260
  notes on, 260
  side effects of, 260
Hepatotoxicity, cimetidine and, 24
Heptavax, 257
Herpes virus, acyclovir for, 184–185
High-pressure liquid chromatography (HPLC), 402
Hirao, M, 368
Hirschmann, 345
Histamine, 2
Hoffman-La Roche, Inc., 355
Hoofnagle, JH, 224
Hookworm, 197, 200
Horner, JL, 215
Hornick, RB, 73
Horowitz, M, 334
Howard, 37
HPLC, 402

Hydrocortisone, 99, 101
  intravenous injection of, 103–104
  topical administration of, 105
Hyperphosphatemia, 10
Hypertrophic hypersecretory gastropathy, 20
Hypoprothrombinemia, vitamin K and, 254, 255, 256

IBS, 305, 323–326
Ileitis, 120
Ileocolitis, 120
Inflammatory bowel disease
  drugs for, 91–96
  metronidazole for, 126
Injection therapy, for gastrointestinal hemorrhage, 365
Insulinoma, somatostatin for, 391
Interferon, for viral hepatitis, 224
Intestinal nematodes, 197–201
Intra-gastric pH values, significance of, 15
Intravenous hyperalimentation, 143
Iodinated contrast agents
  notes on, 381
  prophylaxis of contrast-agent allergy and, 380
  side effects of, 379–380
Iodochlorhydroxyquin, 195
Iodoquinol
  for amebiasis, 195–196
  metronidazole and, 193–194
Irritable bowel syndrome (IBS)
  anticholinergics, 326
  bulk-forming agents and, 305
  calcium channel blockers for, 323
  dicyclomine hydrochloride for, 324–325
Isenberg, JI, 15
Islet cell tumors, somatostatin for, 389–390
Isodorbide dinitrate, 321
Isordil, 321

Jacobsen, E, 262
Jefferys, DB, 25
Jensen, DM, 365, 366
Jensen, RT, 26, 37
Johnson, PC, 294

Kamme, C, 126
Kaolin
  contraindications for, 292
  indications for, 291
  notes on, 292
  pharmacology of, 291
  side effects of, 292
Kaopectate
  contraindications for, 292
  dosage of, 292
  indications for, 291
  notes on, 292
  pharmacology of, 291
Kaplan, HP, 103
Kaplan, MM, 224, 248
Karrar, ZA, 293
Kasof, 313
Kaye, D, 341
Kersh, ES, 267
Kershenobich, D, 248, 249
Ketoconazole, 179–180
  contraindications for, 180
  dosage and administration of, 180
  indications for, 179–180
  pharmacokinetics of, 179
  side effects of, 180
Kingsley, AN, 21
Kingsworth, 392
Klotz, U, 36
Koldinger, RE, 246
Konakion, 255
Korelitz, BI, 92, 119, 120

La Brooy, SJ, 20
Labs, JD, 215
Lactulose
  dosage and administration of, 267
  mechanism of action of, 266–267
  notes on, 268
  side effects of, 267
Lam, SK, 61
Lanza, F, 32, 65
Lavo, B, 294
Laxatives, 287–288
  abuse of, 288
  anthraquinones, 309–314
  bile salt binders as, 298–301
  contact, 309–312
  diphenylmethane derivatives, 311–312
Lebert, PA, 29
Lennard-Jones, JE, 119
Leung, JWC, 367

Levison, ME, 215
Levy, 59
Lewis, JH, 180
Lieberman, DA, 23–24
Lindner, 92
Liquid antacids, 7, 8(t)
Liver disease
  alcoholic, 225, 228
  chronic, ranitidine and, 29
  chronic autoimmune (CALD), 223–224, 225, 227, 230
  drugs for, 223–225
Liver transplants, cyclosporine and, 401
Loeffler's syndrome, 197
Loperamide, 208
  administration of, 294
  contraindications for, 294
  indications for, 293–294
  mechanism of action of, 292–293
  notes on, 294
  pharmacodynamics of, 292
  pharmacokinetics of, 292
  side effects of, 294
Loperamide hydrochloride, 208
Low-dose antacids, 9
Lubarsch, 397
Lubricants
  contraindications for, 315
  dosage of, 315–316
  indications for, 315
  notes on, 316
  pharmacology of, 314–315
  side effects of, 315
Lundgren, 397
Lupid hepatitis. *See* Chronic autoimmune liver disease (CALD)
Lyon, DT, 36

Maalox, 10, 15
Maalox Plus, 10
McCallum, RW, 323
McClung, JH, 291
Maddrey, W, 228
Magnesium-containing antacids, 10
Magnesium hydroxide, 7
Male infertility, sulfasalazine and, 116
Malnutrition, Crohn's disease and, 144–146
Mannitol, 349
Marshall, BJ, 19, 73

Martin, DF, 73
Martin, LF, 23
M1-cholinergic receptor, 2
Mebendazole
  for *Ascaris lumbricoides,* 197
  for hookworm, 200
  for *Strongyloides stercoralis,* 201
Megaloblastic anemia, 116
Menaquinone (vitamin K$_2$), 255
Menetrier's disease (hypertrophic hypersecretory gastropathy), 20
Menguy, RB, 1
Meningitis, 171
Mephyton, 255
6-mercaptopurine, 96, 119–123
Merke, Sharp, and Dohme Research Laboratories, 84, 257
Metamucil, 303
  Sugar-Free, 308
Methylcellulose, 303
Methylprednisolone, 104
  for alcoholic liver disease, 228
  for Crohn's disease, 96
Methysergide
  contraindications for, 399
  dosage of, 399
  indications for, 398–399
  notes on, 399–400
  pharmacology of, 398
  side effects of, 399
Metoclopramide
  administration of, 79–80
  for chemotherapy-induced emesis, 78, 80
  contraindications for, 79
  for diabetic gastroparesis, 78, 79–80
  dosages for, 80–81
  for gastroesophageal reflux, 78, 79–80
  indications for, 78–79
  mechanism of action of, 77
  nonapproved indications for, 79
  notes on, 79–80
  for small-bowel radiographic examination, 79, 80
Metronidazole (Flagyl), 96, 128, 130, 194, 196
  for amebiasis, 193–195
  anticonvulsants and, 131

for bacterial infections, 127–128, 131
cimetidine and, 131
for *Clostridium difficile*–associated colitis, 128
contraindications, 129–130, 194
for Crohn's disease, 126–127, 131
dosage and administration of, 195
for dracunculiasis, 129
drug interactions with, 130–131
for giardiasis, 129, 188, 189, 190
indications for, 126–129, 193–194
for inflammatory bowel disease, 126
mechanism of action of, 126, 193
notes on, 131
pharmacokinetics of, 193
pharmacology of, 125
for protozoal infections, 128–129
for pseudomembranous colitis, 172
side effects of, 129–130, 194
sulfasalazine and, 130–131
for surgical prophylaxis, 128
for ulcerative colitis, 126
warfarin and, 131
Meyer, 103
Midazolam
contraindications for, 361
vs. diazepam, 362–363
dosage and administration of, 362
drug interactions with, 362
indications for, 361
mechanism of action of, 360–361
notes on, 363
pharmacology of, 359–360
side effects of, 361–362
Mineral oil, 314–316
Misoprostol, 4
aspirin-induced duodenal mucosal damage and, 65
cytoprotective properties of, 63–64
gastric ulcer and, 65
indications for, 64–66
mechanism of action of, 64
notes on, 66
pharmacodynamics of, 64
pharmacokinetics of, 64
vs. ranitidine, 65
refractory duodenal ulcer disease and, 65
Mistilis, SP, 227
Mitral valve prolapse, 345
Mitrolan, 304
M1-muscarinic receptor antagonists, 9
Moctanin, 276–277, 280
Modane, 311
Modane Soft, 313
Monooctanoin (Moctanin)
contraindications for, 277
indications for, 277
pharmacology of, 276–277
side effects of, 277, 280
Motidine, 2
Motility disorder drugs, 287–288
Mucosal damage. *See* Stress-related mucosal damage
Mulholland, 23
Mulinos, MG, 315
Muller-Lissner, SA, 334
Mylanta, 10
Mylanta II, 9, 10, 21
Mylanta-like antacids, 7

Nacarato, R, 40
Nakamura, 125
Naloxone hydrochloride
contraindications for, 384–385
dosage of, 384
indications for, 383–384
mechanism of action of, 383
notes on, 385
pharmacology of, 383, 384(t)
side effects of, 384–385
Narcotic-induced respiratory depression, naloxone for, 383–385
National Cooperative Crohn's Disease Study (NCCDS), 95–96, 106
National Cooperative Gallstone Study, 271
Nausea, domperidone for, 331
NCCDS, 95–96, 106
Necator americanus, 200
Nematodes, intestinal, 197–201
Neoloid, 313
Neomycin, 266

Nicholson, 65
Nifedipine, 322, 323–324
Nitrates, gastrointestinal
    disease and, 320–321
Nitroglycerin
    dosage and administration of,
        321
    indications for, 320–321
    mechanism of action of, 320
    notes on, 321–322
    side effects of, 321
Nitroglycerin-vasopressin, 371
    contraindications for, 371
    dosage and administration of,
        371–372
    drug interactions with, 372
    notes on, 372
    side effects of, 372
Nizatidine, 2
    antiandrogenic side effects, 40
    dosages of, 39, 40
    for duodenal ulcer, 38, 39, 40
    indications for, 17(t), 39–40
    mechanism of action of, 39
    notes on, 40
    pharmacodynamics of, 39
    pharmacokinetics of, 39
    side effects of, 40
    structure and formula of, 14(f)
Nonulcer dyspepsia, sucralfate
    and, 61
Norfloxacin
    dosage and administration of,
        207
    mechanism of action of, 206–
        207
    pharmacology of, 206–207
    side effects of, 207
Nutrition and diet therapy, for
    Crohn's disease, 144–146
Nystatin, 178–179
    contraindications for, 179
    dosage and administration of,
        179
    indications for, 178
    pharmacokinetics of, 178
    side effects of, 179

Omeprazole, 3
    carcinogenicity of, 85
    dosages for, 84–85
    for duodenal ulcer disease,
        84–85
    for erosive reflux esophagitis,
        84
    for gastric ulcer disease, 84
    indications for, 84–85
    mechanism of action of, 83
    pharmacodynamics of, 83
    pharmacokinetics of, 83
    side effects of, 85
    for Zollinger-Ellison
        syndrome, 36–37, 83, 84
Onderdonk, AB, 215
Oral rehydration, for diarrhea,
    158
Organ transplants, cyclosporine
    and, 401, 404
Ostro, MJ, 20, 21
Oxazepam, 356

Page, JG, 324
Pancolitis, 93
Pancrealipase
    contraindications for, 283
    dosage of, 283–284
    indications for, 282–283
    notes on, 284–285
    pharmacology of, 282
    side effects of, 283
Pancreatic disease, 223–225,
    282
Pancreatic enzyme replacement,
    282–285
Parasitic Disease Division,
    Centers for Disease Control,
    196
Parasitic infections, 159
Parenteral corticosteroids, 93
Parietal cell acid secretion,
    cimetidine and, 13
PBC. *See* Primary biliary
    cirrhosis
Pectin
    contraindications for, 292
    dosage of, 292
    indications for, 291
    notes on, 292
    pharmacology of, 291
Pederzoli, P, 392
Pedialyte, 158
PEG-ELS. *See* Polyethylene
    glycol electrolyte lavage
    solutions
Penicillamine
    administration of, 243
    indications for, 240–242
    mechanism of action of, 240
    notes on, 243–244
    side effects of, 242–243
    for Wilson's disease, 223–224,
        240–244

Penston, JG, 30
Pentasa, 115, 134, 136
Pepsin
  cimetidine and, 13
  famotidine and, 35
  ranitidine and, 29
  sucralfate and, 60
Peptic ulcer disease, 1
  antacid treatment for, 7–9, 10
  bismuth treatment for, 4
  prostaglandins for, 3
  refractory, 3
  sucralfate and, 60–61
Pepto-Bismol, 72, 73, 74, 206
Pera, A, 61
Perdiem, 303, 308
Perforated duodenal ulcers, cimetidine for, 18
Periactin, 397–398
Peridiverticulitis, 215
Perillo, RP, 224
Peripheral vein feedings, 143
Peterson, WL, 7
Peura, DA, 22, 32
Phenolphthaleins, 311–312, 314
Phillip's Laxcaps, 311
Phytonadione (Vitamin K$_1$), 255
Piperazine citrate, for *Ascaris lumbricoides,* 199
Pirenzepine, 9, 326–327
Pitressin, 369–370
Pleisomonas shigelloides, ciprofloxacin for, 211
Poly-ASA, 115
Polycarophil, 304
Polyethylene glycol electrolyte lavage solutions (PEG-ELS)
  composition of, 350(t)
  contraindications for, 351–352
  dosage and administration of, 350
  efficacy of, 350–351
  mechanism of action of, 349–350
  side effects of, 351–352
Polypectomy, antimotility agents and, 375
Porter, JB, 24
Potter, T, 323
Powell-Tuck, J, 103
Prednisolone, 92, 99, 100, 103
  for alcoholic liver disease, 228
  for chronic autoimmune liver disease, 230, 231
  intravenous injection of, 104
  oral administration of, 103

Prednisolone metasulfobenzoate, 101
Prednisone, 99, 100
  for chronic autoimmune liver disease (CALD), 230
  for Crohn's disease, 95
  intravenous injection of, 104
  oral administration of, 105
  side effects of, 106
  for viral hepatitis, 224, 228
Pregnancy
  chenodiol therapy and, 273
  ciprofloxacin and, 212
  mineral oil and, 316
  relative risks and benefits of drugs during, 407–411(t)
  sucralfate and, 62
Present, DH, 119, 120
Priebe, HJ, 9, 21
Primary biliary cirrhosis (PBC), 224
  azathioprine for, 234–235
  colchicine for, 246–248
  corticosteroids for, 229–230
  D-penicillamine for, 241(t)
Proctitis, 93
Prokinetic agents
  cisapride, 332–335
  domperidone, 330–332
  notes on, 325–326
Prostaglandin dependent mechanisms, 60
Prostaglandin independent mechanisms, 60
Prostaglandins, 3, 63–64
  A type, 63
  E types, 63
  E1 type (misoprostol), 63–64
  E2 type, 3, 63
  F2 type, 63
  I types, 63
  I2 type, 3, 63
Protozoal infections, 159, 188–191
  metronidazole for, 128–129
Proximal signoid disease, 93
Prulet, 311
Pseudomembranous colitis, 158, 171–173, 300
Psyllium hydrophilic colloid, 303, 308
Purgatives
  contraindications of, 351–352
  dosage and administration of, 350

Purgatives—*Continued*
  efficacy of, 350–351
  mechanism of action of, 349–350
  notes on, 352
  side effects of, 351–352
Pyrantel pamoate
  for *Ascaris lumbricoides*, 197–199
  for hookworm, 200
  for *Strongyloides stercoralis*, 201
Pyridoxine, for Wilson's disease, 242

Quinacrine (Atabrine), for giardiasis, 188–189, 190

Radioimmunoassay (RIA), 402
Ranitidine, 2, 3
  acute gastric ulcers and, 30–31
  administration of, 33–34
  Barrett's esophagus and, 32
  central nervous system toxicities and, 34(t)
  continuous infusion of, 35
  for duodenal ulcer disease, 18, 30, 32
  gastric acid and, 31–32
  gastroesophageal reflux disease and, 31
  indications for, 17(t), 30–32
  mechanism of action of, 29
  vs. misoprostol, 65
  notes on, 35
  vs. omeprazole, 84
  pepsin secretion and, 29
  pharmacokinetics of, 29–30
  potency of, 35
  side effects of, 33
  stress-related mucosal bleeding and, 32
  structure and formula of, 14(f)
  Zollinger-Ellison syndrome and, 31
Rankin, FW, 215
Ransohoff, DF, 249
Read, AE, 229
Recombivax HB, 257
Refractory duodenal ulcer disease, misoprostol and, 65
Refractory peptic ulcer disease, 3
Refractory proctitis, 93

Rehydration therapy
  for cholera, 167–169
  recipe for, 168–169
Reid, SR, 32
Renal disease
  cimetidine and, 25
  nizatidine and, 40
Renal failure, chronic
  antacid treatment for, 9–10
  cimetidine dosage and, 28
Retroperitoneal fibrosis, Sansert and, 398–399
Reusser, P, 32
Reynolds, JC, 36
RIA, 402
Ricci, DA, 78
Richter, JE, 322–323
Ricinoleic acid
  contraindications for, 313
  dosage of, 313
  mechanism of action of, 312
Rigaud, D, 31
Rompalo, 184, 185
Rosch, W, 334
Rotaviruses, 164, 203
Roundworm, 197–199
Rudnick, MR, 25
Rydning, A, 9

Saccharomyces cerevisias, 257–258
Saeed, ZA, 19–20
Salmonella, 159, 164, 203
  ciprofloxacin for, 211, 212
  clinical entities of, 161
  notes on, 163–164
  treatment of, 162–163
  transmission of, 161–162
Salmonella cholerasuis, 161
Salmonella enteritidis, 161
Salmonella paratyphi, 161, 163
Salmonella typhi, 161, 163
  ciprofloxacin for, 211
Salofalk, 134, 136
Salomon, 73
Sondheimer, JM, 315
Sandhu, BK, 293
Sandostatin, 288–394
Sansert, 398–399
SAS. *See* Sulfasalazine
Savarino, V, 64
Scheinberg, IH, 243
Schiller, LR, 293
Schistosoma japonicum, 157

Schneider, JS, 62–63
Schuster, M, 326
Sclerosants
  absolute alcohol, 367
  epinephrine, 367–369
  mechanism of action of, 365
  nitroglycerin-vasopressin, 371–372
  sodium morrhuate, 366–367
  sodium teradecyl sulfate (STS), 365–366
  vasopressin, 369–370
  vasopressin analogues, 370–371
Sclerotherapy, antimotility agents and, 375
Scott, J, 240
Searle Research and Development, 64
Senna, 310
Sepsis, 23
  cimetidine and, 29
Septicemia, 168, 171
Shaffer, JA, 101
Shaldon, S, 228
Sherlock, S, 228, 230
Shigella, 158, 161, 163, 164–166, 203
Shigella flexneri, 211
Shigella sonnei, 211
Shigellosis
  notes on, 166
  pathogenesis of, 164–165
  transmission of, 164, 166
  treatment of, 165
Shreeve, DR, 74
Siepler, J, 20, 32
Sigmoidoscopy, 158
Silvis, SE, 30
Simethicone, 9
Simon, B, 33, 36, 40
Simpson, CJ, 18
Singh, 293
Singleton, JW, 95
Sinus bradycardia, cimetidine and, 25
Sippy diet, 1
Sircus, W, 17–18
Small-bowel radiographic examination, metoclopramide and, 78
Smoking
  cimetidine and, 18
  ranitidine and, 31

Smooth-muscle relaxants
  antimuscarinics, 325–327
  belladonna, 325–327
  calcium channel-blocking agents, 322–324
  dicyclomine hydrochloride, 324–325
  nitroglycerin, 320–322
Sodium azo-disalicylate, 115
Sodium bicarbonate, 7
Sodium morrhuate
  contraindications for, 367
  dosage and administration of, 366
  notes on, 372
  side effects of, 366
Sodium sulfate, 349
Sodium tetradecyl sulfate (STS)
  dosage and administration of, 365–366
  side effects of, 366
Sohendra, 368
Soloway, RD, 235
Somatostatin, 288
  contraindications for, 393
  dosage and administration of, 393
  indications for, 389–393
  notes on, 393–394
  pharmacology of, 389
  side effects of, 393
Sontag, S, 18
Sphincter of Oddi dysfunction, 321
  antimuscarinics for, 326
  calcium channel blockers for, 323
  nitroglycerin and, 321, 322
Spiramycin, for cryptosporidiosis, 191
Staphyococcal infection, *Salmonella* and, 163
Stellon, AJ, 223, 235
Sternlieb, I, 243
Steroids. *See also* Corticosteriods
  for Crohn's disease, 94–96
  rectally-administered, 102
  for typhoid fever, 163
Stool culture, 158, 166
  for *Campylobacter*, 171
Streptomyces nodosus, 181
Streptomyces noursei, 178
Stress-related mucosal damage
  causal factors of, 22(f)

Stress-related mucosal damage—*Continued*
 cimetidine and, 20–23, 29
 famotidine and, 37
 natural history of, 21(t)
 prevention of, 9
 ranitidine and, 32
 sucralfate and, 61
Stress ulcer bleeding rates, 23(t)
Strickland, 240
Strongyloides stercoralis, 197, 200–201
STS, 355–356
Substituted benzimidazole omeprazole. *See* Omeprazole
Sucralfate, 3
 bile reflux gastritis and, 61
 vs. cimetidine, 61
 dosage and administration of, 62–63
 drug-induced gastritis and, 61
 drug interactions with, 62
 gastroesophageal reflux disease and, 61
 indications for, 60–62
 laboratory abnormalities of, 62
 mechanism of action of, 59–60
 nonulcer dyspepsia and, 61
 notes on, 63
 peptic ulcer disease and, 60–61
 pharmacology of, 59
 pregnancy and, 62
 side effects of, 62
 stress-related mucosal damage and, 61
Sucrose octasulfate, 59
Sugar-Free Metamucil, 308
Sulfamethoxazole (SXT)
 for shigellosis, 165, 166
 for typhoid fever, 162–163
Sulfapyridine, 112, 113, 134
Sulfasalazine (SAS), 94
 absorption, 112
 analogues of, 115
 for Crohn's disease, 95, 113
 distribution of, 112
 dosage of, 113–114
 drug interactions with, 115
 indications for, 113
 mechanism of action of, 112–113
 metabolism, 112
 metronidazole and, 130–131
 notes on, 116
 patient desensitization for, 114–115
 side effects of, 114
 for ulcerative colitis, 113
Sulfonamide, 112
Surfak, 313
Surgery, on ulcers, 1–2
Surgical prophylaxis, metronidazole for, 128
Sutton, DR, 74
Svartz, Nana, 112
SXT, 162–63, 165, 166

Tanner, AR, 74, 101
TDB, 72–73
Teasley, DG, 128
Tedesco, FJ, 172–173
Terruzzi, V, 26
Tetracycline
 antacids and, 10
 for *Campylobacter,* 170
 for cholera, 167
 for enteritis, 170
 for septicemia, 168
 for shigellosis, 165
Theophylline levels
 cimetidine and, 26
 factors affecting, 27(f)
Thiabendazole, for *Strongyloides stercoralis,* 201
Thistle, JL, 276
Tixocortol pivalate, 101
T-lymphocytes, 91–92
TMP. *See* Trimethoprim (TMP)
TMP/SMX. See Trimethoprim-sulfamethoxazole (TMP/SMX)
Tong, 230
Toskes, PP, 283
Total parenteral nutrition (TPN)
 administration of, 146–152
 catheter-related complications and, 153
 central vein feedings, 144
 complications of, 153–154
 history of, 143
 indications for, 143–144
 inflammatory bowel disease and, 144–146
 metabolic complications of, 153
 monitoring, 149–152
 ordering solutions of, 148–149
 organ-related complications of, 154
 peripheral vein feedings, 143

potential modulation of, 150–151(t)
TPN. *See* Total parenteral nutrition (TPN)
Tranquilizers
  benzodiazepines, 355
  diazepam, 355–359, 362–363
  midazolam, 359–363
Transaminase elevation, cimetidine and, 24
Traube, M, 323
Traveler's diarrhea, 203–208. *See also* Diarrhea
  bismuth subsalicylate for, 205–206
  chemoprophylaxis of, 202–208
  ciprofloxacin for, 211, 212
  doxycycline for, 204–205
  loperamide for, 294
  norfloxacin for, 206–207
  preventing, 207–208
  risk factors for, 207
  TMP/SMX for, 203–204
Triamcinolone acetonide dental paste, 105
Triamcinolone hexacetonide, 105
Trichinella spiralis, 157
Trichuris trichiura, 197, 199
Trimethoprim (TMP)
  for shigellosis, 165, 166
  for typhoid fever, 162–163
Trimethoprim-sulfamethoxazole (TMP/SMX), 208
  dosage and administration of, 204
  mechanism of action of, 203–204
  pharmacology of, 203–204
  side effects of, 204
  for traveler's diarrhea, 203–204
Tripotassium dicitrato bismuthate (TDB), 72–73
Truelove, SC, 93
Turnberg, LA, 293
Typhoid fever (enteric fever)
  Salmonella and, 161
  transmission of, 161–162
  treatment of, 162–163

Ulcerative colitis, 91, 92–94
  corticosteroids for, 92–94, 103–104
  metronidazole for, 126
  sulfasalazine for, 113

Ulcers, 1–4. *See also* Duodenal ulcer disease; Gastric ulcer disease; Peptic ulcer disease
Upper intestinal hemorrhage, ranitidine and, 31
Urbain, JL, 334
Ursing, B, 126, 127
Ursodeoxycholic acid (Ursodiol)
  dosage of, 276
  pharmacology of, 275–276
  side effects of, 276
Ursodiol, 275–276

Vaccination agents, 257–260
Valium, 355–359, 363
Vancomycin, 346
  for pseudomembranous colitis, 172–173
VanTrappen, G, 74
Variceal bleeding, injection therapy for, 365
Vasopressin
  contraindications for, 370
  dosage and administration of, 369–370
  indications for, 369
  mechanism of action of, 369
  nitroglycerin and, 371–372
  side effects of, 370
Vasopressin analogues, 370–371
Verapamil, 323
Verlinden, M, 334
Verner-Morrison syndrome, somatostatin for, 390
Vesikar, T, 293
Vibrio cholera, 166–169
Vibrio parahemolyticus, 163, 168, 211
Vibrio vulnificus, 168
Villeneuve, JP, 24
Villous adenoma, 158
Vince, A, 266
VIPoma, somatostatin for, 390
Viral hepatitis, 224
  corticosteroids for, 228–229
Viral infections, 159
  acyclovir for, 184–185
  ganciclovir for, 185–186
Vitamin K
  dosage and administration of, 255
  indications for, 254–255
  mechanism of action of, 254
  notes on, 256
  side effects of, 255
Vitamin K_1, 254–255

Vitamin K$_2$, 254–256
Vivonex, 145
Vomiting, domperidone for, 331

Wald, J, 262
Waldenstrom, 227, 397
Walker, John, 271, 291
Walshe, 240
Warfarin
   cimetidine and, 27
   metronidazole and, 131
Warnes, TW, 248
Warren, JR, 73
Weber, FL, 267
Weiner, N, 322
Welage, LS, 37
Welch, CE, 215
Wiesner, RH, 248
Wille-Jorgensen, P, 293
Wilson's disease
   D-penicillamine for, 240–244
   penicillamine for, 223–224, 240–244
   pyridoxine for, 242

Woffler, 2
Wolf, AM, 229
World Health Organization, 167
Wormsley, KG, 30
Wren, Sir Christopher, 143
Wright, 30–31

Yellolax, 311
Yersinia enterocoliticus, ciprofloxacin for, 211
Yokoya, H, 18, 19
Young, EL, 215

ZES. *See* Zollinger-Ellison syndrome (ZES)
Zimmerman, TW, 31
Zollinger-Ellison syndrome (ZES)
   cimetidine for, 19–20
   famotidine for, 37
   omeprazole for, 83, 84
   ranitidine for, 31
   somatostatin for, 390